ANNALS OF
THE NEW YORK ACADEMY
OF SCIENCES

Volume 975

EDITORIAL STAFF

Executive Editor
BARBARA M. GOLDMAN

Managing Editor
JUSTINE CULLINAN

Associate Editor
JOYCE HITCHCOCK

The New York Academy of Sciences
2 East 63rd Street
New York, New York 10021

THE NEW YORK ACADEMY OF SCIENCES
(Founded in 1817)

BOARD OF GOVERNORS, September 2002–September 2003
TORSTEN N. WIESEL, *Chairman of the Board*
JOHN T. MORGAN, *Treasurer*
ELLIS RUBENSTEIN, *Chief Executive Officer* [ex officio]

Honorary Life Governors
WILLIAM T. GOLDEN   JOSHUA LEDERBERG

Governors

ELEANOR BAUM	KAREN E. BURKE	LAWRENCE B. BUTTENWIESER
PRAVEEN CHAUDHARI	BRIAN FERGUSON	GERALD FISCHBACH
JOHN H. GIBBONS	MICHAEL GOLDEN	RONALD L. GRAHAM
MARNIE IMHOFF	JACQUELINE LEO	BRUCE McEWEN
PAUL MARKS	RONAY MENSCHEL	JOHN F. NIBLACK
SANDRA PANEM	PETER RINGROSE	JOHN J. ROCHE
LEE VANCE		DEBORAH WILEY

HELENE L. KAPLAN, *Counsel* [ex officio]

MICROARRAYS, IMMUNE RESPONSES, AND VACCINES

ANNALS OF THE NEW YORK ACADEMY OF SCIENCES
Volume 975

MICROARRAYS, IMMUNE RESPONSES, AND VACCINES

Edited by
Luc Aujame, Nicolas Burdin,
Betty Dodet, and Marissa Vicari

The New York Academy of Sciences
New York, New York
2002

Copyright © 2002 by the New York Academy of Sciences. All rights reserved. Under the provisions of the United States Copyright Act of 1976, individual readers of the Annals *are permitted to make fair use of the material in them for teaching and research. Permission is granted to quote from the* Annals *provided that the customary acknowledgment is made of the source. Material in the* Annals *may be republished only by permission of the Academy. Address inquiries to the Permissions Department (permissions@nyas.org) at the New York Academy of Sciences.*

Copying fees: *For each copy of an article made beyond the free copying permitted under Section 107 or 108 of the 1976 Copyright Act, a fee should be paid through the Copyright Clearance Center, Inc., 222 Rosewood Drive, Danvers, MA 01923 (www.copyright.com).*

∞ *The paper used in this publication meets the minimum requirements of American National Standard for Information Sciences—Permanence of Paper for Printed Library Materials. ANSI Z39.48-1984.*

Library of Congress Cataloging-in-Publication Data

Microarrays, immune responses, and vaccines / edited by Luc Aujame ... [et al.].
    p. ; cm. — (Annals of the New York Academy of Sciences ; v. 975)
Includes bibliographical references and index.
    ISBN 1-57331-446-3 (cloth : alk. paper) — ISBN 1-57331-447-1 (paper : alk. paper)
    1. Immune response—Congresses. 2. DNA microarrays—Congresses. 3. Vaccines—Congresses.
    [DNLM: 1. Oligonucleotide Array Sequence Analysis—Congresses. 2. Immunity—Congresses. 3. Vaccines—Congresses. QZ 52 M626 2002] I. Aujame, Luc. II. Series.
    Q11 .N5 vol 975
    [QR186]
    500 s—dc21
    [616.07

2002151074
CIP

K-M Research/PCP
Printed in the United States of America
ISBN 1-57331-446-3 (cloth)
ISBN 1-57331-447-1 (paper)
ISSN 0077-8923

ANNALS OF THE NEW YORK ACADEMY OF SCIENCES

Volume 975
December 2002

MICROARRAYS, IMMUNE RESPONSES, AND VACCINES

Editors
LUC AUJAME, NICOLAS BURDIN,
BETTY DODET, AND MARISSA VICARI

Conference Organizer
FONDATION MÉRIEUX

Scientific Committee
LUC AUJAME, BRIAN BARBER, NICOLAS BURDIN,
BETTY DODET, AND BERNARD MALISSEN

This volume is the result of a conference entitled **Microarrays, Immune Responses and Vaccines**, held May 26–29, 2002, in Les Pénsieres, Veyrier-du-Lac, Annecy, France, and organized by the Mérieux Foundation with the support of Aventis Pasteur and Mérial.

CONTENTS

Preface: Microarrays, Immune Responses, and Vaccines. *By* MARISSA VICARI AND BETTY DODET	ix
How Microarrays Can Improve Our Understanding of Immune Responses and Vaccine Development. *By* LUC AUJAME, NICOLAS BURDIN, AND MARISSA VICARI	1
Historical Background and Anticipated Developments. *By* BERTRAND JORDAN	24

Part I. Transcription Profiles in Lymphoid Tissues

Analysis of B Cell Memory Formation Using DNA Microarrays. *By* CAROLA G. VINUESA, MATTHEW C. COOK, MICHAEL P. COOKE, IAN C. M. MACLENNAN, AND CHRISTOPHER C. GOODNOW	33
IL-15 Is a Growth Factor and an Activator of CD8 Memory T Cells. *By* NAN-PING WENG, KEBIN LIU, MARTA CATALFAMO, YU LI, AND PIERRE A. HENKART	46
A Genomic View of Helper T Cell Subsets. *By* LARS ROGGE	57

Gene Profiling Approach to Establish the Molecular Bases for Partial versus Full Activation of Naïve CD8 T Lymphocytes. *By* GRÉGORY VERDEIL, DENIS PUTHIER, CATHERINE NGUYEN, ANNE-MARIE SCHMITT-VERHULST, AND NATHALIE AUPHAN-ANEZIN 68

Complexity of Inflammatory Responses in Endothelial Cells and Vascular Smooth Muscle Cells Determined by Microarray Analysis. *By* OLGA BANDMAN, ROGER T. COLEMAN, JEANNE F. LORING, JEFFREY J. SEILHAMER, AND BENJAMIN G. COCKS.. 77

Integrated Genomic and Proteomic Analysis of Signaling Pathways in Dendritic Cell Differentiation and Maturation. *By* JOHN RICHARDS, FRANÇOIS LE NAOUR, SAMIR HANASH, AND LAURA BERETTA 91

CD30—Governor of Memory T Cells? *By* ECKHARD R. PODACK, NATASA STRBO, VLATKA SOTOSEC, AND HIROMI MUTA 101

Stronger Correlation of bcl-3 than bcl-2, bcl-x_L, Costimulation, or Antioxidants with Adjuvant-Induced T Cell Survival. *By* THOMAS C. MITCHELL, T. KENT TEAGUE, DAVID A. HILDEMAN, JEREMY BENDER, WILLIAM A. REES, ROSS M. KEDL, BRAD SWANSON, JOHN W. KAPPLER, AND PHILIPPA MARRACK 114

Additional Invited Paper
A Short Domain within Bcl-3 Is Responsible for Its Lymphocyte Survival Activity. *By* THOMAS C. MITCHELL, BRUCE S. THOMPSON, JOHN O. TRENT, AND CAROLYN R. CASELLA....................... 132

Molecular Characterization of Antigen-Induced Lung Inflammation in a Murine Model of Asthma. *By* MASSOUD DAHESHIA, NIAN TIAN, TIMOTHY CONNOLLY, AMAR DRAWID, QUIYAN WU, JEAN-GUY BIENVENU, JEAN CAVALLO, RAY JUPP, GEORGE T. DE SANCTIS, AND ANNE MINNICH.. 148

Part II. Pathogens and Host–Cell Interactions

Unlocking the Mysteries of Virus–Host Interactions: Does Functional Genomics Hold the Key? *By* MARCUS J. KORTH AND MICHAEL G. KATZE 160

Genetic Determinants of Coxsackievirus B3 Pathogenesis.
By BRUCE M. MCMANUS, BOBBY YANAGAWA, NANA REZAI, HONGLIN LUO, LYDIA TAYLOR, MARY ZHANG, JANE YUAN, JONATHAN BUCKLEY, TIMOTHY TRICHE, GEORGE SCHREINER, AND DECHENG YANG 169

A Functional Genomics Approach to Kaposi's Sarcoma. *By* ASHLEE V. MOSES, MICHAEL A. JARVIS, CAMILO RAGGO, YOLANDA C. BELL, REBECCA RUHL, B.G. MATTIAS LUUKKONEN, DIANA J. GRIFFITH, CECILY L. WAIT, BRIAN J. DRUKER, MICHAEL C. HEINRICH, JAY A. NELSON, AND KLAUS FRÜH...................................... 180

Chlamydiae Host Cell Interactions Revealed Using DNA Microarrays.
By JAMES B. MAHONY 192

Gene Expression Profile in *Neisseria meningitidis* and *Neisseria lactamica* upon
Host–Cell Contact: From Basic Research to Vaccine Development.
By R. GRIFANTINI, E. BARTOLINI, A. MUZZI, M. DRAGHI, E. FRIGIMELICA,
J. BERGER, F. RANDAZZO, AND G. GRANDI 202

Part III. Immune Responses in Cancer

Prognosis of Breast Cancer and Gene Expression Profiling Using DNA Arrays.
By FRANÇOIS BERTUCCI, RÉMI HOULGATTE, SAMUEL GRANJEAUD,
VALÉRY NASSER, BÉATRICE LORIOD, EMMANUEL BEAUDOING,
PASCAL HINGAMP, JOCELYNE JACQUEMIER, PATRICE VIENS,
DANIEL BIRNBAUM, AND CATHERINE NGUYEN. 217

Identifying Immunotherapeutic Targets for Prostate Carcinoma through the
Analysis of Gene Expression Profiles. *By* PETER S. NELSON 232

Index of Contributors 247

The New York Academy of Sciences believes it has a responsibility to provide an open forum for discussion of scientific questions. The positions taken by the participants in the reported conferences are their own and not necessarily those of the Academy. The Academy has no intent to influence legislation by providing such forums.

Preface

Microarrays, Immune Responses, and Vaccines

DNA microarrays, or DNA chips, have been heralded as being one of the most important emerging technologies for biological research. With the power to measure the differential expression of up to 400,000 genes in one experiment, microarrays are furthering our understanding of cell development, differentiation, and function as well as our understanding of disease. The objective of the symposium **Microarrays, Immune Responses and Vaccines**, organized by the Fondation Mérieux in Veyrier-du-Lac, France, 27–29 May 2002, was to focus on how microarray technology has improved our understanding of immune responses, and more specifically, how it is being used to further vaccine development.

The meeting opened with a historical look at DNA arrays, followed by a session devoted to transcription profiles in lymphoid tissues. Pathogen–host cell interactions were then explored, looking at how microarrays are being used to better understand the mechanisms of infection and crosstalk between host cells and viruses (coxsackievirus B3, Kaposi's sarcoma), bacteria (*Chlamydia*, *Helicobacter*), and parasites (*Toxoplasma*, *Plasmodium*). The meeting closed with a session on immune responses in cancer.

A unique feature of this meeting is that all speakers, from various fields, were asked not only to present their unique experiences and data, but also to address the following common questions:

- What microarray technological improvements remain to be achieved?
- What are the current biological limitations in generating new insights?
- In which areas should emphasis be placed in order to move ahead faster?
- How can the enormous amount of data generated be shared most effectively?
- Can we expect to monitor antigen-specific immune responses?
- If so, what would be needed to do so?
- What will the impact of this technology be on vaccine development?

These common threads were present and alive throughout the meeting, in the presentations and in the discussions; and we now invite the reader to discover them in the proceedings.

We are grateful to all those who participated in the meeting, to the authors of the manuscripts, and to the staff of NYAS for their kind collaboration in publishing the Symposium proceedings. We would like to thank Aventis Pasteur and Mérial for their financial support. Our sincere gratitude is conveyed to the Scientific Committee for their kind help in the preparation of the program, with special thanks to Luc Aujame and Nicolas Burdin for their work on this publication.

MARISSA VICARI, PROJECT MANAGER
BETTY DODET, SCIENTIFIC DIRECTOR
*FONDATION MÉRIEUX, 17, RUE BOURGELAT,
BP 2021, 69227 LYON, FRANCE*

How Microarrays Can Improve Our Understanding of Immune Responses and Vaccine Development

LUC AUJAME, NICOLAS BURDIN, AND MARISSA VICARI

Campus Mérieux, 69280 Marcy l'Etoile, France

KEYWORDS: transcriptome; gene profiling; immune response; host-pathogen interaction; cancer; vaccine

The international symposium **Microarrays, Immune Responses and Vaccines** held in Veyrier du Lac, France, 26–29 May 2002, is the first to our knowledge to assess the impact of DNA microarray technology in the fields of immunology and vaccinology. It was based on the premise that the unfolding field of functional genomics has already proven its ability to provide new approaches that could be used to better unravel the complexity of immunology, with the challenge of extending it to vaccine development. Furthermore, it was felt that enough data have accumulated to serve as a basis for a fruitful discussion between scientists from different fields.

The last two decades have seen a revolution in molecular biology due essentially to large scale DNA sequencing and gene expression profiling (measurement of the transcriptome, or the regulation of mRNA levels at the genomic level) and the development of tools which have facilitated the analysis of complex data. While several high-throughput methods are available for measuring gene expression, including qRT-PCR, SAGE, and DNA microarrays, the later offers the advantage of simplicity, at least in theory (microarrays are the reverse of Southern blots), sensitivity (down to the single cell level), flexibility (regarding the choice of genes to be analyzed), and power of analysis (in combination with bioinformatic tools). Robotics has now made it possible to array tens of thousands of distinct spots of DNA, each corresponding to a single gene, on glass slides or other supports such that complete genomes can be explored. With the description of the human genome, the way is now open for the creation of arrays covering the full spectrum of the human transcriptome. Among other things, this should open the way to:

- a more complete description of gene expression in different cells and tissues, and the subsequent analysis of differential gene patterns or signatures in normal and disease states; and

- a fuller understanding of host-pathogen interactions, and the comparison of host and pathogen gene expression during infection, latency, pathology, and recovery.

Address for correspondence: Luc Aujame, Building X, Campus Mérieux, 1541 Avenue Marcel Mérieux, 69280 Marcy l'Etoile, France. Voice: 33 4 37 37 36 56; fax: 33 4 37 37.
Luc.Aujame@aventis.com

GENE PROFILING AND THE IMMUNE SYSTEM

Gene expression profiling analysis should have a tremendous impact on our understanding of the immune system. A more comprehensive and integrated view of an immune response can be achieved by going from hypothesis-driven strategies using experimental models to the multigenic discovery approach, which we hope will ultimately lead us to generate a complete list of proteins involved in immune functions. For example, the compilation of one million measurements using the human lymphochip, performed on multiple normal or pathological immune cells in different states of activation, can unravel analogies of gene regulation between different models.[1]

Immunology is particularly well-adapted to gene profiling studies. The different subsets of immune cells are well-characterized, can be easily purified, and different culture conditions have been developed to grow them and even to induce their differentiation into various effector cells. Naturally occurring pathologies caused by dysfunctions of the immune system (autoimmune disorders, immunodeficiencies, tumors) and sophisticated genetic engineering in mice (knock-in and knock-out) provide *in vitro* and *in vivo* experimental models that are particularly well formatted for genomics approaches. In the past five years, a growing list of reports using microarray technologies have identified new genes and/or new pathways involved in various aspects of the immune response (for general reviews see refs. 2–7).

DEVELOPMENT AND ACTIVATION/TOLERIZATION OF IMMUNOCOMPETENT CELLS

Many reports have already shown how microarrays can be powerful tools to identify and characterize gene regulation in the ontogeny, differentiation, and activation of immune cells. A nonexhaustive list of such studies is provided in TABLE 1. Studies presented at the symposium are identified in **bold** in this table. Differential gene expression between activated and tolerized B cells was investigated in some of the first studies.[8,9] It appears that the summation of numerous small changes in the expression of stimulatory and inhibitory genes are the molecular basis of cell fate decisions leading either to anergy/tolerization of B lymphocytes on the one hand, or to their activation on the other. The global molecular profiles obtained in this study illustrate how quiescence and anergy are actively maintained in circulating B cells, how these states are switched to clonal expansion, and how they could be better emulated by protolerogenic drugs, offering potential therapeutic approaches. The work of Carola G. Vinuesa *et al.* (this volume) also demonstrates how microarray analysis combined with a conventional approach (an experimental model of induction of either T cell–dependent or –independent germinal centers in mice) can provide a great opportunity for investigating the genetic signals that control memory B cell differentiation.

Similarly, gene profiling of T lymphocytes in resting versus activated states has been studied in a "pioneer" report.[10] The authors found that resting T cells express a surprisingly large diversity of genes and that this pattern of gene expression considerably changed within 8 hours of T cell activation but returned back to a "resting-like" state within 48 hours of exposure to antigen. Nathalie Auphan-Anezin *et al.*

TABLE 1. Gene profiling of immune cells using microarray analysis (table continues on next four pages)

Immune cells		Experimental conditions	Arrays	Genes	Comments/ observations	Ref.
Dendritic Cells (DCs):	Differentiation Maturation:	CD14- derived DCs: IL-4+GM-CSF+/- TNFα	Affimetrix	6,300 human	**Combined arrays and proteomic approaches.**	43
		Effect of Gram negative-bacteria on bone marrow like DC cell line D1	**Affimetrix 11,000 genes**	11,000 mouse	**3,000 differentially expressed genes unexpected finding: IL-2.**	12
	Activation:	Maturation of a mouse bone marrow like DC cell line D1 by LPS versus TNFα	Affimetrix	6500 mouse	Diverse modulation of gene expression depending on the stimulus.	44
		Maturation of CD14-derived DCs by either E. coli, C. albicans or influenza virus and derived components	Affimetrix	6,800 human	A shared core response and pathogen specific programs of gene expression.	13
		Differentiation and activation (by a glycolipid antigen) of human monocyte derived DCs	Micromax cDNA	2,400 human	28 upregulated genes: ribonuclease, collapsin	45,46
		Other analysis of gene profiling on DC differentiation and/or maturation	cytokine array (R&D)	mouse	Upregulation of cytokines and chemokines.	47–51

TABLE 1/continued 1.

Immune cells		Experimental conditions	Arrays	Genes	Comments/Observations	Ref.
T cells:	Th1/Th2 polarization	Development of T helper cells from cord blood Th0 cells	Affimetrix Roche Pa-1 Oligo.	6,000 human 517 human	**Th1 versus Th2: 215 differentially expressed genes.**	52
		Same approach			**Differential expression of several death and apoptosis-related genes.**	53
		Differential gene expression in both CD4 and CD8 Type 1 and Type 2 T cells	Affimetrix	11,000 mouse	100 differentially expressed genes: similar program of type1:type polarization between CD4 and CD8.	54
		Profiling of differential gene expression in allergen specific human Th2 cells	cDNA arrays Genome Systems	100 human	15 sequences with selected expression in allergen specific Th2 cells.	55
	Naive versus memory:	Memory versus naive CD4 T lymphocytes	cDNA array (Incyte Genomics)	54,768 human	A set of 200 clones are more highly upregulated in memory than in naive cells upon activation.	56
	Activation:	Activation of CD8 T cells: IL-15 versus anti-CD3	cDNA array (Research Genetics)	**4,604 human**	**IL-15 and TCR signaling: similar responses, less than 20% of differentially expressed genes.**	57
		Genomic expression program and integration of CD28 triggering	cDNA microarray	18,000 human	CD28 signaling: increases the amplitude of TCR-induced transcriptional response (NFAT-related)	58

TABLE 1/continued 2.

Immune cells	Experimental conditions	Arrays	Genes	Comments/observations	Ref.
	CD30 signaling in a cytotoxic T cell line	Unigen Microarray	4,000 human	**Inhibition of cytotoxicity: downregulation of cytotoxic effector genes.**	59
	Effect of other compounds on T lymphocytes	Customized cDNA arrays, Affimetrix or cDNA Lymphochip	Human: 2,000, 6,300 or 15,000	Determination of subsets of genes specifically regulated by chemokines, cytokines or other immunomodulators. Identification of calcium-dependent gene expression.	60–63
	Activation of T cells *in vivo* using adjuvants	Affimetrix genes	6,400 mouse	**Identification of Bcl-3 as an adjuvant-induced survival factor for T cells.**	42
Unconventional T cells:	CD4 CD25 regulatory T cells: gene profiling	Affymetrix	11,000 mouse	Set of genes specific for regulatory T cells. Most are signaling antagonists.	64
	Gene expression in NKT cells	Affimetrix	12,000 human	**41 genes specific for NKT cells compared to conventional CD4 or CD8 cells: target for therapy?**	65, 66
	Intestinal intraepithelial γδ T lymphocytes (IEL)	Affymetrix	6,352 mouse	γδ IEL are constitutively activated effectors and use different cascade than CD8 cells.	67

TABLE 1/continued 3.

Immune cells	Experimental conditions	Arrays	Genes	Comments/observations	Ref.
B cells:					
Ontogeny, regulation and differentiation	Gene expression profiles of 5 consecutive stages of B cell development	Affimetrix	13,104 mouse	Differential expression of 10.7% of all genes during B cell development: balance between cell division and apoptosis.	68
	Transcriptomic of activated versus anergic B cells	Affymetrix	6,500 mouse	Molecular footprint of the mechanism of peripheral self tolerance.	8
B lymphocyte disorders:	Gene expression profiling in germinal center B cells	Customized cDNA array	588 human	Profiling of normal GC B cells compared to neoplastic follicular lymphomas.	69
	Expression profiling in EBV transformed human B cells	Atlas cDNA Affymetrix	588 and 12,500 human	Identification of a gene subset influenced by Bruton kinase mutations.	70
	B cell isotype control in atopy and asthma in humans	Atlas cDNA 609 genes	609 human	Differentially expressed genes between atopic and normal subjects.	71
Activation:	CD40-mediated activation of primary murine B cells...	Affymetrix Atlas cDNA	6,500 mouse 588 human	Induction of genes involved in survival, growth and germinal center formation.	72
	...or B cell lines			Identification of the NFκB induced PIM-1 kinase.	73

TABLE 1/continued 4.

Immune cells		Experimental conditions	Arrays	Genes	Comments/observations	Ref.
Monocytes Macrophages	**Activation:**	Transcriptomic of monocytes activated by LPS or RANTES	Affimetrix	5,600 human	RANTES and LPS induced distinct gene profiling: migratory versus phagocytic programs respectively.	74
		LPS-inducible genes on macrophage cell line RAW264	cDNA array (Research Genetics) or Atlas cDNA	3,700 mouse 588 mouse	Probability of activation of LPS-inducible genes depends on cell subclones. A core of genes induced by LPS are also upregulated upon bacterial infection.	75 76
		Cholesterol (LDL) induced gene expression in THP-1 macrophage cell line	cDNA (Research Genetics)	6,805 human	Subset of modulated genes involved in growth, survival, inflammation and matrix remodeling.	77, 78
Other cells:	**Neutrophils:**	LPS-Activation of neutrophils	Affymetrix	7,070 human	100 upregulated genes, poor concordance with proteomic results.	79
	Polymorphonuclear cells:	Changes in gene expression during receptor-mediated phagocytosis	Affymetrix	12,561 human	279 genes are regulated upon CR- or FcR-mediated phagocytosis, including 30 apoptosis-related genes.	80

(this volume) have further investigated the molecular basis of T cell activation by comparing gene profiling obtained on purified murine CD8 T cells activated by either a partial or a full agonist peptide. They conclude that partial T cell activation upon suboptimal stimulation is regulated at the transcriptional level and is caused by transient mRNA expression versus stable induction in fully activated cells. Several reports have also compared gene profiles between Th1 and Th2 polarized T cells, in humans and in mice (for review, see ref. 3). Such studies have confirmed markers already identified specific for either Th1 or Th2 cells, but they also have revealed new, sometimes unexpected, genes that were differentially expressed between the two subsets. Th1 cells express higher activation-induced cell death (AICD) related genes (TRAIL, BAK, Caspase 8...) suggesting that they are more susceptible to apoptosis. Differences in expression of homing and adhesion molecules between Th1 and Th2 cells could explain why these cell subsets are not similarly distributed in the body. Adhesion and extravasion of Th1 cells are more frequently observed in inflamed tissues while Th2 cells have preferential homing to mucosal sites.[11]

Antigen-presenting cells (APCs), especially dendritic cells (DCs), have also been investigated at the molecular level using microarray approaches. Transcription profiles of monocytes undergoing DC differentiation, and of different subsets of human or murine DCs have already been analyzed.[3] Using this approach, P. Ricciardi Castagnoli et al. have identified that an initial burst of IL-2 could be produced by DCs and is critical for T cell priming.[12] Many reports have also tried to determine whether pathogens or derived compounds (heat-inactivated microbes, LPS...), inflammatory cytokines (TNFα) or synthetic immunostimulatory molecules induce specific gene expression signatures in DCs. It usually appears that a shared core response is induced by all these stimuli but some pathogen-specific programs are also identified. This suggests that diverse microbes elicit different gene expression patterns in DCs which then subsequently drive specific and appropriate immune responses.[13]

Taken together, these results show that microarrays present a profound advantage over other techniques in the probing and characterization of new genes and/or novel pathways playing key roles in many different immune processes such as lineage commitment, cell differentiation and maturation, growth, apoptosis, phagocytosis, homing, energy metabolism, angiogenesis, and signaling.[2,7] This should ultimately lead to a molecular map of immune cell homeostasis connecting surface receptor-ligand pairs involved in cell-cell contact as well as soluble factor-mediated signaling, with intracellular proteins involved in the regulation of cell activation, survival or death.

COMPREHENSIVE UNDERSTANDING OF IMMUNOLOGICAL DISORDERS

Such discoveries will considerably improve our understanding of the immune system, but will also provide even more appropriate molecular targets, thus offering new hopes of therapy for various pathologies caused by immunological disorders: autoimmune syndromes, immunodeficiencies, and cancers (for review, see ref. 1).

Autoimmunity

Autoimmune diseases have been investigated using gene profiling. Microarray analysis of multiple sclerosis lesions have revealed some complex regulations of the inflammatory gene response[14] and differential gene regulation of GM-CSF, which is induced in acute lesions but not in "silent" uninflamed lesions.[15] This latter study yielded new targets further validated in a mouse model of autoimmune encephalomyelitis. Similarly, several other reports have investigated gene signatures of various autoimmune diseases: diabetes,[16] Sjogren syndrome,[17] alopecia areata,[18] experimental autoimmune encephalomyelitis,[19] and others.[5] In fact, combining microarray approaches with murine models of congenic strains may help unravel the genetic basis of susceptibility to autoimmune disorders by identifying both defective genetic variants and the pathways they control.[20]

Inflammatory Disease

Similarly, transcriptome analysis of pathogenesis associated with exacerbated inflammation will uncover the molecular basis of such dysregulation. An early attempt to dissect inflammatory disease was reported in 1997 for rheumatoid arthritis and inflammatory bowel disease.[21] More recently, other pathologies such as psoriasis or colitis and Crohn's disease have been investigated.[22–24] Signatures for lethal type 1 and type 2 cytokine-mediated inflammatory reactions in responses to infections have also been looked at.[25]

Cancer

The applications of microarray technology in the field of cancer are numerous (for review, see refs. 26 and 27) and, although it is beyond the scope of this paper to review the vast use of gene profiles in cancer research, it is important to note some examples of what is being done. Gene profiling is providing a wide variety of information that can be applied to yield a more accurate classification of cancers, better-defined diagnosis, and novel approaches for therapy. Comparisons of gene expression patterns between normal and malignant or premalignant cells, as well as between different tumor samples, are being used to further our understanding of oncogenesis, to identify specific genes involved in hereditary cancer, and to refine cancer subtypes into prognostic classes that may reflect on treatment decisions.

An example of this in the field of breast cancer is the contribution by François Bertucci et al. (this volume), in which they pursue a particularly critical objective: the identification of new prognostic subclasses of breast cancers currently unrecognized by classical parameters. Using microarray-based studies, they revealed a set of genes with differential expression patterns that correlate with groups of patients presenting different survival outcomes after adjuvant chemotherapy. This allowed them to then refine the classification of the tumors, distinguishing three classes each with significantly different long-term survival.

Gene profiling is being applied in a similar way to better characterize immune cell cancers, as well as to monitor the immune response to different tumors and identify tumor antigens for use as therapeutic vaccines (immunotherapy). A study by Alizadeh et al., for example, identified two molecularly distinct forms of diffuse large B cell lymphoma, which corresponded to different stages of B cell differentiation, as well as different overall patient survival.[28] In this case, gene profiling opened the way to the observation of a new clinical subtype of lymphoma.

In this volume, Peter Nelson explains how microarray studies have been used to identify possible targets for therapeutic vaccination in prostate carcinoma. Here again, microarray-based studies have repeatedly allowed for the refinement of tumor classification, revealed novel features, and provided predictive prognostic correlations. In addition, differential expression studies are being used to identify genes with expression restricted to the prostate gland that could act as appropriate tumor antigens. Such is the case with prostase/KLK4, a serine protease whose expression is highly restricted to normal and neoplastic prostate cells, and which is currently being evaluated as a possible vaccine candidate.

INFECTOMICS: MICROARRAY ANALYSIS OF GENE EXPRESSION DURING HOST/PATHOGEN INTERACTIONS

Another major topic addressed by the symposium was that of host-pathogen interactions. TABLE 2 summarizes efforts carried out in this area to date. The number of viruses and bacteria that are being examined has increased significantly in the last few years, and studies are now being extended to parasites. Pathogens of all three types covered by contributors to this volume or speakers at the meeting have been highlighted in bold in TABLE 2. Thus far, most studies have concentrated on host responses initially limiting themselves to cataloguing genes with the largest change in gene expression (most often upregulated genes) under defined conditions (generally upon infection of cell lines derived from tissues which are normally infected in the host). Sometimes rather small arrays are used (although the trend is towards more complete arrays), and in some cases unexpected and clearly significant aspects of the immune response have been revealed. This was already the case with one of the first studies by Zhu et al.[29] using a 6.6K human array to analyze cytomegalovirus (CMV) infection of human foreskin fibroblasts: here a displayed upregulation in cytosolic phopholipase A2 and COX2 leading to the subsequent increase of the proinflammatory mediator PGE2, was revealed as a means by which CMV attracts a reservoir of monocytes: this is hypothesized to facilitate spreading of the infection.

Similarly, Klaus Früh (Moses et al., this volume) discusses the use of microarrays to analyze infection of human DMEVC cells by Kaposi-associated herpes virus (or Herpes virus 8). This work extends that of Poole et al.,[30] who employed essentially the same model with a more limited set of arrayed genes, to focus on the role of c-kit in cellular transformation, demonstrating the key role of this receptor tyrosine kinase in Kaposi's sarcoma.[31] Other contributions in this issue that cover viral host interactions include those of James Mahony on chlamydia and Bruce McManus et al. on coxsackievirus B3, the primary etiological agent of viral myocarditis. More recent studies have now been extended to parasites such as T. cruzi and T. gondii.

Another approach is to compare the immune response to a number of pathogens and determine both common and unique themes developed by each pathogen so as to understand how the proinflammatory response develops as well as the strategies used by the pathogens to enhance or optimize their survival. This was proposed a few years back by Manger and Relman,[32] and one such study has now been published by this group[33] (see TABLE 2) in which the response to infection to at least 3 pathogens (heat-killed *S. aureus*, *B. pertussis,* and *E. coli*) was examined at the level of PBMCs. The data generally argue for the convergence of specialized responses to each pathogen, whereby similar profiles could arise from separate sensors (which can be distinguished in particular at lower doses). This strongly suggests that an analysis of host expression patterns may be able to distinguish infection by different pathogens. Huang *et al.*[13] have taken a similar approach looking at a unique cell population, mainly dendritic cells, generating both a core response as well as specific responses in which unique subsets of genes are up- or downregulated. Among the contributors to this volume, Michael Katze has investigated flu, HCV, SIV, and HIV with a view to constructing a "viral compendium," a centralized catalogue of events that occur upon viral infection.

The reciprocal approach to host-pathogen interactions is to look at bacterial or viral genes and how their expression is modulated by host contact or upon infection. Again, examples can be found in TABLE 2. Among bacteria, *H. pylori* and *N. meningitidis* group B (MenB) have been the most studied, for a number of reasons: the complete genomic sequences of a number of strains of each have been published, they infect hundreds of millions of individuals (for *H. pylori*, this is probably half the world population), they have severe pathological consequences, and there are no vaccines for either of them. The case of MenB exemplifies the potential application of the technology to the discovery of new vaccine antigens. Guido Grandi (Grifantini *et al.*, this volume), extending previous work of the same team on genome mining which had already identified a number of potential vaccine candidates,[34] has now compared bacteria interacting with epithelial cells to that grown in culture in order to identify which MenB genes are affected by host cell contact. Two aspects of these results should be noted: first, a high proportion of the genes identified as being regulated by host-pathogen interaction are presumed to code for surface-associated proteins, suggesting substantial remodeling of the bacterial membrane. Second, a number of the potential vaccine antigens (on the basis of their bactericidal properties) were not identified by the genome-mining approach and indeed were not predicted to be membrane associated by available algorithms.

FUTURE EVOLUTION AND IMPACTS OF MICROARRAYS ON VACCINE DEVELOPMENT

As microarray technology is still developing, contributors were also asked to respond to a series of questions addressing the issue of the future evolution and potential impacts of the technology, specifically: What microarray technological improvements remain to be achieved? What are the current biological limitations in generating new insights? In which areas should emphasis be placed in order to move ahead faster? How can the enormous amount of data generated be shared most effectively? Can we expect to monitor antigen-specific immune responses? If so what would be needed to do so? What will the impact of this technology be on vaccine development?

Readers may judge to what extent each contribution has been able to answer the questions and issues raised above. However, we wish to provide our own critical

TABLE 2. Microarray analysis of host-pathogen interactions (table continues on next three pages)

Pathogen	Model	Experimental conditions	Array	Genes	Comments/Observations	Ref.
Viruses						
Coxsackie B3	Mouse Hela	3, 9 and 30 d post-infection analysis of heart RNA infection	PCR, glass Oligo, glass	4,200 rat human	619 differentially expressed genes.	81
CMV	Human foreskin fibroblasts	infection	Affymetrix	6.6K human	258 cellular genes differentially expressed.	29
	Human fibroblast	lytic infection	Oligo, glass	207 CMV genes	Temporal map of all viral genes.	82
	Human foreskin fibroblasts	Infection and γB incubation	PCR, glass	about 9,000 human	Major role of γB in HCMV-regulated cell transcription profile.	83
HIV	Human T cell	2–3 d infection	PCR, glass	1,500 human	Differential regulation of T-cell signaling, subcellular trafficking and transcriptional regulation.	84
Influenza	Human lung epithelial cells	WT and NS1⁻ infection	PCR, glass	13K human	NS1⁻ = upregulation of IFN and NFκB.	85
KSHV/Human herpes 8	primary effusion lymphoma (PEL)-derived cell line/ BCBL-1	Latency and TPA–induced lytic expression	PCR, nylon	about 90 viral genes	Confirmation of temporal expression of lytic genes; identification of novel ORFs.	86, 87
	Human Dermal microvascular endothelial	Infection ± TPA	PCR, nylon PCR, glass	2,350 and 9,180 human	Regulation of IFN-responsive genes, chemokines and adhesion factors.	30

TABLE 2/continued 1.

Pathogen	Model	Experimental conditions	Array	Genes	Comments/Observations	Ref.
	Human DMVEC	**Infection**	**PCR, glass, oligo, glass**	**4,165 human 39 K human**	**Role of c-kit in cellular transformation.**	**31**
HPV31	keratinocytes	Transfected expanded culture	PCR, glass	7,075 human	Downregulation of three groups of genes: regulation of cell growth; keratinocyte-specific; IFN-stimulated (Stat-1).	88
HSV1	HEL /H1299 (p53-/-lung fibroblast)	infection with HSV-1 ICP0	PCR, nylon	588 human	p53 responsive genes induced, including in p53- cells	89
	HLF	Infection with WT and $\gamma_1 34.5$ gene	PCR, nylon	588 human	Accumulation of transcripts representing mostly transcriptional factors.	90
	HeLa	Infection, 2,4, and 8 h p.i. ± CHX or PAA/ α27 mutant	Oligos, glass	99 HSV 57 human stress response	Role of a27 in modulation of IE viral transcripts and host cell protein synthesis.	91
Measle virus	Human PBMC	Infection	PCR, nylon	3,000 human	Upregulation of ER stress response.	92
Bacteria						
B. pertussis	Human PBMCs	Heat-killed bacteria	PCR, glass	about 7.6K human	Common induced and repressed genes by Bp *E. coli* and *S. aureus*.	33

TABLE 2/continued 2.

Pathogen	Model	Experimental conditions	Array	Genes	Comments/Observations	Ref.
Borrelia burgdorferi	Mouse	Infection of CH3 and SCID mice	PCR, glass	137 Bb lipoproteins	Early transcription of most Lp genes, downregulation at later stage.	93
Chlamydia pneumoniae	**Human endothelial cells**	**Infection**	**cDNA, nylon**	**268 human**	**Cytokines, chemokines, growth factors and kinases upregulated.**	**94**
E. coli	Dendritic cells	Coculture/adhesion	Oligo	6.8K human	Identification of common upregulated inflammatory genes (with *C. albicans* and flu).	13
	Human PBMC	Heat-killed bacteria	PCR, glass	about 7.6K human	Common induced and repressed genes by Bp *E. coli* and *S. aureus*.	33
H. pylori[a]	Mongolian gerbils AGS gastric epithelial cells	*In vivo* infection Adhesion	cDNA, glass	1,660 Hp	Differences in cag island gene expression.	95
	Gnotobiotic transgenic mice	Clinical isolates			Role of type I and II R-M systems in host response.	96
	Kato 3 gastric epithelial cell line	Cag + or − infection	cDNA and oligos, nylon	about 58K human genes	Cag-dependent differential expression.	97
Meninge B	**Human bronchial epithelial cell line**	**Adhesion assay**	**PCR, glass**	**2,100 Men B**	**5/12 adhesion-induced surface Ags induce bactericidal Abs.**	**98**
Pseudomonas	Human lung pneumocytes	Coculture/adhesion assay	PCR, glass	1,056 human	Upregulation of IRF-1.	99

TABLE 2/continued 3.

Pathogen	Model	Experimental conditions	Array	Genes	Comments/Observations	Ref.
Salmonella	Human monocytes	PhoP-Vs PhoP+ comparison	PCR, glass	22K human	Role of PhoP in human macrophage death.	100
	Human colorectal/colon epithelial cells	Infection	PCR, nylon	4.3 K human	Regulation of proinflammatory cytokines chemokines and cellular factors.	101
Staphylococcus aureus	Human monocytes	Co-culture/ adhesion	PCR, nylon	588 human	Proinflammatory mediators upregulated.	29
	Human PBMCs	Heat-killed bacteria	PCR, glass	about 7.6K human	Common induced and repressed genes by *B. pertussis*, *E. coli*, and *S. aureus*.	33
Eukaryotes						
C. albicans	Dendritic cells	Coculture	Oligo, glass	6.8K human	As above/ *E. coli*.	13
Toxoplasma gondii[a]	*Human foreskin fibroblasts*	*Infection (24 h p.i.)*	*cDNA, glass*	*18-27K human*	*Early upregulation of immune response genes not requiring infection; later regulation of cell processes dependent on parasite.*	*102*
Trypanosoma cruzi	Human foreskin fibroblasts	Infection (2-24h p.i.)	cDNA, glass	27K human	Few changes during initiation of infection.	103

[a]Presented at the conference, but not in this volume; see references.

assessment, based on both the contributions presented here and the recent literature, in relation to these questions.

1. What microarray technological improvements remain to be achieved?

Bertrand Jordan reflects on this question in his contribution. Issues that can be raised are as follows. First, there is an urgent need for the full sequencing and annotation of major eukaryotic and prokaryotic genomes to open the way to complete arrays (including arrays with both host and pathogen represented on the same support). Second, while a survey of the contributions presented at this meeting might infer that the use of nylon membranes and ^{32} or ^{33}P-labeled probes predominates, this is biased owing to the fact that, except for Affymetrix's Genechip® (oligonucleotides on a glass slide), a large number of experiments presented in Veyrier du Lac made use of commercial arrays on nylon (mainly from Clontech). However, a shift to either cDNA or long oligonucleotides on glass (the later apparently preferred by an increasing number of array suppliers), raises the issue of sensitivity. One of the current solutions seems to be reflected in the move to three-dimensional arrays, which by increasing the amount of DNA spotted, up to 100-fold compared to planar arrays, allows for a corresponding increase in sensitivity. Other approaches are being developed to decrease background as well (Zeptosens/Qiagen's SensoChip, for example). The use of long oligonucleotides (50- to 60-mers), while allowing for automation and flexibility (as exemplified by geniom®one from the German company Febit) raises the issue of the appropriate choice of oligonucleotides (are the softwares currently employed adequate?).

2. What are the current biological limitations in generating new insights?

In the final analysis, one would want to understand what happens in an organism. This is true of both immune responses and host pathogen interactions. While *ex vivo* or *in vitro* work will yield a wealth of information, they cannot substitute for the ultimate understanding of what goes on *in vivo*. Some challenges for the future are discussed below.

- The capacity to purify small samples and work from a limited amount of RNA is a limiting factor. Laser microdissection now makes it possible to isolate extremely small biological samples (hundreds of cells). At the same time, flow sorting can give access to highly purified cell populations numbering in the thousands. Thus, the major concern is being able to work with a limited amount of RNA: current hybridization procedures still call for fairly large amounts of total RNA (at least for fluorescence) and, while there are amplification procedures (T7 polymerase or PCR), bias introduced by such techniques has to be critically assessed[35] and could lead to mistaken interpretations.

- Natural variability should be taken into account. This has been addressed specifically by Peter Nelson[36] as well as Boldrick *et al.*[33] Interestingly, it appears that some of the most variable genes are involved in the immune response (this is true in both humans and mice), especially in responses to viruses. This can in part be explained by the relative cell populations in the peripheral blood and accompanying variability of basal levels of some key cytokines. This raises the issue of the reproducibility of experiments performed *in vivo*, and of the proper statistical analysis, but could also apply to *in vitro* analyses of cell lines (with respect to the host-pathogen interaction, for example). In the case of monitoring immune responses, this becomes a serious challenge as it might prove difficult to set a basal reference level for a given gene or set of genes.

- There is more to life than RNA. Limitations of DNA microarrays were raised by a number of speakers and are addressed in some of the contributions presented here (Baretta, Katze, but see also Daniel Carucci[37]). As obvious as it may seem, posttranslational modifications, which affect protein expression, cannot be addressed by DNA arrays. As indicated by Michael Katze (this volume), for example, viruses are well known for their capacity to regulate host protein synthesis at the translational level.

3. How can the enormous amount of data generated be shared most effectively? Among the issues that need to be addressed are:

- *Information:* this concerns the information which should be reported concerning any microarray experiment so as to ensure interpretability. This is being considered by the MIAME (Minimal Information About a Microarray Experiment) working group, which has already issued a draft of specifications (version 1.1 draft 6 can be found on their web site: http://www.mged.org/Annotations-wg/index.html).

- *Format:* different formats must be compatible for sharing. As groups either develop their own tools, or use diversely available commercial ones, this could be a stumbling block. Efforts towards the standardization of storage and exchange of data are ongoing,[38] but still require general acceptance.

- Centralized data bank: this in fact is in the works as a number of databases are available: Gene Expression Omnibus (GEO) (http://www.ncbi.nlm.nih.gov/geo) by the NCBI to which data may be submitted and an accession number provided, ArrayExpress (http://www.ebi.ac.uk/arrayexpress/) by EBI, GeneX (http://www.ncgr.org/research/genex/) by the National Centre for Genome resources and the DNA data bank of Japan (http://www/ddbj.nig.ac.jp/). What is needed is a unique database recognized by the scientific community, equivalent to Genebank for DNA sequences.

However, one major caveat to the constitution and usefulness of such a database is the fact that different platforms yield results that may not be correlated to one another. This has been observed by Kuo *et al.*,[39] who compared Stanford type cDNA and Affymetrix oligonucleotide microarrays. Their results suggest a poor correlation between the two platforms with various gene-specific and probe-specific factors differently influencing the two types of array measurements.

4. Can we expect to monitor antigen-specific immune responses? If so what would be needed to do so?

This question was not even addressed. It is likely that it is too early to respond, as the answer will indeed require complete genome analysis. Nevertheless, if one considers the results described above by Boldrick *et al.* and Huang *et al.*,[13,33] which define both common and unique responses to pathogens at either the level of PBMCs or dendritic cells, the profiles corresponding to Th1 or Th2 cells (contribution of Ben

Cocks *et al.*, this volume) and other specific immune cell types, a positive answer seems possible.

5. What will be the impact of this technology be on vaccine development?

The contribution by Guido Grandi *et al.* already provides a positive answer to this question.[40] The approach of analyzing host-pathogen interactions from the point of view of the invading microbe can be applied to any number of other pathogens where experimental models exist. This is already being done for *H. pylori* (see TABLE 2).

More generally, for the rational design of new vaccines, genomics should offer the opportunity to increase our chances of success of more rapidly identifying correlates of protection in different models (for review, see ref. 41). The foreseeable opportunity of being able to simultaneously analyze the crosstalk between responsive immunocompetent cells and either pathogens or tumor cells will represent a major step towards the development of new vaccines. This should facilitate the discovery of new vaccine antigens (virulence factors or other unexpected proteins induced at specific stages of the infection process).

Transcriptome analysis will also help unravel new host cell pathways that must be stimulated in order to drive accurate and protective immunity. In keeping with this, formulating the antigen with adjuvants plays a major role in the induction of an appropriate response (humoral versus cell-mediated, Th1 versus Th2 polarization...) and it is likely that microarrays will be useful in the assessment and rational selection of new vaccine adjuvants. This was illustrated during the meeting by Thomas Mitchell *et al.* with the identification of Bcl-3 as a key survival factor for T cells, specifically induced by adjuvants such as LPS, CD40L or vaccinia viruses.[42]

Therefore, genomics will considerably improve exploratory investigations at the research level, but we can anticipate that microarray technology might also be ultimately applied to improve the industrialization processes of production and validation of vaccine batches.

It is our hope that bringing together such a diverse group of researchers will spur novel synergistic investigations and further contribute to the use of DNA microarray technology in the field of immunology and vaccine research.

REFERENCES

1. STAUDT, L.M. 2001. Gene expression physiology and pathophysiology of the immune system. Trends Immunol. **22:** 35–40.
2. ALIZADEH, A.A. & L.M. STAUDT. 2000. Genomic-scale gene expression profiling of normal and malignant immune cells. Curr. Opin. Immunol. **12:** 219–225.
3. GRANUCCI, F., P.R. CASTAGNOLI, L. ROGGE & F. SINIGAGLIA. 2001. Gene expression profiling in immune cells using microarray. Int. Arch. Allergy Immunol. **126:** 257–266.
4. LOY, A.L. & C.C. GOODNOW. 2002. Novel approaches for identifying genes regulating lymphocyte development and function. Curr. Opin. Immunol. **14:** 260–265.
5. MAAS, K., S. CHAN, J. PARKER, *et al.* 2002. Cutting edge: molecular portrait of human autoimmune disease. J. Immunol. **169:** 5–9.
6. STAUDT, L.M. & P.O. BROWN. 2000. Genomic views of the immune system. Annu. Rev. Immunol. **18:** 829–859.
7. SHAFFER, A.L., A. ROSENWALD, E.M. HURT, *et al.* 2001. Signatures of the immune response. Immunity **15:** 375–385.
8. GLYNNE, R., S. AKKARAJU, J.I. HEALY, *et al.* 2000. How self-tolerance and the immunosuppressive drug FK506 prevent B-cell mitogenesis. Nature **403:** 672–676.

9. GLYNNE, R., G. GHANDOUR, J. RAYNER, et al. 2000. B-lymphocyte quiescence, tolerance and activation as viewed by global gene expression profiling on microarrays. Immunol. Rev. **176:** 216–246.
10. TEAGUE, T.K., D. HILDEMAN, R.M. KEDL, et al. 1999. Activation changes the spectrum but not the diversity of genes expressed by T cells. Proc. Natl. Acad. Sci. USA **96:** 12691–12696.
11. BONECCHI, R., G. BIANCHI, P.P. BORDIGNON, et al. 1998. Differential expression of chemokine receptors and chemotactic responsiveness of type 1 T helper cells (Th1s) and Th2s. J. Exp. Med. **187:** 129–134.
12. GRANUCCI, F., C. VIZZARDELLI, N. PAVELKA, et al. 2001. Inducible IL-2 production by dendritic cells revealed by global gene expression analysis. Nat. Immunol. **2:** 882–888.
13. HUANG, Q., D. LIU, P. MAJEWSKI, et al. 2001. The plasticity of dendritic cell responses to pathogens and their components. Science **294:** 870–875.
14. BARANZINI, S.E., C. ELFSTROM, S.Y. CHANG, et al. 2000. Transcriptional analysis of multiple sclerosis brain lesions reveals a complex pattern of cytokine expression. J. Immunol. **165:** 6576–6582.
15. LOCK, C., G. HERMANS, R. PEDOTTI, et al. 2002. Gene-microarray analysis of multiple sclerosis lesions yields new targets validated in autoimmune encephalomyelitis. Nat. Med. **8:** 500–508.
16. EAVES, I.A., L.S. WICKER, G. GHANDOUR, et al. 2002. Combining mouse congenic strains and microarray gene expression analyses to study a complex trait: the NOD model of type 1 diabetes. Genome Res. **12:** 232–243.
17. AZUMA, T., M. TAKEI, T. YOSHIKAWA, et al. 2002. Identification of candidate genes for Sjogren's syndrome using MRL/lpr mouse model of Sjogren's syndrome and cDNA microarray analysis. Immunol. Lett. **81:** 171–176.
18. CARROLL, J.M., K.J. MCELWEE, E. KING, et al. 2002. Gene array profiling and immunomodulation studies define a cell-mediated immune response underlying the pathogenesis of alopecia areata in a mouse model and humans. J. Invest. Dermatol. **119:** 392–402.
19. BECHER, B., B.G. DURELL & R.J. NOELLE. 2002. Experimental autoimmune encephalitis and inflammation in the absence of interleukin-12. J. Clin. Invest. **110:** 493–497.
20. LYONS, P. 2002. Gene-expression profiling and the genetic dissection of complex disease. Curr. Opin. Immunol. **14:** 627.
21. HELLER, R.A., M. SCHENA, A. CHAI, et al. 1997. Discovery and analysis of inflammatory disease-related genes using cDNA microarrays. Proc. Natl. Acad. Sci. USA **94:** 2150–2155.
22. LAWRANCE, I.C., C. FIOCCHI & S. CHAKRAVARTI. 2001. Ulcerative colitis and Crohn's disease: distinctive gene expression profiles and novel susceptibility candidate genes. Hum. Mol. Genet. **10:** 445–456.
23. OESTREICHER, J.L., I.B. WALTERS, T. KIKUCHI, et al. 2001. Molecular classification of psoriasis disease-associated genes through pharmacogenomic expression profiling. Pharmacogenomics J. **1:** 272–287.
24. BOWCOCK, A.M., W. SHANNON, F. DU, et al. 2001. Insights into psoriasis and other inflammatory diseases from large-scale gene expression studies. Hum. Mol. Genet. **10:** 1793–1805.
25. HOFFMANN, K.F., T.C. MCCARTY, D.H. SEGAL, et al. 2001. Disease fingerprinting with cDNA microarrays reveals distinct gene expression profiles in lethal type 1 and type 2 cytokine-mediated inflammatory reactions. FASEB J. **15:** 2545–2547.
26. STAUDT, L.M. 2002. Gene expression profiling of lymphoid malignancies. Annu. Rev. Med. **53:** 303–318.
27. HANASH, S.M. 2001. Global profiling of gene expression in cancer using genomics and proteomics. Curr. Opin. Mol. Ther. **3:** 538–545.
28. ALIZADEH, A.A., M.B. EISEN, R.E. DAVIS, et al. 2000. Distinct types of diffuse large B-cell lymphoma identified by gene expression profiling. Nature **403:** 503–511.
29. ZHU, H., J.P. CONG, G. MAMTORA, et al. 1998. Cellular gene expression altered by human cytomegalovirus: global monitoring with oligonucleotide arrays. Proc. Natl. Acad. Sci. USA **95:** 14470–14475.

30. POOLE, L.J., Y. YU, P.S. KIM, et al. 2002. Altered patterns of cellular gene expression in dermal microvascular endothelial cells infected with Kaposi's sarcoma-associated herpesvirus. J. Virol. **76:** 3395–3420.
31. MOSES, A.V., M.A. JARVIS, C. RAGGO, et al. 2002. Kaposi's sarcoma-associated herpesvirus-induced upregulation of the c-kit proto-oncogene, as identified by gene expression profiling, is essential for the transformation of endothelial cells. J. Virol. **76:** 8383–8399.
32. MANGER, I.D. & D.A. RELMAN. 2000. How the host 'sees' pathogens: global gene expression responses to infection. Curr. Opin. Immunol. **12:** 215–218.
33. BOLDRICK, J.C., A.A. ALIZADEH, M. DIEHN, et al. 2002. Stereotyped and specific gene expression programs in human innate immune responses to bacteria. Proc. Natl. Acad. Sci. USA **99:** 972–977.
34. PIZZA, M., V. SCARLATO, V. MASIGNANI, et al. 2000. Identification of vaccine candidates against serogroup B meningococcus by whole-genome sequencing. Science **287:** 1816–1820.
35. PUSKAS, L.G., A. ZVARA, L. HACKLER, JR. & P.VAN HUMMELEN. 2002. RNA amplification results in reproducible microarray data with slight ratio bias. Biotechniques **32:** 1330–1340.
36. PRITCHARD, C.C., L. HSU, J. DELROW & P.S. NELSON. 2001. Project normal: defining normal variance in mouse gene expression. Proc. Natl. Acad. Sci. USA **98:** 13266–13271.
37. CARUCCI, D.J. 2001. Functional genomic technologies applied to the control of the human malaria parasite, Plasmodium falciparum. Pharmacogenomics **2:** 137–142.
38. SPELLMAN, P.T., M. MILLER, J. STEWART, et al. 2002. Design and implementation of microarray gene expression markup language (MAGE-ML). Genome Biol. **3:** RESEARCH0046-1-0046.9.
39. KUO, W.P., T.K. JENSSEN, A.J. BUTTE, et al. 2002. Analysis of matched mRNA measurements from two different microarray technologies. Bioinformatics **18:** 405–412.
40. GRIFANTINI, R., E. BARTOLINI, A. MUZZI, et al. 2002. Previously unrecognized vaccine candidates against group B meningococcus identified by DNA microarrays. Nat. Biotechnol. **20:** 914–921.
41. DHIMAN, N., R. BONILLA, D.J. O'KANE & G.A. POLAND. 2001. Gene expression microarrays: a 21st century tool for directed vaccine design. Vaccine **20:** 22–30.
42. MITCHELL, T.C., D. HILDEMAN, R.M. KEDL, et al. 2001. Immunological adjuvants promote activated T cell survival via induction of Bcl-3. Nat. Immunol. **2:** 397–402.
43. LE NAOUR, F., L. HOHENKIRK, A. GROLLEAU, et al. 2001. Profiling changes in gene expression during differentiation and maturation of monocyte-derived dendritic cells using both oligonucleotide microarrays and proteomics. J. Biol. Chem. **276:** 17920–17931.
44. GRANUCCI, F., C. VIZZARDELLI, E. VIRZI, et al. 2001. Transcriptional reprogramming of dendritic cells by differentiation stimuli. Eur. J. Immunol. **31:** 2539–2546.
45. LAPTEVA, N., M. NIEDA, Y. ANDO, et al. 2001. Gene expression analysis in human monocytes, monocyte-derived dendritic cells, and alpha-galactosylceramide-pulsed monocyte-derived dendritic cells. Biochem. Biophys. Res. Commun. **289:** 531–538.
46. LAPTEVA, N., Y. ANDO, M. NIEDA, et al. 2001. Profiling of genes expressed in human monocytes and monocyte-derived dendritic cells using cDNA expression array. Br. J. Haematol. **114:** 191–197.
47. CHEN, Z., J.R. GORDON, X. ZHANG & J. XIANG. 2002. Analysis of the gene expression profiles of immature versus mature bone marrow-derived dendritic cells using DNA arrays. Biochem. Biophys. Res. Commun. **290:** 66–72.
48. CHEN, Z., S. DEHM, K. BONHAM, et al. 2001. DNA array and biological characterization of the impact of the maturation status of mouse dendritic cells on their phenotype and antitumor vaccination efficacy. Cell Immunol. **214:** 60–71.
49. SUCIU-FOCA, C.N., F. PIAZZA, E. HO, et al. 2001. Distinct mRNA microarray profiles of tolerogenic dendritic cells. Hum. Immunol. **62:** 1065–1072.

50. MOSCHELLA, F., A. MAFFEI, R.P. CATANZARO, et al. 2001. Transcript profiling of human dendritic cells maturation-induced under defined culture conditions: comparison of the effects of tumour necrosis factor alpha, soluble CD40 ligand trimer and interferon gamma. Br. J. Haematol. **114:** 444–457.
51. BALTATHAKIS, I., O. ALCANTARA & D.H. BOLDT. 2001. Expression of different NF-kappaB pathway genes in dendritic cells (DCs) or macrophages assessed by gene expression profiling. J. Cell. Biochem. **83:** 281–290.
52. ROGGE, L., E. BIANCHI, M. BIFFI, et al. 2000. Transcript imaging of the development of human T helper cells using oligonucleotide arrays. Nat. Genet. **25:** 96–101.
53. HAMALAINEN, H., H. ZHOU, W. CHOU, et al. 2001. Distinct gene expression profiles of human type 1 and type 2 T helper cells. Genome Biol. **2:** RESEARCH0022.1-0022.11
54. CHTANOVA, T., R.A. KEMP, A.P. SUTHERLAND, et al. 2001. Gene microarrays reveal extensive differential gene expression in both CD4(+) and CD8(+) type 1 and type 2 T cells. J. Immunol. **167:** 3057–3063.
55. LI, X. D., D.M. ESSAYAN, M.C. LIU, et al. 2001. Profiling of differential gene expression in activated, allergen-specific human Th2 cells. Genes Immun. **2:** 88–98.
56. LIU, K., Y. LI, V. PRABHU, et al. 2001. Augmentation in expression of activation-induced genes differentiates memory from naive CD4+ T cells and is a molecular mechanism for enhanced cellular response of memory CD4+ T cells. J. Immunol. **166:** 7335–7344.
57. LIU, K., M. CATALFAMO, Y. LI, et al. 2002. IL-15 mimics T cell receptor crosslinking in the induction of cellular proliferation, gene expression, and cytotoxicity in CD8+ memory T cells. Proc. Natl. Acad. Sci. USA **99:** 6192–6197.
58. DIEHN, M., A.A. ALIZADEH, O.J. RANDO, et al. 2002. Genomic expression programs and the integration of the CD28 costimulatory signal in T cell activation. Proc. Natl. Acad. Sci. USA **99:** 11796–11801.
59. MUTA, H., L.H. BOISE, L. FANG & E.R. PODACK. 2000. CD30 signals integrate expression of cytotoxic effector molecules, lymphocyte trafficking signals, and signals for proliferation and apoptosis. J. Immunol. **165:** 5105–5111.
60. LI, Z., L. HE, K. WILSON & D. ROBERTS. 2001. Thrombospondin-1 inhibits TCR-mediated T lymphocyte early activation. J. Immunol. **166:** 2427–2436.
61. SUZUKI, Y., M. RAHMAN & H. MITSUYA. 2001. Diverse transcriptional response of CD4(+) T cells to stromal cell-derived factor (SDF)-1: cell survival promotion and priming effects of SDF-1 on CD4(+) T cells. J. Immunol. **167:** 3064–3073.
62. GROLLEAU, A., J. BOWMAN, B. PRADET-BALADE, et al. 2002. Global and specific translational control by rapamycin in T cells uncovered by microarrays and proteomics. J. Biol. Chem. **277:** 22175–22184.
63. FESKE, S., J. GILTNANE, R. DOLMETSCH, et al. 2001. Gene regulation mediated by calcium signals in T lymphocytes. Nat. Immunol. **2:** 316–324.
64. MCHUGH, R.S., M.J. WHITTERS, C.A. PICCIRILLO, et al. 2002. CD4(+)CD25(+) immunoregulatory T cells: gene expression analysis reveals a functional role for the glucocorticoid-induced TNF receptor. Immunity **16:** 311–323.
65. WILSON, S.B. & M.C. BYRNE. 2001. Gene expression in NKT cells: defining a functionally distinct CD1d-restricted T cell subset. Curr. Opin. Immunol. **13:** 555–561.
66. WILSON, S.B., S.C. KENT, H.F. HORTON, et al. 2000. Multiple differences in gene expression in regulatory Valpha 24Jalpha Q T cells from identical twins discordant for type I diabetes. Proc. Natl. Acad. Sci. USA **97:** 7411–7416.
67. FAHRER, A.M., Y. KONIGSHOFER, E.M. KERR, et al. 2001. Attributes of gammadelta intraepithelial lymphocytes as suggested by their transcriptional profile. Proc. Natl. Acad. Sci. USA **98:** 10261–10266.
68. HOFFMANN, R., T. SEIDL, M. NEEB, et al. 2002. Changes in gene expression profiles in developing B cells of murine bone marrow. Genome Res. **12:** 98–111.
69. HUSSON, H., E.G. CARIDEO, D. NEUBERG, et al. 2002. Gene expression profiling of follicular lymphoma and normal germinal center B cells using cDNA arrays. Blood **99:** 282–289.

70. ISLAM, T.C., J. LINDVALL, A. WENNBORG, et al. 2002. Expression profiling in transformed human B cells: influence of Btk mutations and comparison to B cell lymphomas using filter and oligonucleotide arrays. Eur. J. Immunol. **32:** 982–993.
71. BRUTSCHE, M.H., I.C. BRUTSCHE, P. WOOD, et al. 2001. B-cell isotype control in atopy and asthma assessed with cDNA array technology. Am. J. Physiol. Lung Cell. Mol. Physiol. **280:** L627–L637.
72. DADGOSTAR, H., B. ZARNEGAR, A. HOFFMANN, et al. 2002. Cooperation of multiple signaling pathways in CD40-regulated gene expression in B lymphocytes. Proc. Natl. Acad. Sci. USA **99:** 1497–1502.
73. ZHU, N., L.M. RAMIREZ, R.L. LEE, et al. 2002. CD40 signaling in B cells regulates the expression of the Pim-1 kinase via the NF-kappa B pathway. J. Immunol. **168:** 744–754.
74. LOCATI, M., U. DEUSCHLE, M.L. MASSARDI, et al. 2002. Analysis of the gene expression profile activated by the CC chemokine ligand 5/RANTES and by lipopolysaccharide in human monocytes. J. Immunol. **168:** 3557–3562.
75. RAVASI, T., C. WELLS, A. FOREST, et al. 2002. Generation of diversity in the innate immune system: macrophage heterogeneity arises from gene-autonomous transcriptional probability of individual inducible genes. J. Immunol. **168:** 44–50.
76. ROSENBERGER, C.M., M.G. SCOTT, M.R. GOLD, et al. 2000. *Salmonella typhimurium* infection and lipopolysaccharide stimulation induce similar changes in macrophage gene expression. J. Immunol. **164:** 5894–5904.
77. MIKITA, T., G. PORTER, R.M. LAWN & D. SHIFFMAN. 2001. Oxidized low density lipoprotein exposure alters the transcriptional response of macrophages to inflammatory stimulus. J. Biol. Chem. **276:** 45729–45739.
78. SHIFFMAN, D., T. MIKITA, J.T. TAI, et al. 2000. Large scale gene expression analysis of cholesterol-loaded macrophages. J. Biol. Chem. **275:** 37324–37332.
79. FESSLER, M.B., K.C. MALCOLM, M.W. DUNCAN & G.S. WORTHEN. 2002. A genomic and proteomic analysis of activation of the human neutrophil by lipopolysaccharide and its mediation by p38 mitogen-activated protein kinase. J. Biol. Chem. **277:** 31291–31302.
80. KOBAYASHI, S.D., J.M. VOYICH, C.L. BUHL, et al. 2002. Global changes in gene expression by human polymorphonuclear leukocytes during receptor-mediated phagocytosis: cell fate is regulated at the level of gene expression. Proc. Natl. Acad. Sci. USA **99:** 6901–6906.
81. TAYLOR, L.A., C.M. CARTHY, D. YANG, et al. 2000. Host gene regulation during coxsackievirus B3 infection in mice: assessment by microarrays. Circ. Res. **87:** 328–334.
82. CHAMBERS, J., A. ANGULO, D. AMARATUNGA, et al. 1999. DNA microarrays of the complex human cytomegalovirus genome: profiling kinetic class with drug sensitivity of viral gene expression. J. Virol. **73:** 5757–5766.
83. SIMMEN, K.A., J. SINGH, B.G. LUUKKONEN, et al. 2001. Global modulation of cellular transcription by human cytomegalovirus is initiated by viral glycoprotein B. Proc. Natl. Acad. Sci. USA **98:** 7140–7145.
84. GEISS, G.K., R.E. BUMGARNER, M.C. AN, et al. 2000. Large-scale monitoring of host cell gene expression during HIV-1 infection using cDNA microarrays. Virology **266:** 8–16.
85. GEISS, G.K., M. SALVATORE, T.M. TUMPEY, et al. 2002. Cellular transcriptional profiling in influenza A virus-infected lung epithelial cells: the role of the nonstructural NS1 protein in the evasion of the host innate defense and its potential contribution to pandemic influenza. Proc. Natl. Acad. Sci. USA **99:** 10736–10741.
86. PAULOSE-MURPHY, M., N.K. HA, C. XIANG, et al. 2001. Transcription program of human herpesvirus 8 (kaposi's sarcoma-associated herpesvirus). J. Virol. **75:** 4843–4853.
87. JENNER, R.G., M.M. ALBA, C. BOSHOFF & P. KELLAM. 2001. Kaposi's sarcoma-associated herpesvirus latent and lytic gene expression as revealed by DNA arrays. J. Virol. **75:** 891–902.

88. CHANG, Y.E. & L.A. LAIMINS. 2000. Microarray analysis identifies interferon-inducible genes and Stat-1 as major transcriptional targets of human papillomavirus type 31. J. Virol. **74:** 4174–4182.

89. HOBBS, W.E. & N.A. DELUCA. 1999. Perturbation of cell cycle progression and cellular gene expression as a function of herpes simplex virus ICP0. J. Virol. **73:** 8245–8255.

90. KHODAREV, N.N., S.J. ADVANI, N. GUPTA, et al. 1999. Accumulation of specific RNAs encoding transcriptional factors and stress response proteins against a background of severe depletion of cellular RNAs in cells infected with herpes simplex virus 1. Proc. Natl. Acad. Sci. USA **96:** 12062–12067.

91. STINGLEY, S.W., J.J. RAMIREZ, S.A. AGUILAR, et al. 2000. Global analysis of herpes simplex virus type 1 transcription using an oligonucleotide-based DNA microarray. J. Virol. **74:** 9916–9927.

92. BOLT, G., K. BERG & M. BLIXENKRONE-MOLLER. 2002. Measles virus-induced modulation of host-cell gene expression. J. Gen. Virol. **83:** 1157–1165.

93. LIANG, F.T., F.K. NELSON & E. FIKRIG. 2002. Molecular adaptation of *Borrelia burgdorferi* in the murine host. J. Exp. Med. **196:** 275–280.

94. COOMBES, B.K. & J.B. MAHONY. 2001. cDNA array analysis of altered gene expression in human endothelial cells in response to *Chlamydia pneumoniae* infection. Infect. Immun. **69:** 1420–1427.

95. ISRAEL, D.A., N. SALAMA, C.N. ARNOLD, et al. 2001. *Helicobacter pylori* strain-specific differences in genetic content, identified by microarray, influence host inflammatory responses. J. Clin. Invest. **107:** 611–620.

96. BJORKHOLM, B.M., J.L. GURUGE, J.D. OH, et al. 2002. Colonization of germ-free transgenic mice with genotyped *Helicobacter pylori* strains from a case-control study of gastric cancer reveals a correlation between host responses and HsdS components of type I restriction-modification systems. J. Biol. Chem. **277:** 34191–34197.

97. COX, J.M., C.L. CLAYTON, T. TOMITA, et al. 2001. cDNA array analysis of cag pathogenicity island-associated *Helicobacter pylori* epithelial cell response genes. Infect. Immun. **69:** 6970–6980.

98. GRIFANTINI, R., O. FINCO, E. BARTOLINI, et al. 1998. Multi-plasmid DNA vaccination avoids antigenic competition and enhances immunogenicity of a poorly immunogenic plasmid. Eur. J. Immunol. **28:** 1225–1232.

99. ICHIKAWA, J.K., A. NORRIS, M.G. BANGERA, et al. 2000. Interaction of *Pseudomonas aeruginosa* with epithelial cells: identification of differentially regulated genes by expression microarray analysis of human cDNAs. Proc. Natl. Acad. Sci. USA **97:** 9659–9664.

100. DETWEILER, C.S., D.B. CUNANAN & S. FALKOW. 2001. Host microarray analysis reveals a role for the *Salmonella* response regulator phoP in human macrophage cell death. Proc. Natl. Acad. Sci. USA **98:** 5850–5855.

101. ECKMANN, L., J.R. SMITH, M.P. HOUSLEY, et al. 2000. Analysis by high density cDNA arrays of altered gene expression in human intestinal epithelial cells in response to infection with the invasive enteric bacteria *Salmonella*. J. Biol. Chem. **275:** 14084–14094.

102. BLADER, I.J., I.D. MANGER & J.C. BOOTHROYD. 2001. Microarray analysis reveals previously unknown changes in *Toxoplasma gondii*-infected human cells. J. Biol. Chem. **276:** 24223–24231.

103. DE AVALOS, S.V., I.J. BLADER, M. FISHER, et al. 2002. Immediate/early response to *Trypanosoma cruzi* infection involves minimal modulation of host cell transcription. J. Biol. Chem. **277:** 639–644.

Historical Background and Anticipated Developments

BERTRAND JORDAN

Marseille-Génopole, Case 901, 13288 Marseille, France

ABSTRACT: Expression profiling using DNA arrays is often believed to have appeared during the second half of the 1990s, and to be based exclusively on nonisotopic methods. In fact, the first article describing the application of cDNA arrays to expression analysis was published in 1992, relied on radioactive labeling, and was a new development of "high-density" membranes used until then essentially for efficient screening of libraries. Several papers described the use of this technology for simultaneous expression measurement of thousands of genes at the time when the first glass microarrays were published. Simultaneously, oligonucleotide chips, originally developed for resequencing and mutation detection applications, were shown to be capable of expression measurement as well. The three approaches have developed over the years and still coexist, as each of them has specific advantages (and drawbacks); the major issues have become those of data quality, data analysis and storage (ideally in a common public database). Meanwhile, the technology continues to evolve. The most obvious trend is a shift towards using arrays of relatively long oligonucleotides that combine most of the advantages of very long (cDNA) and very short (25-mer) DNA segments. The search for better detection methods, ideally without labeling of the sample, is continuing, although it seems difficult to reach the required sensitivity. New materials for microarray manufacture and new implementations of existing methods have appeared. In addition, the field is progressively becoming segmented into high gene number, low volume (research) applications on the one hand, and low gene number, high throughput (diagnostic) uses on the other.

KEYWORDS: DNA arrays; expression; history; trends

HISTORICAL BACKGROUND

DNA arrays consist of a series of DNA segments regularly arranged on a support, and the expression measurement involves hybridizing the whole array with a labeled nucleic acid sample. The essential feature is parallel processing: in a single experiment, information is obtained on the expression level for each of the thousands of genes represented on the array. This parallelism has made the technology essential at a time when many megabases of genome sequence need to be understood in functional terms.

Address for correspondence: Bertrand Jordan, Marseille-Génopole, Case 901, 13288 Marseille, France. Voice: 33 (0)4 91 82 94 70; fax: 33 (0)4 91 82 94 71.
jordan@genopole.univ-mrs.fr

Early DNA Arrays for Homology Studies and Library Access

DNA arrays already existed in the seventies as dot blots[1] and slot blots that allowed for homology determination or expression analysis on a series of samples, with radioactive labeling in almost all cases. A major change in the field came with the development in the late 1980s of robotic devices ("gridding robots") that made it possible to array bacterial colonies in compact and regular patterns. The resulting "high-density filters" contained typically 10,000 spots on a square $22 \times 22\,cm^2$ surface, corresponding to a "pitch" (center to center spacing) of approximately 2 millimeters (see FIGURE 1). These arrays were essentially used for library access, providing an efficient approach to genome analysis,[2,3] at a time when the path taken

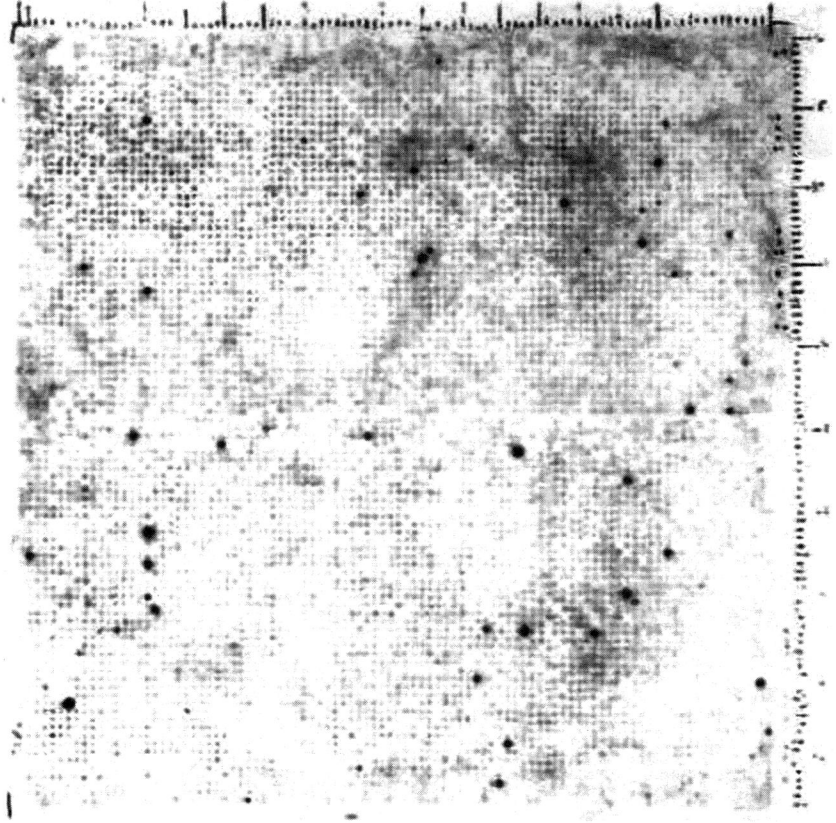

FIGURE 1. Early DNA array: 10,000 bacterial colonies containing DNA segments cloned in cosmids spotted on a 22 by $22\,cm^2$ nylon membrane. Hybridization with a radioactive probe prepared from the insert of a cDNA clone reveals positive spots indicating the corresponding genomic clones. The whole grid is visible because of light background hybridization. Successive hybridizations to search for various genomic clones are performed on the same membrane without stripping (to avoid loss of material), hence the large number of "positive" spots.

in the USA relied instead on PCR screening of cleverly arranged pools of clones.[4,5] Several resource centers accumulated various genomic and cDNA libraries and distributed them to laboratories as high-density membranes. When the user had identified a positive spot using a probe for a gene of interest, the center then provided the corresponding clone, an important advance at a time when library access was difficult and sequence information very meager.

Beginnings of Expression Analysis

The use, for expression analysis, of unordered or ordered colony filters containing cDNA clones began in the early 1980s with differential screening. Duplicate membranes, containing clones from conventional or subtracted cDNA libraries, were hybridized in parallel with complex labeled cDNA mixtures prepared from two different samples. The goal, of course, was to pin-point genes whose expression was different in the two conditions. Using radioactivity and X-ray film detection, the method was necessarily qualitative; it was also cumbersome and suffered from a number of technical problems, but it was nevertheless instrumental in isolating several important genes such as those coding for the T cell receptor[6] or the CTLA (Cytotoxic T Lymphocyte-Associated transcript) series of molecules.[7]

The concept of using imaging plate systems for quantitative acquisition of hybridization signals, allowing for more refined analysis of expression patterns, was discussed as early as 1990, with a first publication reporting actual data in 1992.[8] The full implementation of the technology took some time, however, as expression measurement with DNA arrays involves the quantification of very weak signals if data for genes expressed at very low levels is required. Artefacts leading to spurious data (especially with the unsequenced cDNA libraries of that period) had to be identified and eliminated,[9] and the fairly primitive image analysis programs of the period required serious improvement—a task made easier by increases in the computing power available to scientists. Automation of PCR and standardization of the plasmid vectors used for cDNA libraries led to a shift from colony filters to membranes on which amplified DNA was deposited.

High-Density Membranes, alias Macroarrays

During the first half of the 1990s, several groups worked out the methods, published proof-of-principle papers[9–11] and began accumulating expression data in different systems. Some of this work was performed in "gene discovery" mode, i.e., measuring the expression level in a number of conditions for a large set of genes, to highlight those that are the most relevant with regard to the biological question approached. Expression measurement was also done in an "expression profiling" mode, in which the set of genes (often more restricted) was chosen *a priori* and usually well known, and the objective was to obtain information on the samples: analysis of the expression profile for a series of tumors, for instance, in the hope of obtaining prognostic and therapeutic information (see, e.g., ref. 12). In this case the genes are used as tools to derive information on the samples. The high-density filter (under the more trendy name of "macroarray") is still widely used: for experiments of moderate scope, it performs quite adequately, requires only small samples, and blends well with existing laboratory equipment.

Miniaturization: cDNA Microarrays ...

In the mid-1990s, miniaturization became a major issue in the further development of DNA arrays, with the aim of increasing the number of genes assayed in a single experiment, and also of reducing sample usage—although most current systems still require microgram amounts of messenger RNA (or a recourse to RNA amplification), a major limitation in practice. One avenue involved scaling down cDNA arrays, using optical detection methods (fluorescence) because of their superior resolution, and depositing the DNA spots on very planar supports (glass slides) to allow intensity measurement with confocal optics in order to achieve the required sensitivity. First published in 1995,[13] this approach has now been applied to many important studies. The use of fluorescence allows for dual labeling, simplifying comparisons and facilitating standardization of series of experiments; good sensitivity has been obtained, although sample requirements remain high. Microarrays can be constructed in the laboratory; the necessary equipment is commercially available, although the expense and logistics are not trivial. Ready-made arrays have appeared on the market, although this has been a relatively slow process owing to the time taken to build up the necessary logistics as well as to intellectual property issues.

Microarrays can also be produced on nylon membranes. Because of the intrinsic fluorescence of all nylon supports (so far), detection must be performed by enzymatic means that are convenient and affordable, but relatively insensitive,[14] or with (^{33}P) radioactive labeling, using high-resolution detectors that provide sufficient resolution to quantify arrays with 400 micron pitch. In this form the method makes possible expression profiling at reasonable sensitivity with very small biological samples.[15]

... and Oligonucleotide Chips

The other, competing approach is that of oligonucleotide chips, pioneered by the firm Affymetrix. These glass chips comprise hundreds of thousands of small (currently $18 \times 18 \mu^2$) "features," each containing several million copies of a given oligonucleotide (20 to 25-mer). These arrays were originally developed for "quasi-sequencing" (mutation detection) applications.[16] They also allow for expression measurement, at the expense of assaying each gene with several (20 to 40) oligonucleotides and controls, in order to average out signal and background artefacts due to the vagaries of short oligonucleotide hybridization.[17] The manufacturing process, very similar to that of microelectronic devices, promises further miniaturization beyond the present chips that contain 500,000 features. Based solely on sequence knowledge, they do not require the cumbersome logistics of cDNA clone storage and PCR amplification, in contrast to cDNA arrays. However, this approach lacks flexibility; the arrays were initially very expensive and, accordingly, their use in the academic sector has developed slowly. Alternative approaches to oligonucleotide chips (notably different synthesis methods), and lower prices stemming from increasing competition, are increasing the popularity of this technology.

Data Acquisition, Storage, and Mining

The importance of software issues in expression measurement was not immediately recognized, but quickly became apparent as more and more data began to flow from these experiments. It includes a number of aspects, from verification of the validity of measurements to sophisticated data mining through data representation and storage issues. Although available computing power has increased dramatically in the last decade, these issues are still far from being satisfactorily solved. An accessible and comprehensive account of this field has recently been published.[18]

Data Validation, Quality, and Statistical Issues

Many of the initial papers on expression analysis using DNA arrays relied on data whose validity was not proven. A number of issues have arisen, for example, errors in the cDNA collections used to produce the PCR products that are supposed to represent specific genes,[19] or in the sets of sequences used by manufacturers to derive oligonucleotide chips. The practice of systematically replicating measurements and of providing a statistical estimate of the variability in the data set has become general only recently.[20] Software suites dedicated to data acquisition and validation now exist, and publication criteria have become more strict; efforts are being made to define the information that should be provided with microarray results in order to make these usable by others, for example the MIAME (Minimum Information on A Microarray Experiment) system developed by the European Bioinformatics Institute together with a wide group of users.[21]

LIKELY DEVELOPMENTS

Whole-Genome Chips?

With the completion of the human (and other) sequences, the race to higher density towards a "whole-genome" chip or microarray allowing for simultaneous measurement of the expression of complete sets of genes for a given organism will continue. Current limitations to minimum spot size and spacing for spotted arrays mean that the highest attainable densities remain below 5,000 spots per cm^2; thus the human or murine complement of genes is covered, at this time, by a set of several microarrays rather than a single array. Changes in spotting mechanisms and surface chemistry may allow for closer spacing, but in any case the future of very complex cDNA microarrays is probably limited because of the difficulty and expense involved in producing such large numbers of PCR products.

Concerning oligonucleotide chips, devices currently marketed by Affymetrix contain more than 500,000 short (20-mer) oligonucleotides on a single chip. However, because more than 20 oligonucleotides (including mismatched controls) are used for each gene, the latest "Human Genome U133" set from this firm requires two arrays to assay approximately 39,000 transcripts. The relatively poor yield of the photochemical on-chip synthesis process used does not allow (so far) for the manufacture of long oligonucleotides that would provide the same specificity with fewer "features." Increasing the chip density and placing one or a few million "features" on the surface of a microscope slide is probably feasible, although the resolution and sensitivity of reading devices would then have to be improved. In summary, assessing all human genes with a single Affymetrix chip will eventually be possible but may represent the limit of this technology. New on-chip synthesis approaches allowing for the production of long oligonucleotides (see below) could remove this limitation.

In any case "full human genome" chips will definitely be expensive, and problems in data acquisition, storage and analysis, because of the sheer volume of data, will be a deterrent to their use. Smaller, specialized arrays are likely to remain attractive for many purposes.

From "Clone-Based" to "Sequence-Based Arrays"

DNA arrays based on the use of cDNA clones suffer from the difficulty, expense and tedium involved in assembling collections of thousands of verified cDNA clones and in producing sufficient amounts of purified DNA of each of them by PCR. Oligonucleotide chips do not suffer from the same problem. They completely eliminate the recourse to clones since they are based solely on sequence information—which is already vast for many organisms and is increasing at an explosive rate. In addition, economies of scale can be considerable, and will be reflected in the prices if competition increases—this is already the case to a certain extent.

A number of laboratories and firms are developing "on-chip" oligonucleotide synthesis techniques that rely, for example, on the fast dispensing of synthesis reagents to individual sites on the chip by print head-like devices; some of them have already begun to market their processes or products. Such procedures allow for the use of classical synthesis chemistry (rather than the less efficient photochemical method), making possible the manufacture of much longer oligonucleotides (40–60-mers) that in turn reduce the need for redundancy in the chip because of their higher specificity. This makes it easier to represent many genes on a chip since only one or a few (long) oligonucleotides are needed to assay each of them. In addition, these approaches are inherently more flexible that the Affymetrix photochemical method. The fabrication of a different chip simply involves reprogramming the dispensing of reagents, rather than the manufacture of a complete new series of precision masks for the photochemical procedure. Other firms offer arrays made with pre-synthesized (long) oligonucleotides. The development of these technologies will not depend solely on scientific and engineering advances, as intellectual property in this field is already a hotly contested issue. Hopefully, these conflicts will be resolved in a fashion that opens up competition.

Altogether, it is certain that sequence-based DNA chips will be increasingly used in the future, certainly for "standard" sets and possibly, depending on methods development, for more specialized arrays.

From "Home-Brew" to Commercial Chips

A definite shift towards the purchase of commercially manufactured devices is apparent. It does not make economic sense for individual groups or even research institutes to invest large resources in the construction of standard microarrays, a task that can be handled more efficiently by industry or, in some cases, by public resource centers. This is not to say that the manufacture of microarrays will disappear from the research environment: custom arrays allowing for the assay of limited, specialised sets of genes will remain useful in many cases, and maximum flexibility can be achieved by making them "in house." Alternately, some manufacturers may undertake to produce such custom arrays, while others provide sets of "ready-to-spot" PCR products or oligonucleotides. The end result is likely to be a mixed situation in which large or standard sets of genes are assessed with commercial oligonucleotide chips or microarrays, while custom arrays are made in various academic-corporate arrangements. Of course in this context it is very important to standardize detection systems so that each type of industry-produced DNA array does not require its own proprietary scanning device.

From "Stand Alone" Array to Integrated "Lab-on-a-Chip"

Biochip technology is not limited to DNA arrays. The integration of a number of functionalities within chips whose dimensions are measured in centimeters is well underway; such devices can perform filtration, fluid handling, and reagent mixing, PCR reactions and even capillary electrophoresis. Their development is strongly stimulated by the need of pharmaceutical companies to perform literally millions of tests in the course of screening compounds for activities ("high throughput screening"), and by the requirement to do these assays very quickly, in a highly parallel mode and with the smallest possible amount of reagents.[22] At least for industrial and clinical systems, expression measurement (probably assessing limited numbers of genes) is likely to be packaged into such systems. This is for example the form in which expression measurement will penetrate in the clinical oncology laboratories—if indeed the clinical utility of such data is confirmed.

Detection without Labeling?

Fluorescent labeling is relatively cumbersome, interferes by steric hindrance with hybridization, and requires high-end, expensive detection systems; radioactive labelling is undesirable in many environments, and provides limited resolution even with high-performance (and costly) detectors. It would be very advantageous to achieve detection of the fact that a given location in the array has hybridized, and to quantify the extent of hybridization, by some other method. This should preferably involve the measurement of an electrical signal, and would, ideally, require no modification of the sample before hybridization. Much effort is devoted by many groups towards achieving this.[23,24] The approaches explored range from the detection of some subtle change of electrical properties upon hybridization to very exotic methods: microbalances "weighing" the extra mass of the hybridized material, or determination of the number of double-stranded (thus hybridized) molecules by atomic force microscopy. Proof of principle has been obtained for some of these approaches; it remains to be seen whether they can achieve the required sensitivity and throughput. If successful, they are likely to have an impact first in applications of DNA arrays such as bacterial identification or mutation detection, where a "yes/no" answer is often sufficient, rather that in expression measurement where accurate quantification is required.

More Sophisticated Data Interpretation and (Hopefully) Public Expression Databases

Software and bioinformatics development is a very important aspect that was not sufficiently taken into account at the beginning of the "DNA array revolution." Even today, the type of analysis performed on expression results remains relatively unsophisticated. In addition, much of the actual data is still unavailable outside of the originator's laboratory and the selected data sets provided by some groups on their websites lack a common format making them directly usable by others. Great efforts are being made to develop better analysis software including both extensive statistical, correlation and clustering analysis, and direct links to current, constantly updated information available on the Web. In addition, serious attempts are underway to define a standard data format that would make it possible to store expression data in the way in which DNA sequences have been archived, and to make it thus generally available and useful to the research community. A number of repositories already exist (for up-to-date lists see http://www.ncgr.org/genex/ and http://www.biologie .ens.fr/en/genetiqu/puces/bddeng.html), but so far there is no unified system comparable to the Genbank and EMBL sequence databases. Of course the problem of data format and standardization is much more complex for expression data than for sequence information.... The "MIAME" standard developed at the European Bioinformatics Institute[21] and already referred to shows how far we still have to go.

Expression Measurement Is Here to Stay

This is an easy prediction to make. Undoubtedly other methods able to add functional significance to gigabases of DNA sequence will be streamlined, made more efficient and more amenable to large-scale implementation: protein interaction studies, proteomics in general, gene inactivation experiments in various model systems are bound to become faster, easier, cheaper. However large-scale expression measurement, enhanced by general availability of sequence data and boosted by technical development of DNA arrays, will certainly remain a major approach in fundamental and applied biology for quite a long time.

REFERENCES

1. KAFATOS, F.C., C.W. JONES & A. EFSTRATIADIS. 1979. Determination of nucleic acid sequence homologies and relative concentrations by a dot hybridization procedure. Nucleic Acids Res. **7:** 1541–1552.
2. LENNON, G.G. & H. LEHRACH. 1991. Hybridization analyses of arrayed cDNA libraries. Trends Genet. **7:** 314–317.
3. HOHEISEL, J.D., G.G. LENNON, G. ZEHETNER & H. LEHRACH. 1991. Use of high coverage reference libraries of *Drosophila melanogaster* for relational data analysis. A step towards mapping and sequencing of the genome. J. Mol. Biol. **220:** 903–914.
4. OLSON, M., L. HOOD, C. CANTOR & D. BOTSTEIN. 1989. A common language for physical mapping of the human genome. Science **245:** 1434–1435.
5. GREEN, E.D. & M.V. OLSON. 1990. Systematic screening of yeast artificial-chromosome libraries by use of the polymerase chain reaction. Proc. Natl. Acad. Sci. USA **87:** 1213–1217.
6. HEDRICK, S.M., D.I. COHEN, E.A. NIELSEN & M.M. DAVIS. 1984. Isolation of cDNA clones encoding T cell-specific membrane-associated proteins. Nature **308:** 149–153.
7. BRUNET, J.F., F. DENIZOT & P. GOLSTEIN. 1988. A differential molecular biology search for genes preferentially expressed in functional T lymphocytes: the CTLA genes. Immunol. Rev. **103:** 21–36.
8. GRESS, T.M., J.D. HOHEISEL, G.G. LENNON, *et al.* 1992. Hybridization fingerprinting of high-density cDNA-library arrays with cDNA pools derived from whole tissues. Mamm. Genome **3:** 609–619.

9. NGUYEN, C., D. ROCHA, S. GRANJEAUD, et al. 1995. Differential gene expression in the murine thymus assayed by quantitative hybridization of arrayed cDNA clones. Genomics **29:** 207–215.
10. ZHAO, N., H. HASHIDA, N. TAKAHASHI, et al. 1995. High-density cDNA filter analysis: a novel approach for large-scale, quantitative analysis of gene expression. Gene **156:** 207–213.
11. PIETU, G., O. ALIBERT, V. GUICHARD, et al. 1996. Novel gene transcripts preferentially expressed in human muscles revealed by quantitative hybridization of a high density cDNA array. Genome Res. **6:** 492–503.
12. BERTUCCI, F., S.VAN HULST, K. BERNARD, et al. 1999. Expression scanning of an array of growth control genes in human tumor cell lines. Oncogene **18:** 3905–3912.
13. SCHENA, M., D. SHALON, R.W. DAVIS & P.O. BROWN. 1995. Quantitative monitoring of gene expression patterns with a complementary DNA microarray. Science **270:** 467–470.
14. CHEN, J.J., R. WU, P.C. YANG, et al. 1998. Profiling expression patterns and isolating differentially expressed genes by cDNA microarray system with colorimetry detection. Genomics **51:** 313–324.
15. BERTUCCI, F., K. BERNARD, B. LORIOD, et al. 1999. Sensitivity issues in DNA array-based expression measurements and performance of Nylon microarrays for small samples. Hum. Mol. Genet. **8:** 1715–1722.
16. FODOR, S.P., J.L. READ, M.C. PIRRUNG, et al. 1991. Light-directed, spatially addressable parallel chemical synthesis. Science **251:** 767–773.
17. WODICKA, L., H. DONG, M. MITTMANN, et al. 1997. Genome-wide expression monitoring in *Saccharomyces cerevisiae*. Nat. Biotechnol. **15:** 1359–1367.
18. BRAZMA, A., A. ROBINSON & J. VILOO. 2001. Gene expression data mining and analysis *In* DNA Microarrays: Gene Expression Applications. B. Jordan, Ed.: 106–129. Springer-Verlag. Berlin.
19. HALGREN, R.G., M.R. FIELDEN, C.J. FONG & T.R. ZACHAREWSKI. 2001. Assessment of clone identity and sequence fidelity for 1189 IMAGE cDNA clones. Nucleic Acids Res. **29:** 582–588.
20. LEE, M.L., F.C. KUO, G.A. WHITMORE & J. SKLAR. 2000. Importance of replication in microarray gene expression studies: statistical methods and evidence from repetitive cDNA hybridizations. Proc. Natl. Acad. Sci. USA **97:** 9834–9839.
21. www.ebi.ac.uk/microarray/
22. TALARY, M.S., J.P. BURT & R. PETHIG. 1998. Future trends in diagnosis using laboratory-on-a-chip technologies. Parasitology **117** (Suppl.) :S191–S203.
23. SOUTEYRAND, E., J.P. CLOAREC, J.R. MARTIN, et al. 1997. Direct detection of the hybridization of synthetic homo-oligomer DNA sequences by field effect. J. Phys. Chem. B **101:** 2980–2985.
24. WANG, J., A. JIANG & B. MUKHERJEE. 1999. New label-free DNA recognition based on doped nucleic-acid probes within conducting polymer films. Anal. Chim. Acta **402:** 7–12.

Analysis of B Cell Memory Formation Using DNA Microarrays

CAROLA G. VINUESA,[a] MATTHEW C. COOK,[b] MICHAEL P. COOKE,[c] IAN C. M. MACLENNAN,[d] AND CHRISTOPHER C. GOODNOW[a]

[a]*Medical Genome Centre, John Curtin School of Medical Research, Australian National University, ACT, Australia*

[b]*Department of Immunology, The Canberra Hospital, Woden, ACT, Australia*

[c]*Genomics Institute of the Novartis Research Foundation, San Diego, California, USA*

[d]*MRC Centre for Immune Regulation, University of Birmingham, Edgbaston, UK*

ABSTRACT: DNA microarray analysis of B cell subsets has identified comprehensive programs of gene expression that distinguish B cells at discrete stages of differentiation. The next task is to identify key genetic signals within these complex programs that regulate the dynamic cellular events during B cell activation *in vivo*. After stimulation with antigen, naïve B cells proliferate and differentiate, and then produce antibodies. Crucial qualitative differences in antibody responses are observed depending on whether or not B cells receive T cell help during activation. Proteins, lipopolysaccharides, and polysaccharides stimulate T-dependent (TD), T-independent type 1 (TI-1), and type 2 (TI-2) antibody responses, respectively. Only TD responses generate somatically mutated antibody-forming (plasma) cells and memory B cells, which produce high affinity anamnestic responses to subsequent antigen challenge. Somatic mutation of immunoglobulin genes occurs during B cell proliferation in germinal centres (GC), which are typical in TD responses but rare in TI responses. However, we have described a model, which is exceptional because numerous large GC form in response to a model TI-2 antigen, (4-hydoxy-3-nitrophenyl) acetyl (NP)-Ficoll. Significantly, these GC undergo involution before memory B cells are generated. This model provides an opportunity to investigate the genetic signals that drive memory cell formation, and we have compared global gene expression in TI and TD GC to identify a relatively small number of genes that are differentially expressed between the two prototypic B cell responses. This model demonstrates how genome-scale technology can be adapted to investigate specific aspects of B cell biology.

KEYWORDS: B cells; germinal centers; memory; microarray

INTRODUCTION

DNA microarray analysis and the availability of human and mouse genome sequences promise new ways of addressing long-asked fundamental questions of immunology. Already, the data generated by microarray analysis of lymphocyte subsets have revealed functional clusters of genes controlling cell division, apoptosis, and

Address for correspondence: Carola Vinuesa, Medical Genome Centre, John Curtin School of Medical Research, ANU, Australia 2600. Voice: +61 2 6125 4576.
carola.vinuesa@anu.edu.au.

cytoskeletal reorganization that are activated during T and B cell differentiation.[1,2] Genome-scale analysis has provided evidence that genes for proteins that perform broadly related functions are sometimes physically clustered within the genome. For the immune system, regions surrounding the major histocompatibility complex (MHC) and the antigen receptor genes for T, B and NK cells are rich in genes that become expressed in immune cells.

Proof-of-principle evidence for genome-scale approaches to identify otherwise indistinguishable subsets of B cells in disease has come from analysis of highly purified diffuse large cell lymphoma B cells. In a patient population that is homogeneous by conventional diagnostic tests yet heterogeneous with regard to outcome, microarray data have identified subtypes that predict prognosis.[3] Nevertheless, converting enormous amounts of genomic information into knowledge of B cell differentiation remains a substantial task. Rapidly evolving bioinformatics provides one tool to tackle the problem. Another approach is to apply the technology to models that can identify small numbers of key genetic signals that propagate the complex genetic programs observed in fully differentiated cells.[2] Here, we describe such an approach to investigate key signals regulating memory B cell formation.

Immunological memory is a hallmark of the adaptive or recombinant immune system. Acquired resistance to infectious disease was recognized in antiquity. Two centuries ago, Jenner provided empirical evidence that this phenomenon could be manipulated to powerful effect when he showed that cowpox provided long-lasting protection from smallpox. Manipulating memory B cell responses underpins all effective vaccination strategies currently in widespread use. These strategies have eradicated smallpox and provide protection against potentially fatal diseases such as tetanus and polio.

B cell memory accounts for the accelerated kinetics of secondary antibody production, which bind antigen with higher affinity than antibodies produced in the primary response. Accounting for this observation was central to the successful formulation of the clonal selection theory.[4] Since then, the sequence of events that leads to memory B cell formation has been largely resolved at the cellular level and remains in accord with the clonal selection theory. However, the fundamental molecular mechanisms that propagate and maintain memory B cells during immune responses remain uncertain.

Memory B cells and long-lived plasma cells are both products of terminal B cell differentiation.[5] Antigen-stimulated B cell differentiation begins when B cells bind antigen and migrate to the T zone areas of secondary lymphoid organs, such as spleen and lymph nodes, where they can potentially elicit help from primed T cells. If cognate T-B cell interaction takes place, a small number of B cells are induced to enter the follicles where they undergo rapid exponential growth and differentiate into proliferating centroblasts.[6] During centroblast expansion, somatic hypermutation of immunoglobulin (Ig) variable region genes changes the affinity of encoded Ig molecules for the original antigen. Since this is a stochastic process, most centroblasts acquire mutations that diminish Ig affinity for antigen, but for a small proportion, binding affinity is enhanced. According to the prevailing model of germinal centers, B cells that acquire advantageous mutations are selected for survival and further differentiation.

Competition between B cells expressing antigen receptors with different affinities takes place in GC after centroblasts exit the cell cycle to become centrocytes and is thought to depend on registration of two signals. The first signal is delivered when BCR bind to antigen held in immune complexes on the surface of follicular dendritic cells,[7] and the second when B cells process and present antigen to GC T cells and elicit help.[8,9] Once selected, centrocytes can differentiate into memory B cells, long-lived plasma cell precursors, or they can re-enter the centroblast pool to undergo further rounds of somatic mutation.[10–12]

Consistent with this model, gene expression profiles from GC B cells have identified high levels of expression of genes involved in regulating the G_2/M phase of the cell cycle. In addition, GC B cells also downregulate clusters of ribosomal subunit genes and genes that regulate energy production via glycolysis. Interestingly, GC B cells fail to upregulate NF-κB target genes.[1,13] Since many of these participate in antiapoptotic pathways, this suggests that GC B cells are biased towards programmed cell death. The transcriptional repressor Bcl-6 is a key regulator of gene expression in GC B cells. Bcl-6 downregulates a host of genes involved in BCR-mediated activation, including a cluster of genes expressed by plasma cell precursors.[14,15] In particular, Bcl-6 downregulates Blimp-1, which is a key promoter of plasma cell differentiation.[15,16] It is clear from these analyses that reprogramming for differentiation into either plasma cells or GC B cells is comprehensive. However, the signals that propagate memory cell differentiation are difficult to identify using this approach and remain unknown. We have begun to address this question using a unique model that enables investigation of the final stage of memory B cell differentiation from GC B cells.

MODEL

B cell responses are classified according to their dependence on T cell help. Immune responses to protein antigens only proceed when T cell help is available. By

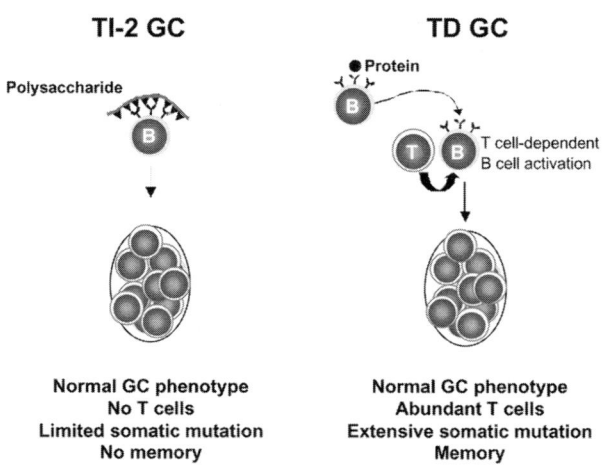

FIGURE 1. Comparison of characteristics of TD and TI-2 germinal centers.

contrast, bacterial polysaccharides and lipopolysaccharides can stimulate antibody production in the absence of T cell help (see FIGURE 1). Formation of GC and memory B cells characterizes immune responses to T-dependent (TD) (protein) antigens, and T cells are required for both the establishment and maintenance of GC in TD responses.[9] While GC are rare in response to T-independent (TI) antigens, we have previously reported that in quasimonoclonal (QM) mice, in which the majority of B cells express a transgenic B cell receptor (BCR) specific for the hapten NP, immunization with the model TI-2 antigen, NP-Ficoll generates large GC in virtually every lymphoid follicle.[17] These are genuine TI GC, because they also occur when either CD40-ligand-deficient mice or irradiated athymic recipients are reconstituted with QM-derived fetal liver. Phenotypically, TI and TD GC are indistinguishable (peanut agglutinin $(PNA)^{hi}$, GL-7+, Ki-67+, and Bcl-6+). However, there is a striking difference in the kinetics of TI GC formation and involution. TD GC survive for approximately three weeks, whereas TI GC peak five days after immunization and are undetectable by day six. This is due to massive and synchronized apoptosis of GC B cells. Since this coincides with the normal time of initial centrocyte selection by T cells, it suggests that terminal differentiation of TI GC B cells into memory B cells or long-lived plasma cells does not take place in the absence of T cells.[17] T-independent GC undergo limited somatic mutation, and there is no accumulation of mutations, presumably because of a blockade in centrocyte recycling back to renew the centroblast pool.[18] We have used this model to compare the genetic fingerprints of highly homogeneous B cell subsets purified from productive (TD) and nonproductive (TI) GC in order to identify centrocyte selection/memory differentiation signals.

METHODS

Mice and Immunizations

QM mice have a rearranged $V_H DJ_H$-transgene inserted into the V_H locus that encodes an Ig heavy chain, which can combine with any λ-light chain to form a BCR that binds NP with high affinity.[19] QM mice were generated on an Igκ-deficient background so that all B cells are specific for NP, except those that have undergone receptor editing. For these experiments, QM mice were mated with wildtype C57BL/6 to generate F_1 mice in which only about 20% of B cells bind NP. To generate TI-2 and TD responses, mice were immunized intraperitoneally with either 30 μg of NP-Ficoll or 50 μg alum-precipitated NP-CGG plus 1×10^9 heat-killed *B. pertussis*. For TD responses, one group of mice was primed with 50μg alum-chicken gamma-globulin (CGG) then rechallenged five weeks later with 50μg soluble NP-CGG so that T cell help was not limiting.

B Cell Purification

Single cell suspensions were prepared from spleens and then stained with B220-PE and GL-7 FITC (both obtained from BD biosciences). B cells were maintained at 4°C throughout staining. Cell suspensions were enriched for GC B cells by magnetic cell sorting with anti-FITC-magnetic beads and midiMACS columns (Miltenyi Biotec), according to the manufacturer's instructions. Next, GC B cells (B220+

GL-7^{high}) and resting B cells (B220$^+$ GL-7$^-$) were further purified by fluorescence-activated cell sorting (MoFlo). Purity of sorted cells exceeded 95%.

Analysis of RNA Expression

RNA was extracted from pellets of sorted cells by RNAzol treatment. Total RNA was transcribed *in vitro* and biotin labeled according to the recommended Affymetrix protocol, then hybridized on Affymetrix U74A arrays. Those genes that were differentially expressed by at least two-fold after ANOVA analysis with $P < 0.01$ were studied.

RESULTS

Primary TD GC do not appear until approximately seven days after immunization because of the time taken for T cell priming, whereas TI GC induced in QM mice by immunization with NP-Ficoll peak on day 4–5 and then undergo involution within 24 hours. In order to compare gene expression in GC B cells from TI and TD germinal centers, primary TI GC were compared with TD CG in carrier-primed mice, which develop with similar kinetics to TI GC because T cell help is not limiting. To this end, mice were primed with CGG 6 weeks before immunization with NP-CGG.

Groups of 16 mice were immunized with either NP-Ficoll or NP-CGG and spleens were harvested four days later. To ensure that late differentiation events were not missed in the groups examined four days after immunization, another group was examined at the peak of a true primary TD response to alum-precipitated NP-CGG administered in heat-killed *B. pertussis*. Finally, a group of unimmunized mice was used to provide reference resting B cell gene expression profiles (see FIGURE 2A).

At either four or ten days after immunization, spleens were harvested, and GC B cells were purified according to GL-7 and B220 expression (FIG. 2B). Approximately 25×10^4 GC B cells were obtained from the spleen of each immunized mouse. Since about 2×10^6 cells are necessary to obtain sufficient RNA (1.5 to 2 μg) for hybridization on Affymetrix DNA microarrays, splenocytes from eight mice were pooled for each experiment. Two microarray replicates were performed for each experimental group.

In total, 602 genes were differentially expressed in resting and GC B cells (see FIGURE 3); 180 genes were upregulated and 152 genes were downregulated in both TD and TI GC. Analysis of a subset of genes with known function is shown in TABLES 1 and 2. Interestingly, comparison of mice that were examined 4 days after NP-CGG immunization in CGG-primed mice and those analyzed 10 days after primary NP-CGG immunization in the presence of adjuvant revealed few differences in gene expression (23 genes exclusively regulated on day 10 versus 8 genes only regulated on day 4). These differentially regulated genes probably include those pathways induced by the use of adjuvant (*B. pertussis* and alum) for the primary immunization.

Gene expression data were validated by examining RNA expression of genes already known to be expressed specifically within GC B cells (see FIGURE 4). Even though Bcl-6 is subject to transcriptional and significant posttranslational regulation,

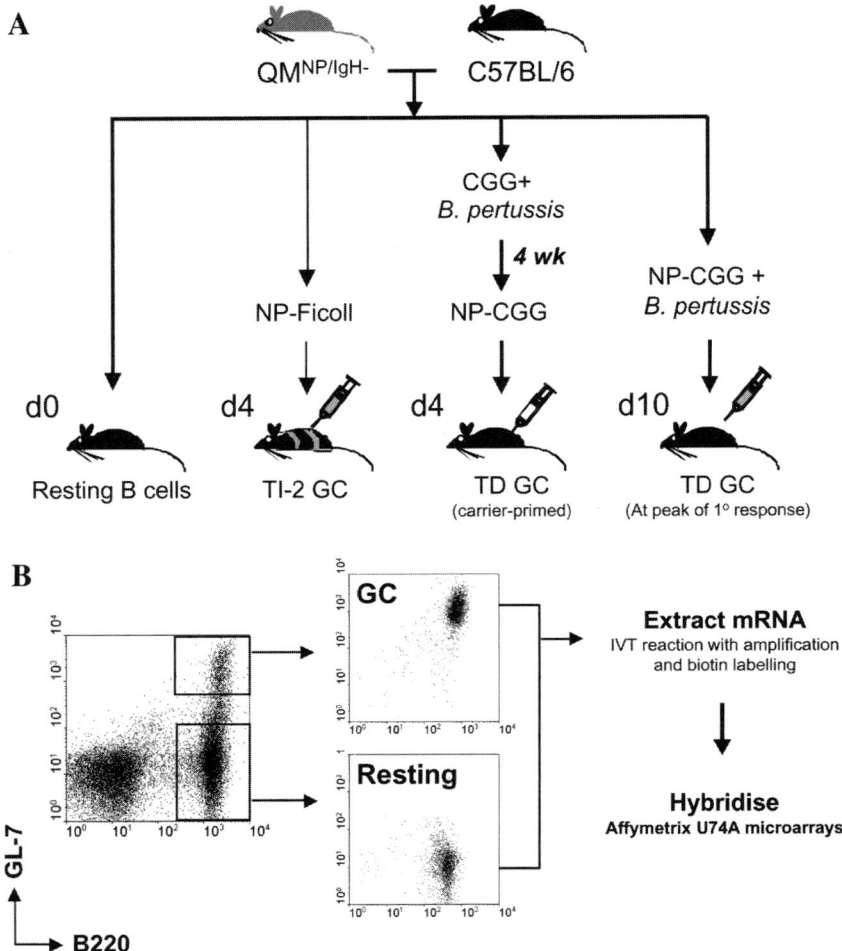

FIGURE 2. Experimental strategy for comparison of TI and TD germinal centers. (QM×C57BL/6) F1 mice were immunized according to three separate protocols to generate TI, primary TD, or secondary TD germinal centers (**A**). GC centers B cells (GL-7^{hi} B220$^+$) were purified by MACS and FACS (**B**). RNA was prepared from purified GC B cells and analyzed on Affymetrix U74A microarrays. RNA from resting B cells was prepared as for reference. See text for further details.

we observed a 3.1-fold increase in Bcl-6 RNA expression in TD GC and a 2.1-fold increase in TI GC. Cell cycle regulators such as such as Ki-67, cyclin B2, and proliferating cell nuclear antigen were increased in all GC. Gcet is a transcript of unknown function that is known to be expressed only by GC B cells.[20] Gcet was upregulated in TD but not TI germinal centers. Consistent with previous reports, the chemokine receptors CXCR5, CCR6 and CCR7 were all downregulated.[21-23]

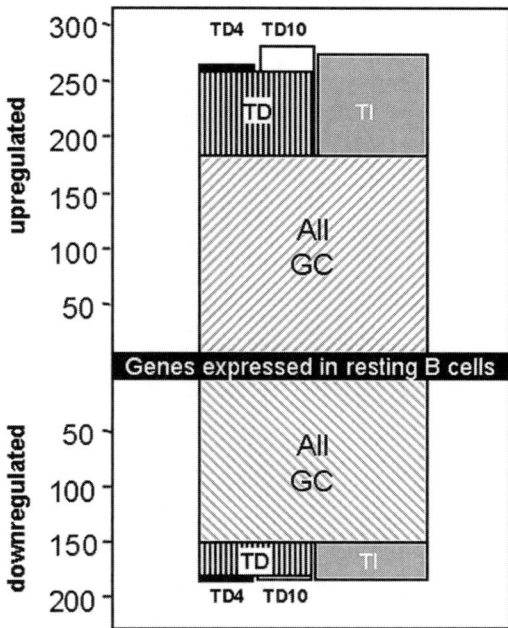

FIGURE 3. Summary of differential gene expression in TI and TD germinal centers. The number of genes whose expression differed between all GC and resting B cells is shown in the hatched boxes. The number of genes selectively up- or downregulated in TI and TD GC is indicated by *grey* or *vertical bars*, respectively.

To validate TI versus TD responses, we examined the pattern of Ig isotype expression (FIG. 4). As predicted, transcription of IgM and IgG3 was higher in TI GC, whereas other IgG isotypes were upregulated in TD GC. Consistent with previous reports, gene clusters controlling cell growth, DNA repair, apoptosis, and cytoskeletal reorganization feature prominently amongst the genes upregulated in GC. A total of nine protein kinases or interacting proteins were differentially expressed in TD GC.

Of the genes selectively regulated in the presence of T cell help, 30 are either unknown or are ESTs. Interestingly, the largest cluster of genes differentially expressed in TD and TI GC comprises 11 genes whose expression has previously only been described in the brain (see FIGURE 5). These genes have been shown to participate in the regulation of dendrite and axonal extension, neuronal differentiation, synaptic plasticity, and memory. This suggests that there may be molecular pathways that are common to formation of both neurological and B cell synapses. Similar evidence is emerging for molecules involved in formation of T cells synapses.[24,25]

We also identified genes exclusively regulated in TI GC (90 genes upregulated and 35 genes downregulated). These include phosphoinositol-3 (PI3)-kinase (alpha subunit), which is known to be crucial for TI-2 responses.[26] We also observed upregulation of genes for immunoglobulin joining (J) chain, immunoglobulin gene

TABLE 1. TD GC-specific gene expression

Function	No. of genes	Function	No. of genes
Upregulated		**Downregulated**	
Protein kinases/interacting proteins	6	Protein kinases/interacting proteins	3
Actin-cytoskeleton	6	Actin-cytoskeleton	2
Nerve growth and differentiation	7	Nerve growth and differentiation	4
Immunoglobulin heavy chains	3	Immunoglobulin heavy chains	2
Transcription factors	6	Cytokines	2
Metabolism	6	Adhesion	2
Hormonal/growth factors	3	Metabolism	2
Cell cycle/cell growth	2	MHC molecules	3
RNA processing/splicing/ribosylation	4	Cell cycle/cell growth	2
Chemokines/receptors	1	BCR co-receptors	2
Adhesion/gap junctions	2	Protein Phosphatases	1
Unknown/ESTs	23	Cathepsins	2
		Unknown/ESTs	7
		Other	3

transcripts, CCR1L (CCR1-like), and CD9. J-chain and immunoglobulin gene transcripts are typically upregulated in plasma cells, and CCR1L and CD9 have been found to be strongly upregulated in human myeloma cells.[27,28] These findings suggest that initial commitment to plasma cells takes place before the TI GC involute.

CONCLUSION

Elucidation of the molecular mechanisms that regulate memory cell formation is fundamental to understanding the adaptive immune response. Until now, two factors have hampered investigation of memory B cells in mice. First, memory B cells represent only about 1–2% of the total peripheral B cell pool.[29] Second, there are no surface markers specific for murine memory B cells, where antigen-specific B cells are otherwise easy to follow.[30] Consequently, investigation of memory formation using gene expression analysis has proceeded by comparison of gene expression profiles from GC B cells and resting naïve B cells, since genes that regulate memory formation must be contained in the list of differentially expressed genes obtained. Genes expressed in memory and GC B cells have been compared in humans, where markers of memory B cells are available. These studies have identified hundreds of differentially expressed genes.[3,31,32] This is not surprising since germinal center B cells undergo a complex process of proliferation, migration, differentiation, somatic hypermutation, isotype switching, selection and final maturation into the three different pathways mentioned above. However, this makes identification of the key signals problematic.

We have taken a different approach, based on comparison of two similar types of immune responses where the key difference is the presence or absence of memory cell formation. Furthermore, we have investigated gene expression in GC when memory cells are propagated. This approach has identified a much smaller number of genes that are likely to play key roles in establishing the more comprehensive programs of memory cell gene expression identified by microarray analysis of fully differentiated cells. Analysis of these genes is the subject of further investigation, but several important findings are apparent already.

A relatively small number of differentially expressed genes was identified. Interestingly, this included 11 genes previously only known to have a function within the brain. The neurological role of these genes includes regulation of dendrite and axonal extension and synaptic plasticity. Their differential expression in TD and TI GC implies that the same molecules are instrumental in memory B cell formation, and suggests that cytoskeletal reorganization, and synapse formation also occurs in GC B cells. This postulate is compatible with the prevailing model of GC reactions, in which centrocytes are thought to compete to capture antigen displayed on follicular dendritic cells in the light zones, where the antigen is held in the form of immune complexes with antibodies generated in the primary response. Somatically

TABLE 2. TI GC-specific gene expression

Function	No. of genes	Function	No. of genes
Upregulated		**Downregulated**	
Carbohydrate metabolism	5	Protein kinases/interacting proteins	9
Lipid/cholesterol metabolism	5	Actin-cytoskeleton	8
Transcriptional repressors/ negative regulators	5	Nerve growth and differentiation	11
Immunoglobulin heavy and light chains	5	Immunoglobulin heavy chains	5
Heat shock proteins	3	Transcription factors	6
Cytoskeleton	3	Metabolism	8
Chemokine receptors	1	Hormonal/growth factors	3
ER/membrane traffic	4	Cell cycle/cell growth	4
Unknown/ESTs	13	RNA processing/splicing/ ribosylation	4
		Chemokines	1
		Adhesion/gap junctions	4
		Cathepsins	2
		BCR co-receptors	2
		Cytokines	2

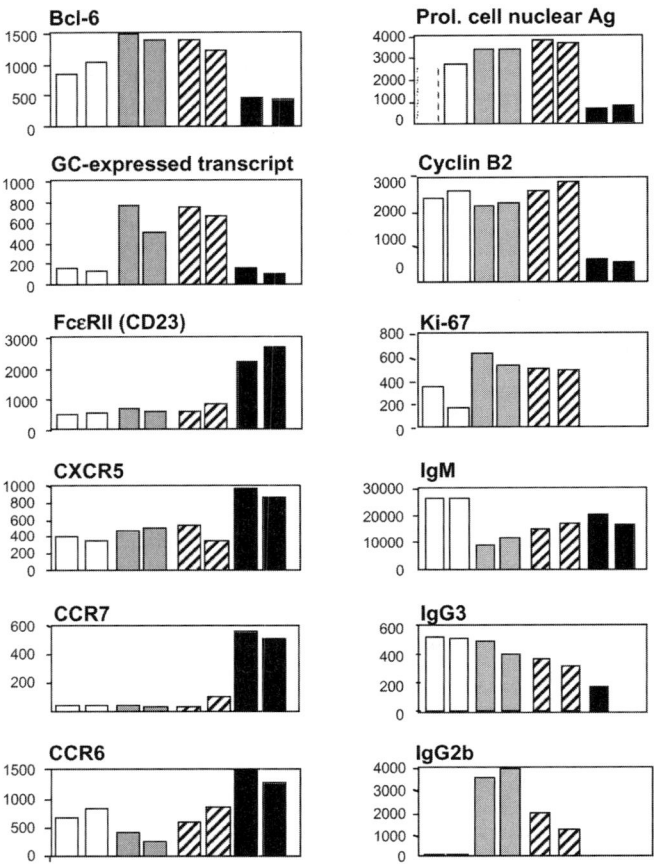

FIGURE 4. Microarray validation. Results of expression analysis for genes known to be selectively upregulated in TD germinal centers or in TI immune responses. TI GC B cells, *white bars*; day10 TD GC B cells, *grey bars*; day 4 TD GC B cells, *hatched bars*; resting B cells, *black bars*.

mutated antibody gives centrocytes an affinity advantage which might facilitate antigen capture; however, cytoskeletal reorganization, BCR clustering in synapses would provide an avidity advantage that would also facilitate antigen capture.

In addition, we have observed upregulation of plasma cell–related genes in both TD and TI GC. This suggests that plasma cells can develop after strong B cell receptor cross-linking in the absence of T cell help not only in extrafollicular areas, but also within the follicular germinal center environment. Current investigations are focussed on the group of genes that are respectively upregulated or downregulated exclusively in TD GC, since these should hold clues to centrocyte selection and the generation of memory B cells.

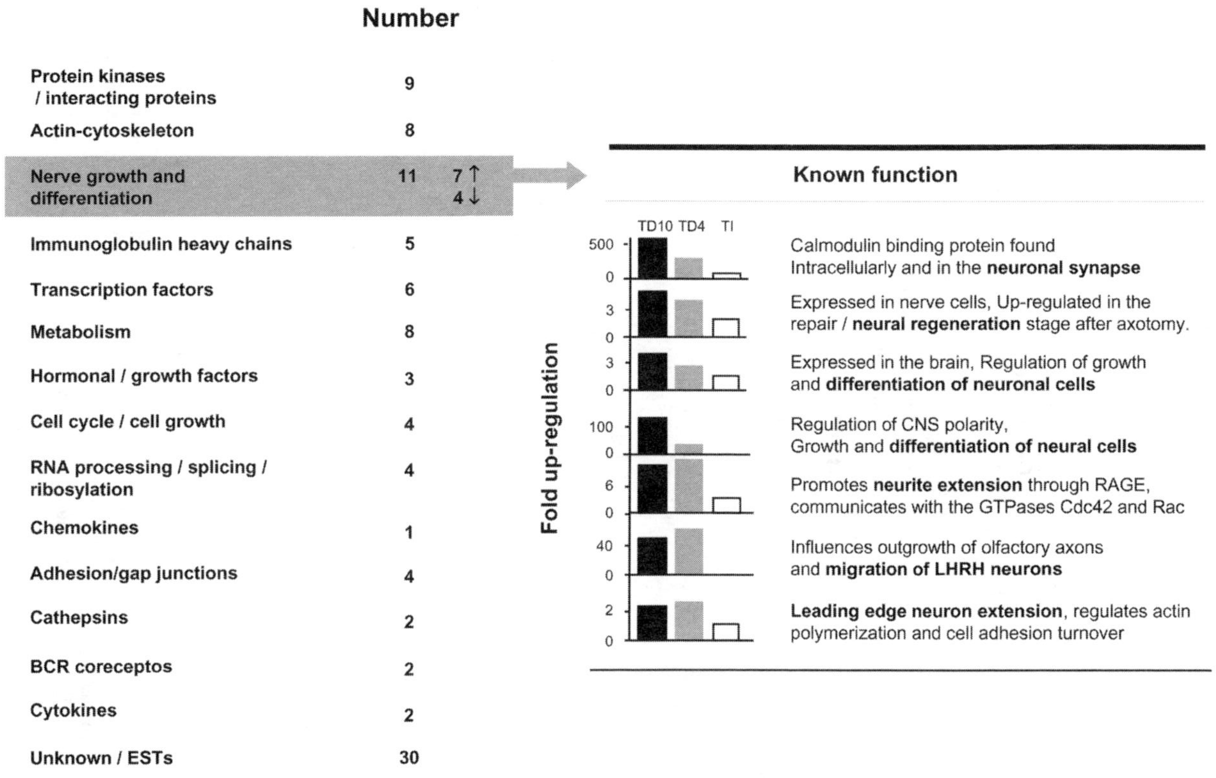

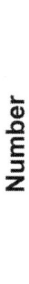

FIGURE 5. Summary of gene clusters selectively upregulated in TD GC. Seven genes previously only demonstrated to be expressed in the brain were selectively upregulated in TD GC. The relative levels of expression of these genes in TI and TD GC B cells are shown.

ACKNOWLEDGMENTS

CGV is a recipient of a Wellcome Trust International Prize Travelling Fellowship. ICMM holds an MRC program grant. MCC is supported by a grant from the Sylvia and Charles Viertel Foundation. We are grateful for the assistance of Susan Sutton.

REFERENCES

1. SHAFFER, A.L. *et al.* 2001. Signatures of the immune response. Immunity **15:** 375–386.
2. GLYNNE, R.J., G. GHANDOUR & C.C. GOODNOW. 2000. Genomic-scale gene expression analysis of lymphocyte growth, tolerance and malignancy. Curr. Opin. Immunol. **12:** 210–214.
3. ALIZADEH, A.A. *et al.* 2000. Distinct types of diffuse large B-cell lymphoma identified by gene expression profiling. Nature **403:** 503–511.
4. BURNET, F.M. 1957. A modification of Jerne's theory of antibody production using the concept of clonal selection. Aust. J. Sci. **20:** 67–69.
5. MCHEYZER-WILLIAMS, M.G. & R. AHMED. 1999. B cell memory and the long-lived plasma cell. Curr. Opin. Immunol. **11:** 172–179.
6. MACLENNAN, I.C.M. 1994. Germinal centres. Annu. Rev. Immunol. **12:** 117–139.
7. KOSCO, M. & D. GRAY. 1992. Signals involved in germinal center reactions. Immunol. Rev. **126:** 63–76.
8. LIU, Y.-J. *et al.* 1989. Mechanism of antigen-driven selection in germinal centres. Nature **342:** 929–931.
9. HAN, S. *et al.* 1995. Cellular interactions in germinal centres. Roles of CD40 ligand and B7-2 in established germinal centres. J. Immunol. **155:** 556–566.
10. COICO, R.F., B.S. BHOGAL & G.J. THORBECKE. 1983. Relationship of germinal centres in lymphoid tissue to immunological memory VI. Transfer of B cell memory with lymph node cells fractionated according to their receptors for peanut agglutinin. J. Immunol. **131:** 2254–2257.
11. KEPLER, T. & A. PERELSON. 1993. Cyclic re-entry of germinal center B cells and the efficiency of affinity maturation. Immunol. Today **14:** 412–415.
12. TARLINTON, D. & K. SMITH. 2000. Dissecting affinity maturation: a model explaining selection of antibody-forming cells and memory B cells in the germinal centre. Immunol. Today **21:** 436–441.
13. DAVIS, R.E. *et al.* 2001. Constitutive nuclear factor kappaB activity is required for survival of activated B cell-like diffuse large B cell lymphoma cells. J. Exp. Med. **194:** 1861–1874.
14. YE, B.H. *et al.* 1997. The Bcl-6 proto-oncogene controls germinal centre formation and Th2-type inflammation. Nature Gen. **16:** 161–170.
15. SHAFFER, A.L. *et al.* 2000. BCL-6 represses genes that function in lymphocyte differentiation, inflammation, and cell cycle control. Immunity **13:** 199–212.
16. TURNER, C.A., D.H. MACK & M.M. DAVIS. 1994. Blimp-1, a novel zinc finger-containing protein that can drive the maturation of B lymphocytes into immunoglobulin-secreting cells. Cell **77:** 297–306.
17. VINUESA, C.G. *et al.* 2000. Germinal centers without T cells. J. Exp. Med. **191:** 485–493.
18. TOELLNER, K.M. *et al.* 2002. Low-level hypermutation in T cell-independent germinal centers compared with high mutation rates associated with T cell-dependent germinal centers. J. Exp. Med. **195:** 383–389.
19. CASCALHO, M. *et al.* 1996. A Quasi-Monoclonal mouse. Science. **272:** 1649–1652.
20. CHRISTOPH, T., R. RICKERT & K. RAJEWSKY. 1994. M17: a novel gene expressed in germinal centers. Int. Immunol. **6:** 1203–1211.
21. WEHRLI, N. *et al.* 2001. Changing responsiveness to chemokines allows medullary plasmablasts to leave lymph nodes. Eur. J. Immunol. **31:** 609–616.
22. BOWMAN, E. *et al.* 2000. Developmental switches in chemokine response profiles during B cell differentiation and maturation. J. Exp. Med. **191:** 1303–1318.

23. YOSHIDA, R. *et al.* 1998. Secondary lymphoid-tissue chemokine is a functional ligand for the CC chemokine receptor CCR7. J. Biol. Chem. **273:** 7118–7122.
24. TORDJMAN, R. *et al.* 2002. A neuronal receptor, neuropilin-1, is essential for the initiation of the primary immune response. Nat. Immunol. **3**(5): 477–482.
25. KHAN, A. *et al.* 2001. Physiological regulation of the immunological synapse by agrin. Science **292:** 1681–1686.
26. FRUMAN, D. *et al.* 1999. Impaired B cell development and proliferation in absence of phosphoinositide 3-kinase p85alpha. Science **283:** 393–397.
27. DE VOS, J. *et al.* 2001. Identifying intercellular signaling genes expressed in malignant plasma cells by using complementary DNA arrays. Blood **98:** 771–780.
28. WANG, Y. *et al.* 2002. Cooperation between heparin-binding EGF-like growth factor and interleukin-6 in promoting the growth of human myeloma cells. Oncogene **21:** 2584–2592.
29. HAYAKAWA, K. *et al.* 1987. Isolation of high-affinity memory B cells: phycoerythrin as a probe for antigen-binding cells. Proc. Natl. Acad. Sci. USA **84:** 1379–1383.
30. MCHEYZER-WILLIAMS, L.J., M. COOL & M.G. MCHEYZER-WILLIAMS. 2000. Antigen-specific B cell memory: expression and replenishment of a novel B220(-) memory B cell compartment. J. Exp. Med. **191:** 1149–1166.
31. HUSSON, H. *et al.* 2002. Gene expression profiling of follicular lymphoma and normal germinal center B cells using cDNA arrays. Blood **99:** 282–289.
32. KLEIN, U. *et al.* 2001. Gene expression profiling of B cell chronic lymphocytic leukemia reveals a homogeneous phenotype related to memory B cells. J. Exp. Med. **194:** 1625–1638.

IL-15 Is a Growth Factor and an Activator of CD8 Memory T Cells

NAN-PING WENG,[a] KEBIN LIU,[a] MARTA CATALFAMO,[b] YU LI,[a] AND PIERRE A. HENKART[b]

[a]*Laboratory of Immunology, National Institute on Aging, National Institutes of Health, Baltimore, Maryland 21224, USA*

[b]*Experimental Immunology Branch, National Cancer Institute, National Institutes of Health, Bethesda, Maryland 20892, USA*

ABSTRACT: Memory lymphocytes, arising from naïve lymphocytes after antigenic stimulation and being long-lived, are the cellular basis for immunological memory. Recent studies of CD8 T cells suggest that generation of CD8 memory T cells requires the engagement of T cell antigen receptors (TCR) with antigen, yet the maintenance of CD8 memory T cells appears to be dependent on cytokines, such as IL-15, independent of TCR. Although considerable progress has been made in understanding the molecular and cellular events of TCR-induced differentiation and proliferation in the past decade, less is known about the mechanisms of IL-15 action. From a kinetic and comparative analysis of the responses of memory phenotype CD8 T cells to IL-15 and TCR stimulation *in vitro*, we found that IL-15 and anti-CD3 induce highly similar responses in memory phenotype CD8 T cells as measured by general gene expression profiles, synthesis of effector molecules (IFNγ, TNFβ, granzyme B and perforin), induction of cytotoxicity, and cellular proliferation. These findings indicate that IL-15 is not only a growth factor but also an antigen-independent activator for CD8 memory T cells.

KEYWORDS: IL-15; memory CD8 T cells; TCR, microarray; cytotoxicity

INTRODUCTION

Upon exposure to infectious agents, antigen-specific naïve T lymphocytes differentiate and proliferate to become effector T cells. The clonal expansion of antigen-specific T cells ensures production of a large number of effector cells and success in defense against pathogens. Once the infectious agents are eliminated, the majority of the effector cells undergo apoptosis, and a few survivors become memory T cells. Memory T lymphocytes are long-lived and are capable of rapid further differentiation and proliferation to become effector cells upon subsequent antigenic encounter.[1,2] These unique features of memory lymphocytes provide the cellular basis for immunological memory, a hallmark of adaptive immunity.

Address for correspondence: Nan-ping Weng, Laboratory of Immunology, National Institute on Aging, NIH, 5600 Nathan Shock Drive, Box 21, Baltimore, MD 21224. Voice: 410 558 8341; fax: 410 558 8284.
  wengn@grc.nia.nih.gov.

Generation of memory lymphocytes is dependent on antigenic stimulation, but the survival of memory lymphocytes appears to be antigen-independent and requires cytokines.[3–5] Several cytokines, such as IL-2, IL-4, IL-7, and IL-15, have been reported in the regulation of lymphocyte homeostasis.[6–9] IL-15 is capable of promoting proliferation and long-term survival of memory phenotype CD8 T cells, but not memory CD4$^+$ T cells in an antigen-independent fashion.[5,8,10]

IL-15 was initially identified by its ability to stimulate proliferation of T cell clones, an activity similar to IL-2.[11] However, in contrast to IL-2, which is produced only by activated T cells, IL-15 is produced by many types of cells including monocytes/macrophages,[12] dendritic cells,[13] keratinocytes,[14] and epithelial cells.[15] The IL-15 receptor consists of a private α-chain and shared IL-2 receptor β (CD122)– and common γ (CD132)–chain that are expressed individually or together to form various functional receptors with different affinities and signaling capabilities.[16] Despite some similarity between IL-15 and IL-2, they appear to have different biological functions.

The interaction of IL-15 with its receptor complex leads to activation of Janus kinases (Jaks) and subsequently to signal transducers and activators of transcription (Stats).[11] The IL-2/IL-15 receptor β chain is associated with Jak1 and Stat3, while the common γ chain is associated with Jak3 and Stat5.[17,18] IL-15 binding leads to phosphorylation of JAKs and subsequently to phosphorylation of the Stats. Phosphorylated Stats translocate to the nucleus, bind to DNA motifs containing a GAS element (TTN5-6AA), and induce gene transcription. In addition, activation of Src typosine kinase and MAPK pathways leads to fos/jun activation, which has also been observed in response to IL-15 signaling.[19]

IL-15 is capable of inducing proliferation of memory CD8 T cells in an antigen-independent fashion.[8,20–22] In the past decade, studies of CD8 T cell activation through the engagement of T cell antigen receptors (TCR) with the MHC class I-peptide complex of the target cells has revealed rich detail about the process of antigen-specific memory CD8 T cell proliferation and differentiation to become effector cells, accompanied by the production of cytokines and effector molecules.[23] Strikingly, despite apparent differences in the initial ligand/receptor interaction, both IL-15 and TCR engagement are capable of inducing CD8 memory T cell proliferation, suggesting that these two pathways share common downstream events. In contrast to the knowledge of TCR-mediated signaling events, the molecular mechanisms underlying IL-15–mediated proliferation and maintenance of CD8 memory T cells are not well understood.

In an effort to analyze the molecular and cellular changes induced by IL-15, and to compare IL-15– and TCR-mediated stimulation, we recently conducted a parallel comparative analysis of genome-scale gene expression, proliferation, effector molecule production, and cytotoxicity in memory phenotype CD8 T cells stimulated *in vitro* with IL-15 or anti-CD3 mAb. Our study reveals several interesting and unexpected findings.

IL-15 INDUCES PROLIFERATION OF MEMORY PHENOTYPE CD8 T CELLS *IN VITRO* SIMILAR TO TCR CROSSLINKING

It is known that IL-15 can selectively and potently stimulate memory phenotype CD8 T cells.[8,20–22] We first examined the ability of various concentrations of recombinant IL-15 to induce of proliferation of memory phenotype CD8 T cells isolated from peripheral blood of normal donors. We found that memory phenotype CD8 T cells proliferated almost at a nearly maximal rate at 100 ng/mL of IL-15 as measured by ^{3}H-thymidine incorporation (see FIGURE 1).[24] Memory phenotype CD8 T cells proliferate at a similar rate in response to either optimal IL-15 or anti-CD3 treatment. In addition, the expression of PCNA, a marker of proliferating cells, was also detected in memory phenotype CD8 T cells at two days after either IL-15 or anti-CD3 stimulation. Thus, IL-15 has a similar effect to TCR crosslinking in induction of proliferation of memory phenotype CD8 T cells.

IL-15 INDUCES GENE EXPRESSION CHANGES IN MEMORY PHENOTYPE CD8 T CELLS

The physiological importance of IL-15 in the homeostasis of CD8 memory T cells has been demonstrated from both *in vivo*[10,25-27] and *in vitro* studies.[8,28] However, the molecular nature of downstream events of IL-15 action has not been characterized. Recently, we analyzed IL-15–induced general gene expression changes in memory phenotype CD8 T cells over a two-day period using a cDNA microarray

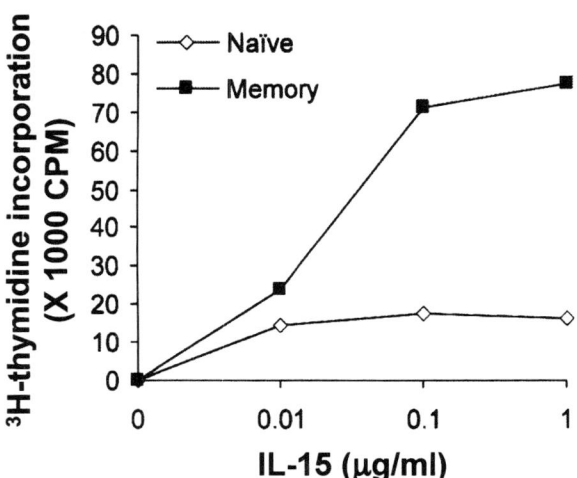

FIGURE 1. IL-15 induces proliferation of memory phenotype CD8 T cells. Recombinant IL-15 at concentration of 10, 100, 1000 ng/mL were used and ^{3}H-thymidine incorporation was analyzed over a four-day period. This is a representative result from three independent donors.

approach.[24] We designed the custom-made cDNA microarray filters consisting of 4,608 cDNA clones that were selected from the initial screening of expression status of over 40,000 unique human clones from resting and activated T cells, as well as from known immune-related genes that were not on the initial screening filters. mRNA was extracted from freshly isolated and stimulated memory phenotype CD8 T cells from normal donors and then pooled for gene expression analysis. The reproducibility between two independent microarray experiments comparing mRNA from the same stimulation conditions was analyzed by linear regression analysis and was found to be highly reproducible (average $R^2 = 0.95 \pm 0.02$).

IL-15 induced a variety of genes in memory phenotype CD8 T cells. We have identified a total of 176 gene/ESTs including 63 down- and 103 upregulated.[24] Functionally, these regulated genes can be divided into several groups:

1. transcriptional regulators (activating transcription factor 4 and HnRNP F),
2. cytokines and receptors (IL-7 receptor, CD74),
3. signaling molecules (cAMP-dependent protein kinase),
4. cell cycle regulators (cyclin-dependent kinase 4, proliferating cell nuclear antigen),
5. effector molecules (IFN-γ, TNF-β),
6. structure and metabolism (actin, glycine dehydrogenase), and
7. genes whose functions are not defined.

In agreement with the recent findings of gene expression analysis in both humans and mice, activation of T cells by IL-15 results in a large group of downregulated genes that are known to prevent cells from entering the cell cycle and apoptosis.[29,30] They include downregulation of genes like B cell translocation gene I and GDP-dissociation inhibitor, both of which are involved in the inhibition of cellular proliferation and activation. Some signal transduction molecules were also downregulated, such as LYN, FYN, FYN-binding protein, Jun B proto-oncogene, IL-1 receptor binding protein, cAMP-dependent protein kinase, NFκBIA, cAMP-specific phosphodiesterase 4B, nucleoside-diphosphate kinase, and protein tyrosine phosphatase type IVA. In addition, IL-15 downregulated several cell surface receptors including IL-7 receptor, CD44, CD69, and CXCR4. The precise roles of those genes in memory CD8 T cell homeostasis are not yet fully understood. Further characterization of their function will help to understand the mechanisms underlying the maintenance of the "resting" status as well as the survival of memory CD8 T cells.

A larger number of genes were upregulated in memory phenotype CD8 T cells after IL-15 treatment. Many of those genes are involved in signal transduction including Rho guanine nucleotide exchange factor 2, tyrosine- and threonine-specific cdc2-inhibitory kinase, v-yes-1, MKP-1 like protein tyrosine phosphatase. Several genes involved in transcription regulation were also identified, such as nuclear transcription factor Y, H2A histone family member O and Y, GA-binding protein transcription factor beta, histone acetyltransferase 1, activating transcription factor 4, cMyc, transcription elongation factor A, and interleukin enhancer binding factor 2. Interestingly, we also found that IL-15 induced expression changes of some activation- and apoptosis-related genes that were observed in antigen-activated T cells. These genes include lymphocyte-specific protein 1, interferon-induced 15 and 56kDa proteins, interferon-induced protein 35, intercellular adhesion molecule 2 and 5, integrin beta-5, and TRAIL, programmed cell death 5, Fas-associated phosphatase, and Apo3/DR3 ligand. Some cytokine and receptor genes were identified such as IFNγ, TNFβ, small inducible cytokine subfamily A, and CCR1 and 2. The enhanced expression of the DNA replication and cell cycle–related genes (proliferation-associated 2G4, proliferating cell nuclear antigen, cyclin-dependent protein kinase, early growth response 2) correlates well with cellular proliferation, suggesting that IL-15 treatment, like TCR crosslinking, is able to effectively turn on the cell cycle machinery in memory phenotype CD8 T cells.

The kinetic assessment of gene expression suggests that downregulation appears to occur early and remain stable over time, while upregulation occurs at all three time points with the number of genes increasing with time.[16,31] Thus, downregulated genes may serve in a maintenance role of the "resting" status, while upregulated genes are critical for proliferation and differentiation of memory CD8 T cells.

IL-15 INDUCES CHANGES OF GENE EXPRESSION SIMILAR TO TCR ENGAGEMENT IN MEMORY PHENOTYPE CD8 T CELLS

It has been reported that activation of T cells through TCR engagement induced enhanced expression of a large number of genes.[29,32–34] IL-15 also induces gene expression changes in memory CD8 T cells. We were surprised to find that these two apparently different stimuli induced remarkably similar overall gene expression changes at three time points over two days (average $R^2 = 0.96 \pm 0.01$).[24]

Among a total of 189 genes/ESTs changed at least 2-fold at one of three time points over a 2-day period in memory-phenotype CD8 T cells after either IL-15 or anti-CD3 treatment, 65 cDNA clones were downregulated and 124 cDNA clones were upregulated. Overall, approximately 77% of cDNA transcripts (145 out of 189) exhibited a similar pattern of changes between IL-15 and anti-CD3 stimulation: 94% of those down- and 68% of upregulated genes exhibited similar expression patterns in response to IL-15 and anti-CD3 treatments (see TABLE 1).[24]

TABLE 1. IL-15 and anti-CD3 induce gene expression changes in memory phenotype CD8 T cells[a]

Gene expression	Down	Up	Total
IL-15+anti-CD3	65	124	189
IL-15=anti-CD3	61	84	145
	(94%)	(68%)	(77%)
IL-15>anti-CD3	2	29	31
	(3%)	(22%)	(16%)
IL-15<anti-CD3	2	11	13
	(3%)	(10%)	(7%)

[a]Memory phenotype CD8 T cells were isolated from peripheral blood of normal donors by an immunomagnetic separation procedure. RNA was extracted from freshly isolated and stimulated cells from different donors and then pooled for gene expression analysis. The gene expression results were derived from two independent microarray hybridizations with a total of six independent measurements of each gene/EST.

Engagement of the TCR leads to a series of changes resulting in proliferation and production of effector molecules including IL-2. Since IL-2 shares two receptor subunits with IL-15 (common β and γ chains), it is necessary to determine whether the observed gene expression after anti-CD3 stimulation could be due to the IL-2R. Although IL-2 protein was not detected in anti-CD3 stimulated memory phenotype CD8 T cells, we cannot rule out the contribution of IL-2/IL-2R–induced gene expression. If there were an IL-2/IL-2R influence, one would expect it to give rise to a similar pattern of gene expression with time after stimulation. However, we observed that gene expression in IL-15 and anti-CD3 stimulated memory CD8 T cells diverged with time as seen by the greater differences in gene expression between anti-CD3 and IL-15 stimulation at 48 hours than at 2 or 12 hours. Therefore, the contribution of IL-2 to the extensive similarities of memory CD8 T cell response to anti-CD3 and IL-15 is likely to be minimal.

IL-15 AND ANTI-CD3 INDUCE SOME DIFFERENTIALLY EXPRESSED GENES IN MEMORY PHENOTYPE CD8 T CELLS

Despite the overall similarity, a few differentially expressed genes/ESTs were identified under IL-15 or anti-CD3 stimulation in memory phenotype CD8 T cells.[24] We have identified a total of 31 genes differentially induced by IL-15 but not by anti-CD3. Two genes, CD44 and Mel-transforming oncogene, were downregulated, and 29 clones were upregulated, which included two interferon-induced proteins (15 KDa and 56 KDa proteins), two chemokine receptors (CCR1 and CCR2), CD26, and CD53, transcriptional regulators (activating transcription factor 4, HnRNP F, and inhibitor of DNA binding 4), and cytoskeleton proteins (actinin alpha 4, profilin1, actin-binding protein 1A, and actin-related protein).

We have also identified genes/ESTs that are differentially regulated only after anti-CD3, but not IL-15 stimulation. Anti-CD3 induced downregulation of two genes, IFN-induced transmembrane protein I and calmodulin-1, and upregulation of 11 genes including CD2, CD83, EGF-response factor 1 and CC-chemokine.

Two of those differentially expressed genes (CD53 and CD2) after IL-15 and anti-CD3 stimulation were also analyzed at the protein level by FACS analysis. We confirmed an increase in CD53 expression only after IL-15 treatment and an increase in CD2 expression only after anti-CD3 treatment in memory phenotype CD8 T cells. As both CD53 and CD2 are involved in signal transduction,[35,36] their differential expression in memory phenotype CD8 T cells in response to IL-15 and anti-CD3 treatment point to the subtle difference between these two stimuli. Therefore, these two cell surface markers may provide valuable tools for further determining the significance of the differences of changes in CD8 memory T cells induced by IL-15 and TCR crosslinking.

IL-15 INDUCES PRODUCTION OF CYTOKINES (IFNγ AND TNFβ) AND EFFECTOR MOLECULES (GRANZYME B AND PERFORIN) IN MEMORY PHENOTYPE CD8 T CELLS

One consequence of CD8 T cell activation is target cell cytotoxicity through the production of certain cytokines and effector molecules.[37] On the basis of cDNA array analysis and subsequently confirmed by RNase protection assay (RPA), two key cytokines, IFNγ and TNFβ, were seen to be upregulated as early as 2 hours after IL-15 and anti-CD3 stimulation in memory phenotype CD8 T cells. Additional analysis of protein expression also confirmed that IFNγ and TNFβ were present only in the supernatant of memory phenotype CD8 T cells two days after stimulation with either IL-15 or anti-CD3 and not in the supernatant of unstimulated cells.

Interestingly, mRNA encoding two key effector molecules, granzymes and perforin, were detected in freshly isolated memory phenotype CD8 T cells and were upregulated in memory phenotype CD8 T cells after IL-15 or anti-CD3 treatment. The magnitude of increase in mRNA levels of these two cytokines did not reach 2-fold increase after stimulation. When the protein levels of granzyme B and perforin in memory phenotype CD8 T cells were measured by Western blot, we found that both granzyme B and perforin protein were detected at very low levels in freshly isolated memory phenotype CD8 T cells, and at 2 and 12 hours after IL-15 and anti-CD3 treatment. A significant increase of both proteins was found at 48 hours after stimulation. Thus, the upregulation of both cytokines and effector molecules at the mRNA and protein levels was evident in memory phenotype CD8 T cells after IL-15 and anti-CD3 stimulation.

IL-15 INDUCES CYTOTOXIC ACTIVITY IN MEMORY PHENOTYPE CD8 T CELLS

Induction of cytotoxic function is predicted to follow the production of effector molecules in memory phenotype CD8 T cells. Although IL-15 induces production of both cytokines and effector molecules in a similar way as anti-CD3 stimulation, it was unknown whether IL-15 was capable of inducing cytotoxic activity in memory phenotype CD8 T cells. We used a redirected cytotoxicity assay to determine if the granule exocytosis cytotoxicity pathway in memory phenotype CD8 T cells is activated by IL-15 treatment.[24] As predicted by the induction of cytokine and effector molecules, IL-15 also induced a significant cytotoxic activity in memory phenotype CD8 T cells after four days of IL-15 treatment. Cytotoxicity was not detected in freshly isolated memory phenotype CD8 T cells and was insignificant in cultured memory phenotype CD8 T cells with IL-2 (10 U/mL). In comparison with anti-CD3 stimulation, IL-15 induced equal or greater levels of cytotoxicity in memory phenotype CD8 T cells from different normal donors. Thus, IL-15–induced upregulation of cytotoxic effector protein correlates as seen by measurement of cytotoxic effector function of memory phenotype CD8 T cells (see FIGURE 2).

In contrast to the findings in a transgenic mouse system,[38] human memory phenotype CD8 T cells freshly isolated from peripheral blood did not show cytotoxic activity. In a remarkably similar way, IL-15 resembles TCR engagement (anti-CD3

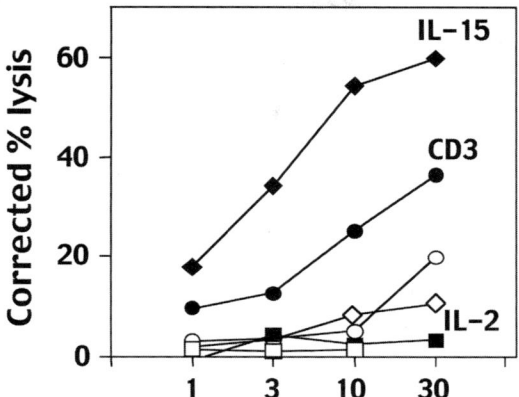

FIGURE 2. IL-15 and anti-CD3 induce cytotoxicity in memory phenotype $CD8^+$ T cells. Memory phenotype $CD8^+$ T cells were cultured with IL-15 or IL-2 for four days, or anti-CD3 for one day, and transferred to fresh wells and cultured without exogenous cytokine for another three days. Cytotoxic activity was then measured on Fas^- L1210 target cells by redirected cytotoxicity assay. Stimulation: IL-15 (*diamonds*), anti-CD3 mAb (*circles*), and IL-2 (*squares*). The presence or absence of biotinylated αCD3 mAb are indicated by closed or open symbols, respectively. This is a representative result from nine independent donors.[24]

stimulation) in inducing cytolytic function in memory phenotype CD8 T cells after a four-day culture. Although cytotoxic T lymphocyte (CTL) mediated killing is generally antigen-induced and specific, innocent bystander killing was also observed.[39,40] The ability of IL-15 to induce cytotoxic activity in memory phenotype CD8 T cells may provide a mechanism for bystander killing *in vivo*.

CONCLUSIONS AND FUTURE DIRECTIONS

The molecular and cellular events of IL-15 on human peripheral blood memory phenotype CD8 T cells have been assessed in parallel with TCR-mediated activation. These new findings point to a remarkable resemblance between IL-15- and anti-CD3–induced changes in memory phenotype CD8 T cells. The IL-15-induced transcriptional responses and cellular changes in memory phenotype CD8 T cells have been identified and analyzed. Together, it is evident that the survival and effector functions of CD8 memory T cells could be maintained by IL-15 in the absence of antigen.

The apparently different initial signaling pathways through IL-15 receptor and the TCR complex deliver significantly overlapping down-stream signals in memory phenotype $CD8^+$ T cells *in vitro*. It remains to be determined at what level these two signals converge, and what molecules are involved in the overlapping processes. Furthermore, it is of great interest to determine the effects of IL-15 on effector as well as naïve CD8 T cells and also to compare IL-15 effects between effector memory and central memory CD8 T cells. In addition, further studies will be needed to explore *in vivo* application of IL-15 in enhancing the lifespan of memory T cells and their effector functions in establishing an efficient long-term immune memory.

ACKNOWLEDGMENTS

We thank Kevin Becker of the DNA Microarray Unit for support the construction of our custom-made filters, the Clinical Core Lab for providing blood, and the Flow-cytometry Unit for technical assistance for FACS analysis at National Institute on Aging, NIH.

REFERENCES

1. AHMED, R. & D.GRAY. 1996. Immunological memory and protective immunity: understanding their relation. Science **272**: 54–60.
2. SPRENT, J. & C.D. SURH. 2001. Generation and maintenance of memory T cells, Curr. Opin. Immunol. **13**: 248–254.
3. UNUTMAZ, D., P. PILERI & S. ABRIGNANI. 1994. Antigen-independent activation of naive and memory resting T cells by a cytokine combination. J. Exp. Med. **180**: 1159–1164.
4. TOUGH, D.F., S. SUN, X. ZHANG & J. SPRENT. 2000. Stimulation of memory T cells by cytokines. Vaccine **18**: 1642–1648.
5. KU, C.C., M. MURAKAMI, A. SAKAMOTO, et al. 2000. Control of homeostasis of $CD8^+$ memory T cells by opposing cytokines. Science **288**: 675–678.
6. WALDMANN, T.A., S. DUBOIS & Y. TAGAYA. 2001. Contrasting roles of IL-2 and IL-15 in the life and death of lymphocytes: implications for immunotherapy. Immunity. **14**: 105–110.
7. SCHLUNS, K.S., W.C. KIEPER, S.C. JAMESON & L. LEFRANCOIS. 2000. Interleukin-7 mediates the homeostasis of naive and memory CD8 T cells in vivo. Nat. Immunol. **1**: 426–432.
8. ZHANG, X., S. SUN, I. HWANG, et al. 1998. Potent and selective stimulation of memory-phenotype $CD8^+$ T cells in vivo by IL-15. Immunity **8**: 591–599.
9. HUANG, L.R., F.L. CHEN, Y.T. CHEN, et al. 2000. Potent induction of long-term $CD8^+$ T cell memory by short-term IL-4 exposure during T cell receptor stimulation, Proc. Natl. Acad. Sci. USA **97**: 3406–3411.
10. LI, X.C., G. DEMIRCI, S. FERRARI-LACRAZ, et al. 2001. IL-15 and IL-2: a matter of life and death for T cells in vivo. Nat. Med. **7**: 114–118.
11. FEHINIGER, T.A. & M.A. CALIGIURI. 2001. Interleukin 15: biology and relevance to human disease. Blood **97**: 14–32.
12. CARSON, W.E., M.E. ROSS, R.A. BAIOCCHI, et al. 1995. Endogenous production of interleukin 15 by activated human monocytes is critical for optimal production of interferon-gamma by natural killer cells in vitro. J. Clin. Invest. **96**: 2578–2582.
13. JONULEIT, H., K. WIEDEMANN, G. MULLER, et al. 1997. Induction of IL-15 messenger RNA and protein in human blood-derived dendritic cells: a role for IL-15 in attraction of T cells, J. Immunol. **158**: 2610–2615.
14. BLAUVEL, T.A., H. ASADA, V. KLAUS KOVTUN, et al. 1996. Interleukin-15 mRNA is expressed by human keratinocytes, Langerhans cells, and blood-derived dendritic cells and is downregulated by ultraviolet B radiation. J. Invest. Dermatol. **106**: 1047–1052.
15. WEILER, M., B. ROGASHEV, T. EINBINDER, et al. 1998. Interleukin-15, a leukocyte activator and growth factor, is produced by cortical tubular epithelial cells. J. Am. Soc. Nephrol. **9**: 1194–1201.
16. TAGAYA, Y., R.N. BAMFORD, A.P. DEFILIPPIS & T.A. WALDMANN. 1996. IL-15: a pleiotropic cytokine with diverse receptor/signaling pathways whose expression is controlled at multiple levels. Immunity **4**: 329–336.
17. MIYAZAKI, T., A. KAWAHARA, H. FUJI, Y. NAKAGAWA, et al. 1994. Functional activation of Jak1 and Jak3 by selective association with IL-2 receptor subunits. Science **266**: 1045–1047.

18. LIN, J.X., T.S. MIGONE, M. TSANG, et al. 1995. The role of shared receptor motifs and common Stat proteins in the generation of cytokine pleiotropy and redundancy by IL-2, IL-4, IL-7, IL-13, and IL-15. Immunity **2:** 331–339.
19. MIYAZAKI, T., Z.J. LIU, A. KAWAHARA, et al. 1995. Three distinct IL-2 signaling pathways mediated by bcl-2, c-myc, and lck cooperate in hematopoietic cell proliferation. Cell **81:** 223–231.
20. RUSSELL, S.M., J.A. JOHNSTON, M. NOGUCHI, et al. 1994. Interaction of IL-2R beta and gamma c chains with Jak1 and Jak3: implications for XSCID and XCID. Science **266:** 1042–1045.
21. BEADLING, C., D. GUSCHIN, B.A. WITTHUHN, et al. 1994. Activation of JAK kinases and STAT proteins by interleukin-2 and interferon alpha, but not the T cell antigen receptor, in human T lymphocytes. EMBO J. **13:** 5605–5615.
22. KANEGANE, H. & G. TOSATO. 1996. Activation of naive and memory T cells by interleukin-15. Blood **88:** 230–235.
23. DOHERTY, P.C. & J.P. CHRISTENSEN. 2000. Accessing complexity: the dynamics of virus-specific T cell responses. Annu. Rev. Immunol. **18:** 561–592.
24. LIU, K., M. CATALFAMO, Y. LI, et al. 2002. IL-15 mimics T cell receptor crosslinking in the induction of cellular proliferation, gene expression, and cytotoxicity in CD8$^+$ memory T cells. Proc. Natl. Acad. Sci. USA **99:** 6192–6197.
25. LODOLCE, J.P., D.L. BOONE, S. CHAI, et al. 1998. IL-15 receptor maintains lymphoid homeostasis by supporting lymphocyte homing and proliferation. Immunity. **9:** 669–676.
26. MARKS-KONCZALIK, J., S. DUBOIS, J.M. LOSI, et al. 2000. IL-2-induced activation-induced cell death is inhibited in IL-15 transgenic mice. Proc. Natl. Acad. Sci. USA **97:** 11445–11450.
27. KENNEDY, Y., M.K., M. GLACCUM, S.N. BROWN, et al. 2000. Reversible defects in natural killer and memory CD8 T cell lineages in interleukin 15-deficient mice. J. Exp. Med. **191:** 771–780.
28. TANCHOT, C., F.A. LEMONNIER, B. PERRANAU, et al. 1997. Differential requirements for survival and proliferation of CD8 naive or memory T cells. Science **276:** 2057–2062.
29. TEAGUE, T.K., D. HILDEMAN, R.M. KEDL, et al. 1999. Activation changes the spectrum but not the diversity of genes expressed by T cells. Proc. Natl. Acad. Sci. USA **96:** 12691–12696.
30. MARRACK, P., T. MITCHELL, D. HILDEMAN, et al. 2000. Genomic-scale analysis of gene expression in resting and activated T cells. Curr. Opin. Immunol. **12:** 206–209.
31. IHLE, J.N. & I.M. KERR. 1995. Jaks and Stats in signaling by the cytokine receptor superfamily. Trends Genet. **11:** 69–74.
32. MARRACK, P., T. MITCHELL, J. BENDER, et al. 1998. T-cell survival. Immunol. Rev. **165:** 279–285.
33. LIU, K., Y. LI, V. PRABHU, L. YOUNG, et al. 2001. Augmentation in expression of activation-induced genes differentiates memory from naive CD4(+) T cells and is a molecular mechanism for enhanced cellular response of memory CD4(+) T cells. J. Immunol. **166:** 7335–7344.
34. ROGGE ,L., E. BIANCHI, M. BIFFI, et al. 2000. Transcript imaging of the development of human T helper cells using oligonucleotide arrays. Nat. Genet. **25:** 96–101.
35. OLWEUS, J., F.LUND-JOHANSEN & V. HOREJSI. 1993. CD53, a protein with four membrane-spanning domains, mediates signal transduction in human monocytes and B cells. J. Immunol. **151:** 707–716.
36. HAHN, W.C., S.J. BURAKOFF & B.E. BIERER. 1993. Signal transduction pathways involved in T cell receptor-induced regulation of CD2 avidity for CD58. J. Immunol. **150:** 2607–2619.
37. HENKART, P.A. 1994. Lymphocyte-mediated cytotoxicity: two pathways and multiple effector molecules. Immunity **1:** 343–346.
38. OPFERMAN, J.T., B.T. BER & P.G. ASHTON-RICKARDT. 1999. Linear differentiation of cytotoxic effectors into memory T lymphocytes. Science **283:** 1745–1748.

39. BURROWS, S.R., A. FERNAN, V. ARGAET & A. SUHRBIER. 1993. Bystander apoptosis induced by CD8+ cytotoxic T cell (CTL) clones: implications for CTL lytic mechanisms. Int. Immunol. **5:** 1049–1058.
40. KUWANO, K. & S. ARAI. 1996. Involvement of two distinct killing mechanisms in bystander target cell lysis induced by a cytotoxic T lymphocyte clone. Cell. Immunol. **169:** 288–293.

A Genomic View of Helper T Cell Subsets

LARS ROGGE

Laboratoire d'Immunorégulation, Département d'Immunologie, Institut Pasteur, 75724 Paris Cedex 15, France

ABSTRACT: Genomic-scale gene expression profiling in combination with the availability of a draft sequence of the human genome is beginning to revolutionize the way immunology is done. The possibility of measuring levels of gene expression for tens of thousands of genes simultaneously and in a quantitative fashion aids in the definition of a comprehensive molecular phenotype of cells and cellular processes of the immune system in health and disease. T helper lymphocytes are an essential element of appropriate immune responses to pathogens. To achieve effective immunity, T helper cells differentiate into at least two specialized subsets that direct type 1 and type 2 immune responses. Here, I discuss recent progress that has been made in our understanding of the genetic program that controls the development and functional properties of helper T cell subsets.

KEYWORDS: T lymphocytes; Th1/Th2 cells; oligonucleotide microarrays; adhesion molecules; cell trafficking; inflammation

INTRODUCTION

The discovery of polarized subsets of CD4+ T cells that differ in their cytokine secretion pattern and effector functions has provided the molecular framework for the understanding of the diversity of T cell-dependent immune responses.[1] The two subsets of differentiated CD4+ T cells, T helper type 1 (Th1) and T helper type 2 (Th2), protect against different microbial pathogens by producing cytokines capable of mobilizing different mechanisms of defense. T helper type 1 (Th1) cells are characterized by secretion of interferon-γ (IFN-γ) and are adept at macrophage activation. Such cells have been demonstrated in numerous infectious disease models to activate appropriate host defenses against intracellular pathogens, including viruses, bacteria, yeast and protozoa. T helper type 2 (Th2) cells produce interleukin (IL)-4, IL-5 and IL-13, and are involved in the development of humoral immunity protecting against extracellular pathogens. Uncontrolled Th1 and Th2 responses can cause chronic inflammatory autoimmune diseases and allergies, respectively. Although individual cells may exhibit a more complex and heterogenous pattern of cytokine production, many naturally occurring and experimentally induced immune responses show patterns of cytokine production and effector reactions that are clearly indicative of Th1 or Th2 dominance.[2,3] Thus, although the diversity of T cell-dependent immune responses cannot always be compressed into the Th1/Th2

Address for correspondence: Lars Rogge, Laboratoire d'Immunorégulation, Département d'Immunologie, Institut Pasteur, 25, rue du Docteur Roux, 75724 Paris Cedex 15, France. Voice: +33-1-4061 3822; fax: +33-1-4061 3204.

lrogge@pasteur.fr

paradigm, understanding the factors and pathways that influence the generation and effector functions of Th1 and Th2 cells is important for the development of therapeutic approaches against a variety of human diseases.[3]

Th1 and Th2 cells develop from a common precursor, the naïve CD4[+] T cell. The differentiation process is initiated by ligation of the T cell receptor (TCR) and directed by cytokines present at the priming of a T cell response. IL-4 promotes Th2 development,[4,5] whereas IL-12 plays a central role in controlling the development of Th1 cells from naïve precursor T cells.[6–8] Bacteria, viruses and intracellular parasites have been described as inducers of the IL-12 heterodimer both *in vitro* and *in vivo*.[6,9,10]

IL-12 is mainly produced by dendritic cells (DCs), the most potent antigen-presenting cells (APC) for naïve T helper cells *in vitro* and *in vivo*.[10,11] After their development in the bone marrow DCs transiently reside in non-lymphoid organs. In the peripheral tissues DCs act as sentinels for pathogen-derived antigens. They then migrate into the lymphoid organs, where they initiate activation of those T cells that are specific for the pathogen-derived antigens. DC migration is initiated by inflammatory stimuli, such as whole bacteria, the microbial cell wall component lipopolysaccharides (LPS), and cytokines such as IL-1, TNF-α. and IFN-α/β. These inflammatory mediators also convert the primarily antigen-capturing mode of the peripheral DCs into a mode specialized for T cell activation after migration into primary lymphoid organs. The recent discovery of subpopulations of DCs with distinct functional properties has further emphasized the importance of the crosstalk between DCs and T cells to direct T helper cell differentiation.[12,13] These observations indicate that DCs are of critical importance not only for the induction, but also for the outcome of primary immune responses.[14,15]

CONTROL OF T HELPER CELL DIFFERENTIATION IN THE PERIPHERY

Work over the past years has begun to unravel the molecular mechanisms that control the differentiation of naïve CD4[+] T cells into polarized Th1 and Th2 cells. One aspect of this work has been the identification and characterization of transcription factors that regulate this process. I will focus here on the control of Th1 cell development. Readers interested in the molecular mechanisms controlling Th2 development are directed to references 14, 16, and 17 for reviews.

Initial studies focused on the characterization of specific signal transducer and activator of transcription (Stat) molecules activated in response to the polarizing cytokines IL-4 and IL-12. IL-12 activates Stat4.[18,19] Accordingly, Stat4-deficient mice have impaired Th1 development.[20,21] The phenotype of Stat4-deficient mice is very similar to the phenotype of mice with targeted deletions of IL-12 or IL-12 receptor subunits[22,23] in that these mice are more susceptible to infection with intracellular pathogens.[11] In contrast, IL-12-, IL-12R- and Stat4-deficient mice are resistant to autoimmune diseases characterized by an uncontrolled Th1 response, such as mouse models of arthritis, insulin-dependent diabetes mellitus (IDDM) and experimental allergic encephalomyelitis (EAE).[24] These findings underline the importance of components of the IL-12 signaling pathway in the generation of type 1 immunity leading to the clearance of intracellular pathogens but also emphasize the necessity of a tight control of Th1 responses in order to avoid chronic inflammation.

IFN-γ has been shown to be an important co-factor for Th1 cell development. IFN-γ primes macrophages and DC for high-level IL-12 production. In addition, IFN-γ has direct effects in particular on mouse T cells such as the induction of the expression of the signaling component of the IL-12R, the IL-12Rβ2 subunit.[25] The direct effects of IFN-γ on mouse T cells have recently been analyzed in more detail using Stat1-deficient mice. This study revealed that Stat1 is required for the development of IFN-γ–producing cells *in vitro* when IL-4 is not neutralized in the cultures. Also the expression of IL-12Rβ2 was dependent on Stat1 under these suboptimal Th1-inducing conditions.[26] Thus, Stat1 is important for Th1 development and IL-12Rβ2 expression in the presence of endogenous IL-4. Although the molecular details still need to be worked out, it is of interest to note that IFN-γ does not appear to be of critical importance for IL-12Rβ2 expression in human cells.[27] In addition, our studies revealed an important function for type I interferon (IFNα/β) in the development of human Th1 cells. IFNα/β strongly induced development of IFN-γ–producing cells, even when IL-4 and neutralizing anti-IL-12 antibodies were present in the cultures.[27] IFNα/β acted directly on human naïve T cells as shown by the fact that IFNα/β induced Th1 differentiation and IL-12Rb2 expression of purified neonatal T cells stimulated with anti-CD3 antibodies.[28] In contrast to human cells, IFNα/β did not induce Th1 differentiation in mouse T cells.[29] We and others have addressed the basis for this interesting species-specificity. Unlike human IFNα/β in human T cells, mouse IFNα/β was unable to activate Stat4 in mouse T cells and consequently unable to induce *in vitro* development of mouse Th1 cells.[28,30] The IFNα/β–induced activation of Stat4 in human but not in mouse T cells has been explained by the finding that Stat4 is recruited to the IFNα/β receptor via the carboxy-terminus of Stat2.[31] Interestingly, Farrar *et al.* found a minisatellite insertion in mouse Stat2 which prevents recruitment of Stat4 to the IFNα/β receptor complex.[32]

In addition to Stat4 and Stat1, the trancription factor T-bet was shown to be of critical importance for the development of Th1 cells.[33] T-bet was isolated in a yeast one-hybrid screen as a factor binding to the IL-2 promoter. T-bet is expressed in Th1 cells but has not been detected in naïve T cells and in Th2 cells. Expression of T-bet in Th2 cells by retrovirus-mediated gene transfer induced IFN-γ production and repression of Th2 cytokine production.[33] The function of T-bet was subsequently analyzed in T-bet-deficient mice. T-bet$^{-/-}$ mice had normal lymphoid development, but exhibited profound defects in mounting Th1 immune responses.[34] Gene disruption of T-bet rendered resistant C57BL/6 mice susceptible to Leishmania major infection, and CD4$^+$ T cells from T-bet$^{-/-}$ animals showed strongly reduced IFN-γ production even when T cells were stimulated in the presence of IL-12.[34] Furthermore, T-bet–deficient mice spontaneously developed multiple inflammatory features characteristic of asthma, such as airway hyperresponsiveness, airway inflammation and airway remodeling.[35] Surprisingly, IFN-γ production by CD8$^+$ was not significantly affected in T-bet-deficient mice.[34] A similar lineage-specific requirement for a transcription factor had previously been reported for Stat4. CD4$^+$ T cells, but not CD8$^+$ T cells from Stat4-deficient mice showed significantly impaired IFN-γ production.[36] These findings leave us with the unexpected notion that IFN-γ production is controlled by independent mechanisms in CD4$^+$ versus CD8$^+$ T cells.

A current controversy concerns the order of events by which IL-12/Stat4, IFN-γ/Stat1 and T-bet induce the development of Th1 cells. Initially, it was suggested that IL-12/Stat4 induce expression of T-bet, which, by its characteristics as a master-regulator of Th1 development, induces expression of IFN-γ and of additional Th1-specific genes.[33] However, this model did not account for the observation that naïve T helper cells do not express detectable levels of IL-12Rβ1 and IL-12Rβ2 and have been reported to be unresponsive to IL-12.[25,27,37] The idea that IL-12/Stat4 were upstream of T-bet was subsequently challenged by Mullen et al. who demonstrated that expression of T-bet was not diminished in Stat4-deficient mice. The authors also reported that retrovirus-mediated expression of T-bet in Stat4$^{-/-}$ T cells induced IFN-γ production, chromatin remodeling of the IFN-γ locus, expression of IL-12Rβ2 and upregulation of endogenous T-bet.[38] The authors concluded that T-bet was upstream of the Stat4 pathway and that IL-12 signaling was only required as a survival signal for Th1 cells and to maximize IFN-γ production. This model was challenged by Afkarian et al. who recently reported that T-bet expression during T helper cell differentiation was strongly dependent on IFN-γ signaling and Stat1 activation, but that it was independent of Stat4.[26] This study also demonstrated that the upregulation of endogenous T-bet mRNA expression following retrovirus-mediated expression of T-bet in T cells is mediated by IFN-γ rather than by T-bet autoregulation.[26] These findings are consistent with a previous report demonstrating that IFN-γ is a potent inducer of T-bet.[39] Thus, more recently, T-bet expression was placed downstream of IFN-γ/Stat1 signaling. One month later, the plot got another twist with the identification of a novel heterodimeric cytokine termed IL-27. IL-27 is composed of the subunits EBI3 and p28. This cytokine is structurally and functionally related to IL-12 but is produced earlier than IL-12 after challenge of APCs with LPS.[40] IL-27 specifically acts on naïve CD4$^+$ T cells to induce their proliferation. Importantly, IL-27 synergizes with IL-12 to induce IFN-γ production and Th1 development in naïve CD4$^+$ T cells. The authors identified the orphan WSX-1/TCCR as a subunit of the IL-27 receptor. WSX-1/TCCR had been cloned by two groups as a type I cytokine receptor with highest homology to the IL-12Rβ2 subunit.[41,42] WSX-1/TCCR is expressed in PBL, thymus and spleen. Highest WSX-1/TCCR mRNA expression levels have been detected in naïve CD4$^+$ T cells but expression appears to be downregulated following T cell activation.[42] WSX-1/TCCR-deficient mice are viable and fertile and show no defects in hematopoietic and lymphoid development.[42,43] One study demonstrated that WSX-1/TCCR$^{-/-}$ mice had impaired Th1 responses as measured by IFN-γ production when challenged with protein antigen *in vivo* and increased susceptibility to infection with an intracellular pathogen, *Listeria monocytogenes*.[42] Interestingly, IL-12Rβ1 and IL-12Rβ2 mRNA expression and cellular responses to IL-12 were not diminished in WSX-1/TCCR-deficient mice, indicating that IL-27–induced signaling does not induce expression of a functional IL-12 receptor after stimulation of naïve CD4$^+$ T cells.[42] More recently, a study by Yoshida et al. confirmed reduced IFN-γ production by CD4$^+$ T cells from WSX-1/TCCR-deficient mice upon primary stimulation under Th1-inducing conditions (Con A, IL-12, anti-IL-4) but found that fully differentiated WSX-1$^{-/-}$ Th1 cells subjected to restimulation produced wild-type levels of IFN-γ.[43] Moreover, although WSX-1-deficient mice exhibited reduced IFN-γ production in the early stages of *L. major* infection and were highly susceptible to the pathogen, IFN-γ production was not reduced during the later phases.[43] The authors conclude that WSX-1/TCCR is critical for the initial production of IFN-γ following infection with an intracellular pathogen, but is not required for the effector functions of Th1 cells.[43] Taken together, these findings are consistent with a model in which APC-derived IL-27 is the "initiator" of Th1 development. Open questions concern the signaling molecules downstream of IL-27/WSX-1/TCCR, the connection of the signaling events induced by IL-27, IFN-γ and IL-12, and whether IL-27 can directly induce expression of T-bet or whether T-bet expression is indirectly induced by IL-27– and IL-12–mediated IFN-γ production. Given the pace of discoveries in this field, it will be interesting to see whether these questions have been answered by the time this manuscript is published.

TRANSCRIPT IMAGINING OF HUMAN AND MOUSE T HELPER CELL SUBSETS

Some time ago, we decided to take an independent approach to study human Th1 and Th2 cells. We wanted to know whether gene expression profiling using high-density oligonucleotides could provide valuable information on the biology of T helper cell subsets. The goals of this study were:

1. to learn more about the functional properties of human Th1 and Th2 cells,
2. to test whether this approach results in the identification of novel molecules regulating the process of T helper cell differentiation, and
3. to identify molecules which could be of interest for pharmacological intervention in chronic inflammatory diseases.

In addition, since substantial progress was made in the understanding of T helper cell differentiation in the course of our study (1997–1999), we could easily assess the robustness of the gene chip technology by comparing our findings to published results. We generated human Th1 and Th2 cells by stimulating cord blood leukocytes with mitogen in the presence of Th1-inducing conditions (IL-12 and neutralizing anti-IL-4 antibodies) or Th2-inducing conditions (IL-4 and neutralizing anti-IL-12 antibodies).[44] Since we were particularly interested in changes of gene expression occurring early in the differentiation process, we purified Th1 and Th2 cells three days after stimulation. Cell purification and subsequent mRNA extraction was performed by negative selection as rapid as possible to avoid possible confounding effects of stimulating antibodies and RNA degradation. In our initial study we used high-density oligonucleotide arrays with the capacity to display transcript levels of 6000 human genes. The analysis of the chip data was performed using software developed in house. After analyzing gene expression data from Th1 and Th2 cells derived from two independent donors, we realized that it was very difficult to discriminate between subset-specific and donor-specific changes in gene expression. We therefore decided to analyze gene expression in Th1 and Th2 cells generated from three additional donors and to analyze the dataset using a statistical algorithm (paired t-test). We found 215 genes to be differentially expressed at a confidence level of 95% and whose change in expression level was at least twofold. The importance of replicate microarray experiments has recently been emphasized in a study addressing the natural differences in mouse gene expression.[45] The authors used a 5406-clone spotted cDNA microarray to quantitate transcript levels in the kidney, liver, and testis from each of 6 normal male C57BL6 mice. ANOVA was used to compare the variance across the 6 mice to the variance among four replicate experiments performed for each tissue. The striking finding was that statistically significant variable gene expression was detected for 3.3%, 1.9%, and 0.8% of the genes in the kidney, testis and liver, respectively.[45] Importantly, many of the transcripts that were found most variable were immune-modulated, stress-induced, and hormonally regulated genes. An overlapping set of genes has recently been identified to be differentially expressed as a result of dietary alterations in a study addressing the effect of aging and caloric restriction on gene expression in the skeletal muscle of male C57BL6 mice.[46] These findings may raise some doubt about the validity of the data reported in reference 46 and in other published microarray studies performed with only one or two replicate experiments. Pritchard *et al.* further point out that genetically diverse populations such as humans are very likely to show an even greater variability in gene expression than inbred mice.[45] This suggests that a meaningful interpretation of global gene expression in humans will require many replicate experiments and/or an extensive characterization of normal variability.

We also analyzed mRNA expression of a selected set of genes in Th1 and Th2 RNA samples using kinetic RT-PCR.[47] As expected, we noticed variability in gene expression changes in cell lines derived from different subjects, but we could confirm differential expression of 28 out of 29 genes in Th1 and Th2 cells generated from two independent donors. Well-established marker genes for Th1 cells, such as IFN-γ and IL-12Rβ2 were found at much higher levels in Th1 than in Th2 cells. In addition, some genes which had previously not been implicated in the process of T helper cell differentiation, such as oncostatin M (OSM), were found to be overexpressed in Th1 cells. In this respect it is of interest to note that Th1 and Th2 cells have very recently been shown to differentially regulate hematopoietic progenitor cell homeostasis.[48] Mice deficient in Stat4 and therefore with defective capacity to efficiently mount Th1 responses had reduced progenitor cell numbers. In contrast, in the absence of Stat6, progenitor cell numbers and cycling status were increased. The phenotype in Stat4-deficient mice correlated with the decreased secretion of OSM by T cells from these mice and *in vivo* injection of OSM into Stat4$^{-/-}$ mice resulted in normal levels of hematopoietic progenitor cell numbers and cycling.[48] Our study is thus one example which illustrates how the availability of large-scale gene expression data can have an impact on the discovery of novel features of a biological system.

The gene expression profiles of Type 1 and Type 2 cells also revealed differential expression of genes encoding transcription factors some of which (GATA3 and IRF-1) have been previously characterized. In addition, several transcription factors that have not been associated with T helper cell polarization were also identified, including ETS-1, RORα2, IRF-7A, and c-fos. Although the target genes of these factors in regulating the gene expression patterns specific to each Th cell subset are not known, it is possible that some of these factors may control individual cytokine gene expression as GATA3 and T-bet control IL-4 and IFN-γ production, respectively.

Th1 cells are more susceptible to activation-induced cell death (AICD), a mechanism for downregulation of an immune response and maintenance of T cell tolerance. Results from our gene expression analysis suggested a potential mechanism for increased susceptibility of Th1 cells to AICD. Th1 cells expressed higher levels of TRAIL than Th2 cells, an apoptosis-inducing molecule; BAK, a proapoptotic Bcl-2 family member; and proapoptotic caspase-8, perforin, and granzyme B. Many of the apoptosis-related genes were further upregulated by additional IL-12 treatment. Indeed, incubation of Th1 cells with IL-12 resulted in an increased proportion of Th1 cells, but not Th2 cells, undergoing AICD. Thus, in addition to promoting Th1 differentiation, by acting on differentiating naïve precursors, IL-12 also affects the phenotype and expression profile of already differentiated Th1 cells.

The functional program of Type 1 and Type 2 T lymphocytes requires these cells to home to different sites. Th1 cells have been shown to preferentially express the chemokine receptor CCR5 and CXCR3, whereas Th2 cells were reported to preferentially express CCR3, CCR4, CCR8, and the chemoattractant receptor CRTh2.[49] Other gene expression changes identified in our study were consistent with previous experiments defining differential recruitment of Th1 and Th2 cells to sites of inflammation. We reported an increased expression of mRNA for fucosyltransferase VII (FucT-VII), which codes for an enzyme that mediates the fucosylation of selectin ligands on the surface of T cells. This fucosylation is required for the first step of lymphocyte adhesion to endothelial cells, "rolling." Recent *in vivo* observations have validated the biological relevance of this finding. FucT-VII was in fact found to be upregulated on T cells infiltrating the inflamed joints of patients affected by either rheumatoid arthritis or juvenile idiopatic arthritis (De Benedetti *et al.*, manuscript submitted). In both diseases, the T cells infiltrating the synovium have a clear Th1 phenotype.

IL-12 also induced two chemokine receptors CCR5 and CCR1, both of which promote increased responsiveness of Th1, but not Th2, cells to MIP-1α or RANTES. The activity of RANTES and other chemokines is regulated by CD26 (dipeptidyl-peptidase IV)-mediated cleavage. The DPP4 (encoding CD26) mRNA was found upregulated in Th1 cells compared to Th2 cells. The inactivation of chemokines by CD26 may contribute to the fine control of chemotactic migration of Th1 cells by providing a stop signal that keeps cells at the site of inflammation. Finally, higher expression on Th1 cells, and further upregulation by IL-12, of integrin α6β1, suggested that adhesion and extravasation of Th1 cells into tissues triggered by inflammatory chemokines might then be mediated by higher surface levels of integrin α6β1 binding to laminin in basal membranes and extracellular matrix. In contrast, mRNA for the integrin α4β7 was increased in Th2 in comparison to Th1 cells. As integrin α4β7 mediates binding of lymphocytes to the mucosal vascular addressing MAdCAM-1, these data predict preferential homing of Th2 cells to mucosal sites.

Of the 215 genes which we found differentially expressed in Th1 and Th2 cells, 157 genes were expressed at higher levels in Th1 cells and 58 genes were overexpressed in Th2 cells (see Table 2 in http://genetics.nature.com/supplementary_info/). There are several possible explanations for the apparent Th1 bias of our study. Previous studies have demonstrated that Th2 cells may require more time to acquire their effector functions than Th1 cells.[50,51] We harvested Th1 and Th2 cells already three days after stimulation, a time point at which the Th2-specific transcriptional program may not have been fully established. In addition, we also cannot rule out the possibility that our protocol of generating polyclonal Th1 and Th2 cell line from cord blood using PHA induces a Th1 bias. Experiments are underway to address this question.

Hamalainen et al. have recently used an oligonucleotide microarray specifically designed to screen for 250 inflammation-related genes in order to identify those differentially expressed in human, cord blood–derived Th1 and Th2 cells.[52] This study focused on the gene expression analysis of established Th1 and Th2 cells which had been restimulated with anti-CD3 and anti-CD28 antibodies two weeks after initial stimulation under Th1- or Th2-inducing conditions. Although the experimental protocol to generate Th1 and Th2 cells used in the study by Hamalainen et al.[52] was quite distinct from our protocol,[44] there was a large overlap of the genes identified in both studies. In addition to the Th1/Th2 signature cytokines such as IFN-γ, IL-4, IL-5 and IL-13, several chemokines (MIP-1α, MIP-1β, RANTES) and chemokine receptors (CCR1, CCR2, CCR4, CCR5) were found differentially expressed in human Th1 and Th2 cells.[52] These results further emphasize the importance of precise positioning of polarized effector T cells to eradicate pathogens.

A subsequent study, Chtanova et al. used high-density oligonucleotide microarrays to analyze gene expression in murine CD4$^+$ Th1 and Th2 cells, as well as CD8$^+$ type 1 and type 2 T cells (Tc1 and Tc2).[53] In contrast to our study where Th1-overexpressed genes predominated,[44] Chtanova et al. identified more type 2-biased genes.[53] It is important to note that different protocols were used to generate polarized T cell subsets in the two studies. Chtanova et al. stimulated purified naïve mouse CD4$^+$ and CD8$^+$ T cells with anti-CD3/CD28 antibodies, IL-2 and IL-6 plus the polarizing cytokine cocktail. Cells were cultured for seven days and then restimulated for 24 hours with anti-CD3 before extracting RNA. A previous report has demonstrated that IL-6 is able to polarize naïve CD4$^+$ T cells into Th2 cells by inducing the initial production of IL-4 in CD4$^+$ T cells.[54] In addition, it has been shown that IL-6 inhibits Th1 differentiation in an IL-4-independent manner through the induction of SOCS1.[55] The addition of IL-6 to the cultures could therefore be a possible explanation for the Th2-bias observed in this study.[53] As expected, CD4$^+$ and CD8$^+$ T cell subsets expressed their signature cytokines. Transcripts levels for IFN-γ were higher in Th1 and Tc1 cells as compared to Th2 and Tc2 cells. Higher levels of IL-4, IL-5, and IL-10 were instead found in Th2 and Tc2 cells. Chtanova et al. found two members of the TNF receptor-associated factor (TRAF) family to be differentially expressed in type 1 and type 2 cells. TRAF4 was expressed at a higher level in type 1 cells while TRAF5 was preferentially expressed in type 2 cells. Members of this family serve as adapter proteins that mediate cytokine signaling, in particular they seem to play a role in TNF and Toll/IL-1 signaling, resulting in activation of transcription factors NF-κB and AP-1. Clearly, much work remains to be done to address the biological relevance of these findings.

Together, the recent results demonstrate the impact of large-scale gene expression profiling on the analysis of biological systems. The analyses of the expression of 6,000 genes in human Th1 and Th2 cells and of 11,000 genes in mouse Th1, Tc1, Th2, and Tc2 cells were first attempts to understand the molecular mechanisms underlying the functional diversity of distinct T cell subsets. The finding that genes regulating key steps in the process of leukocyte extravasation into inflamed tissues are coregulated in human T cell subsets sheds light on the importance of the correct positioning of T cells within tissues to eliminate pathogens. Moreover, many pathological processes including allergies and autoimmune diseases are associated with the presence of specialized subsets of T helper cells at the site of inflammation. Knowledge of the genetic program that controls the functional properties of Th1 versus Th2 cells may therefore provide insight into the pathophysiology of inflammatory diseases.

REFERENCES

1. MOSMANN, T.R. & R.L. COFFMAN. 1989. Th1 and Th2 cells: different patterns of lymphokine secretion lead to different functional properties. Annu. Rev. Immunol. **7**: 145.
2. ABBAS, A.K., K.M. MURPHY & A. SHER. 1996. Functional diversity of helper T lymphocytes. Nature **383**: 787.
3. ROMAGNANI, S. 1994. Lymphokine production by human T cells in disease states. Annu. Rev. Immunol. **12**: 227.
4. SEDER, R.A., W.E. PAUL, M.M. DAVIS & B. FAZEKAS DE ST. GROTH. 1992. The presence of interleukin-4 during in vitro priming determines the lymphokine-producing potential of $CD4^+$ T cells from T cell receptor transgenic mice. J. Exp. Med. **176**: 1091.
5. HSIEH, C.S., A.B. HEIMBERGER, J.S. GOLD, *et al.* 1992. Differential regulation of T helper phenotype development by interleukins 4 and 10 in an alpha beta T cell-receptor transgenic system. Proc. Natl. Acad. Sci. USA **89**: 6065.
6. HSIEH, C.-S., S.E. MACATONIA, C.S. TRIPP, *et al.* 1993. Development of TH1 $CD4^+$ T cells through IL-12 produced by Listeria-induced macrophages. Science **260**: 547.
7. SEDER, R.A., R. GAZZINELLI, A. SHER & W.E. PAUL. 1993. IL-12 acts directly on $CD4^+$ T cells to enhance priming for interferon γ production and diminishes interleukin 4 inhibition of such priming. Proc. Natl. Acad. Sci. USA **90**: 10188.
8. MANETTI, R., P. PARRONCHI, M.G. GIUDIZI, *et al.* 1993. Natural killer cell stimulatory factor (Interleukin 12 [IL-12]) induces T helper 1 type (Th1)-specific immune responses and inhibits the development of IL-4-producing Th cells. J. Exp. Med. **177**: 1199.
9. GAZZINELLI, R.T., S. HIENY, T.A. WYNN, *et al.* 1993. Interleukin-12 is required for the T-lymphocyte-independent induction of interferon-γ by an intracellular parasite and reduces resistance in T-cell deficient hosts. Proc. Natl. Acad. Sci. USA **90**: 6115.
10. TRINCHIERI, G. 1995. Interleukin-12: A proinflammatory cytokine with immunoregulatory functions that bridge innate resistance and antigen-specific adaptive immunity. Annu. Rev. Immunol. **13**: 251.
11. GATELY, M.K., L.M. RENZETTI, J. MAGRAM, *et al.* 1998. The interleukin-12/interleukin-12-receptor system: role in normal and pathologic immune responses. Annu. Rev. Immunol. **16**: 495.
12. RISSOAN, M.C., V. SOUMELIS, N. KADOWAKI, *et al.* 1999. Reciprocal control of T helper cell and dendritic cell differentiation. Science **283**: 1183.
13. CELLA, M., F. FACCHETTI, A. LANZAVECCHIA & M. COLONNA. 2000. Plasmacytoid dendritic cells activated by influenza virus and CD40L drive a potent TH1 polarization. Nat. Immunol. **1**: 305.
14. MURPHY, K.M., W. OUYANG, J.D. FARRAR, *et al.* 2000. Signaling and transcription in T helper development. Annu. Rev. Immunol. **18**: 451.
15. LANZAVECCHIA, A. & F. SALLUSTO. 2001. Regulation of T cell immunity by dendritic cells. Cell **106**: 263.
16. O'GARRA, A. 1998. Cytokines induce the development of functionally heterogenous T helper subsets. Immunity **8**: 275.
17. GLIMCHER, L.H. & K.M. MURPHY. 2000. Lineage commitment in the immune system: the T helper lymphocyte grows up. Genes Dev **14**(14): 1693.

18. JACOBSON, N.G., S.J. SZABO, R.M. WEBER-NORDT, *et al.* 1995. Interleukin 12 signaling in T helper type 1 (Th1) cells involves tyrosine phosphorylation of signal transducer and activator of transcription (Stat)3 and Stat4. J. Exp. Med. **181**(5): 1755.
19. HILKINS, C.M.U., G. MESSER, K. TESSELAAR, *et al.* 1996. Lack of IL-12 signaling in human allergen-specific Th2 cells. J. Immunol. **157**: 4316.
20. THIERFELDER, W.E., J.M. VAN DEURSEN, K. YAMAMOTO, *et al.* 1996. Requirement for Stat4 in interleukin-12-mediated responses of natural killer and T cells. Nature **382**: 171.
21. KAPLAN, M.H., Y.-L. SUN, T. HOEY & M.J. GRUSBY. 1996. Impaired IL-12 responses and enhanced development of Th2 cells in Stat4-deficient mice. Nature **382**: 174.
22. MAGRAM, J., S.E. CONNAUGHTON, R.R. WARRIER, *et al.* 1996. IL-12 deficient mice are defective in IFNγ production and type I cytokine responses. Immunity **4**: 471.
23. WU, C., X. WANG, M. GADINA, *et al.* 2000. IL-12 receptor beta 2 (IL-12R beta 2)-deficient mice are defective in IL-12-mediated signaling despite the presence of high affinity IL-12 binding sites. J. Immunol **165**: 6221.
24. CHITNIS, T., N. NAJAFIAN, C. BENOU, *et al.* 2001. Effect of the targeted disruption of STAT4 and STAT6 on the induction of of experimental autoimmune encephalomyelitis. J. Clin. Invest. **108**: 739.
25. SZABO, S.J., A.S. DIGHE, U. GUBLER & K.M. MURPHY. 1997. Regulation of the interleukin (IL)-12R beta 2 subunit expression in developing T helper 1 (Th1) and Th2 cells. J. Exp. Med. **185**(5): 817.
26. AFKARIAN, M., J.R. SEDY, J. YANG, *et al.* 2002. T-bet is a STAT1-induced regulator of IL-12R expression in naive CD4$^+$ T cells. Nature Immunol. **3**: 549.
27. ROGGE, L., L. BARBERIS-MAINO, M. BIFFI, *et al.* 1997. Selective expression of an interleukin-12 receptor component by human T helper 1 cells. J. Exp. Med. **185**(5): 825.
28. ROGGE, L., D. D'AMBROSIO, M. BIFFI, *et al.* 1998. The role of Stat4 in species-specific regulation of Th cell development by type I IFNs. J. Immunol. **161**(no. 12): 6567.
29. WENNER, C.A., M.L. GÜLER, S.E. MACATONIA, *et al.* 1996. Roles of IFN-γ and IFN-α in IL-12 induced T helper cell-1 development. J. Immunol. **1156**: 1442.
30. CHO, S.S., C.M. BACON, C. SUDARSHAN, *et al.* 1996. Activation of STAT4 by IL-12 and IFN-α. Evidence for the involvement of ligand-induced tyrosine and serine phosphorylation. J. Immunol. **157**: 4781.
31. FARRAR, J.D., J.D. SMITH, T.L. MURPHY & K.M. MURPHY. 2000. Recruitment of Stat4 to the human interferon-alpha/beta receptor requires activated Stat2. J. Biol. Chem. **275**(4): 2693.
32. FARRAR, J.D., J.D. SMITH, T.L. MURPHY, *et al.* 2000. Selective loss of type I interferon-induced STAT4 activation caused by a minisatellite insertion in mouse Stat2. Nat. Immunol. **1**(1):65.
33. SZABO, S.J., S.T. KIM, G.L. COSTA, *et al.* 2000. A novel transcription factor, T-bet, directs Th1 lineage commitment. Cell **100**(6): 655.
34. SZABO, S.J., B.M. SULLIVAN, C. STEMMANN, *et al.* 2002. Distinct effects of T-bet in TH1 lineage commitment and IFN-gamma production in CD4 and CD8 T cells. Science **295**(5553): 338.
35. FINOTTO, S., M.F. NEURATH, J.N. GLICKMAN, *et al.* 2002. Development of spontaneous airway changes consistent with human asthma in mice lacking T-bet. Science **295**(5553): 336.
36. CARTER, L.L. & K.M. MURPHY. 1999. Lineage-specific requirement for signal transducer and activator of transcription (Stat)4 in interferon gamma production from CD4(+) versus CD8(+) T cells. J. Exp. Med. **189**(8): 1355.
37. ROGGE, L., A. PAPI, D.H. PRESKY, *et al.* 1999. Antibodies to the interleukin 12 receptor β2 chain mark human Th1 but not Th2 cells in vitro and in vivo. J. Immunol. **162**: 3926.
38. MULLEN, A.C., F.A. HIGH, A.S. HUTCHINS, *et al.* 2001. Role of T-bet in commitment of Th1 cells before IL-12-dependent selection. Science **292**: 1907.
39. LIGHVANI, A.A., D.M. FRUCHT, D. JANKOVIC, *et al.* 2001. T-bet is rapidly induced by interferon-γ in lymphoid and myeloid cells. Proc. Natl. Acad. Sci. USA **98**: 15137.

40. PFLANZ, S., J.C. TIMANS, J. CHEUNG, et al. 2002. IL-27, a heterodimeric cytokine composed of EBI3 and p28 protein, induces proliferation of naive CD4$^+$ T cells. Immunity **16:** 779.
41. SPRECHER, C.A., F.J. GRANT, J.W. BAUMGARTNER, et al. 1998. Cloning and characterization of a novel class I cytokine receptor. Biochem. Biophys. Res. Commun. **246:** 82.
42. CHEN, Q., N. GHILARDI, H. WANG, et al. 2000. Development of Th1-type immune responses requires the type I cytokine receptor TCCR. Nature **407:** 916.
43. YOSHIDA, H., S. HAMANO, G. SENALDI, et al. 2001. WSX-1 is required for the initiation of Th1 responses and resistance to *L. major* infection. Immunity **15:** 569.
44. ROGGE, L., E. BIANCHI, M. BIFFI, et al. 2000. Transcript imaging of the development of human T helper cells using oligonucleotide arrays. Nat. Genet. **25**(1): 96.
45. PRITCHARD, C.C., L. HSU, J. DELROW & P.S. NELSON. 2001. Project normal: defining normal variance in mouse gene expression. Proc. Natl. Acad. Sci. USA **98:** 13266.
46. LEE, C.-K., R.G. KLOPP, R. WEINDRUCH & T.A. PROLLA. 1999. Gene expression profile of aging and its retardation by caloric restriction. Science **285:** 1390.
47. HIGUCHI, R. & R. WATSON. 1999. Kinetic PCR analysis using a CCD camera and without using oligo nucleotide probes. *In* PCR Applications. M.A. Innis, D.H. Gelfand & J.J. Sninsky, Eds.: 263. Academic Press.
48. BROXMEYER, H.E., H.A. BRUNS, S. ZHANG, et al. 2002. Th1 cells regulate hematopoietic progenitor cell homeostasis by production of oncostatin M. Immunity **16:** 815.
49. SALLUSTO, F., C.R. MACKAY & A. LANZAVECCHIA. 2000. The role of chemokine receptors in primary, effector, and memory immune responses. Annu. Rev. Immunol. **18:** 593.
50. BIRD, J.J., D.R. BROWN, A.C. MULLEN, et al. 1998. Helper T cell differentiation is controlled by the cell cycle. Immunity **9:** 229.
51. LEDERER, J.A., J.S. LIOU, S. KIM, et al. 1996. Regulation of NF-κB activation in T helper 1 and T helper 2 cells. J. Immunol. **156:** 56.
52. HAMALAINEN, H., H. ZHOU, W. CHOU, et al. 2001. Distinct gene expression profiles of human type 1 and type 2 T helper cells. Genome Biol. **2**(7).
53. CHTANOVA, T., R.A. KEMP, A.P. SUTHERLAND, et al. 2001. Gene microarrays reveal extensive differential gene expression in both CD4(+) and CD8(+) type 1 and type 2 T cells. J. Immunol. **167**(6): 3057.
54. RINCON, M., J. ANGUITA, T. NAKAMURA, et al. 1997. Interleukin (IL)-6 directs the differentiation of IL-4-producing CD4+ T cells. J. Exp. Med. **185:** 461.
55. DIEHL, S., J. ANGUITA, A. HOFFMEYER, et al. 2000. Inhibition of Th1 differentiation by IL-6 is mediated by SOCS1. Immunity **13:** 805.

Gene Profiling Approach to Establish the Molecular Bases for Partial versus Full Activation of Naïve CD8 T Lymphocytes

GRÉGORY VERDEIL,[a,c] DENIS PUTHIER,[b,c] CATHERINE NGUYEN,[b] ANNE-MARIE SCHMITT-VERHULST,[a] AND NATHALIE AUPHAN-ANEZIN[a]

[a]*Centre d'Immunologie de Marseille-Luminy, CNRS-INSERM-Univ. de la Méditerranée, Marseille-Luminy, France*

[b]*TAGC, Campus de Luminy, Case 906, 13288 Marseille, Cedex 9, France*

ABSTRACT: When initial antigen encounter involves optimal antigenic and costimulatory stimuli, naïve CD8 T cells undergo a developmental program that leads to their activation, expansion and acquisition of effector functions (including production of IL-2, IFNγ and expression of cytolytic effector molecules). A subset of the activated CD8 T cells thrives as long-lived memory cells. Encounter of tissue-associated, and in particular tumor-associated antigen, may often be suboptimal in terms of antigenicity and costimulation, however. We previously developed a model of naïve CD8 T cells from transgenic mice expressing an alloreactive TCR for which a mutant alloantigen behaved as a partial agonist, inducing only some of the effector functions induced by the native alloantigen. To ascertain the molecular bases for the establishment of divergent fates within the same naïve CD8 T cells, we have used cDNA microarrays to monitor sequential gene expression patterns in conditions of full or partial response of these naïve CD8 T cells. Of the 5000 different genes monitored on the array, 18% showed changes in expression in activated versus naïve CD8 T cells, independent of whether stimulation was with full or partial agonist. These included antigen-induced upregulated as well as downregulated genes. Clusters of genes that were differentially expressed were also identified, being either (i) weakly versus strongly, or (ii) transiently versus stably expressed in response to partial and full agonist, respectively. They included (i) genes encoding costimulatory molecules and (ii) genes controlling cytolytic function, cytokine production, and chemokines. Therefore, the cDNA microarray approach was a sensitive tool to provide an exhaustive picture of T cell activation as it could discriminate quantitative, qualitative and dynamic differences in mRNA expression profiles between fully or partially activated T cells.

KEYWORDS: gene profiling; partial agonist; CD8 T lymphocytes; transcriptional regulation

Address for correspondence: Nathalie Auphan-Anezin, Centre d'Immunologie de Marseille-Luminy, CNRS-INSERM-Univ. Méd., Campus de Luminy, Case 906, 13288 Marseille, Cedex 9, France. Voice: +33 4 91 26 94 06; fax: +33 4 91 26 94 30.
 auphan@ciml.univ-mrs.fr
[c]These authors contributed equally to this work.

INTRODUCTION

Cell-mediated immune responses are critical for the elimination of viral pathogens and tumor cells. The main effector cell population against these two types of aggression consists of the CD8 T cell subset. Therefore, the efficiency of the immune response is dependent on the differentiation of naïve CD8 T cells into CTL effector cells that secrete cytokines and acquire the capacity to kill infected or tumor target cells, and on the expansion of such effectors.

In several pathological situations, an inefficient immune response was linked to the existence of dysfunctional or partially functional CD8 T cells (reviewed by Welsh[1]). Therefore, it is particularly important to understand how dysfunctional or partially functional CD8 T cells arise and what molecular mechanisms underlie partial activation. Examination of the mechanisms responsible for partial T cell responses is difficult to conduct in the nonmanipulated T cell repertoire owing to the low frequency of the specific T cells and the low magnitude of their response. *In vitro*, evidence exists for both CD4 and CD8 partially reactive T cell clones that recognized peptide ligands harboring subtle amino acid changes as compared to the initial peptide ligand.[2,3] The functional outcomes of the recognition of APLs consist in the induction of some functions, but not all, which rely on the corresponding gene transactivation.

We have developed a model of mice transgenic for an alloreactive TCR (tgTCR) specific for an endogenous peptide presented by $H-2K^b$. Naïve CD8 T cells expressing this tgTCR differentiate into potent cytotoxic CTLs that secrete IFNγ and IL-2, and proliferate in response to $H-2K^b$ APC. We have also previously shown that the natural $H-2K^{bm8}$ mutant behaved as a partial agonist, as stimulation of the same naïve CD8 tgTCR population by this altered ligand was able to trigger their differentiation into cytolytic effectors that produce IFNγ but are defective for IL-2 secretion and exhibit weak proliferation. As an approach towards understanding partial signaling at the transcriptional level, we first used transgenic mice expressing a reporter gene under the control of DNA binding sites for AP-1 or NF-κB, two transcription factors involved in the activation-induced regulation of many cytokine genes, including the IL-2 gene. We demonstrated that TCR engagement on naïve CD8 tgTCR cells by the partial agonist was able to transactivate NF-κB, but was not efficient for AP-1 induction. In contrast, stimulation of the same naïve CD8 tgTCR cells by the full agonist drove the activation of both transcription factors.[4] This study was the first evidence that a differential transcriptional control may account for the distinct functional program induced in naïve CD8 T cells by a full versus a partial agonist. It also prompted us to investigate at a large scale, the gene expression patterns in differentially activated homogenous naïve CD8 T cell populations. By the use of cDNA microarray technology and hierarchical clustering, we obtained evidence for different patterns of gene expression in naïve CD8 T cells in response to partial or to full agonist antigen (Verdeil *et al.*, in preparation), which are summarized here. First, a common set of genes was expressed following TCR engagement by a full or a partial agonist that probably reflects a signature of T cell activation. More importantly, we also identified specifically regulated gene clusters that further prove that differential transcriptional control accounts for the distinct functional programs induced in naïve CD8 T cells by a full versus a partial agonist. We observed, furthermore, that the most common profile was stable versus transient gene regulation induced respectively by the full and the partial agonist.

MATERIAL AND METHODS

Cell Culture

Naive CD8 tgTCR cells were isolated from lymph nodes of transgenic mice (described in Auphan *et al.*[5]). They were enriched by magnetic depletion of both CD4 and B lymphocytes using specific monoclonal Abs and Dynabeads coupled to Goat anti-Rat IgGs (Dynal, Oslo, Norway). In all experiments, CD8 T cells represented 90 to 98% of the enriched population. The purified CD8 tgTCR cells were either directly used for RNA extraction (naïve control cells) or cultured for 48 h or 72 h with irradiated T-depleted splenocytes from C57BL/6 (B6) and C57BL/6.C-H-2bm8 (bm8) mice.

cDNA Microarray Preparation

cDNA clones derived from adult mouse thymus, lymph node and spleen were obtained from Soares-thymus-2NbMT, Soares-mouse-lymph-node-NbMLN and Soares-mouse-spleen-3NbMS libraries, respectively. cDNA inserts were homogeneous in size (near 1 kb) and all cloned into pT7T3D vector. The 5228 cDNA clones (see FIGURE 1) were amplified in fifty-five 96-well microtiter plates using a vector-PCR amplification with the following primers 5′-GTGGAATTGTGAGCGGATAA-CA-3′ and 5′-CCAAAAGGGTCAGTCTGCAACA-3′. The microarrays were prepared by spotting PCR products onto Hybond N+ membranes using a microarrayer GMS 417 robot (MWG). The membranes were first hybridized with an [γ-^{33}P]dATP-labeled oligonucleotide corresponding to a vector sequence: LBP9 5′-ACTGGCCGTCGTTTTACA-3′. Quantification of the obtained signals allowed for the estimation of the amount of DNA deposited in each spot. After stripping, the membranes were subsequently used for hybridization with a complex probe.

Complex Probe Preparation

Total RNA was isolated using TriZol reagent (Gibco BRL) and RNA quality was verified on an agarose gel. Complex probes were prepared from 3μg of total RNA from each sample. Retrotranscription was conducted as previously described[6] with [α-^{33}P]dCTP-labeling. The presence of a large excess (8μg) of oligo(dT) primers (dT25) during cDNA synthesis as well as annealing of the labeled probe with poly(dA80) ensured the saturation of poly(A) tails. Hybridizations were conducted for 48 h at 68°C in a volume of 0.5 mL. After washes, arrays were exposed to phosphoimaging plates, which were than scanned with a FUJI BAS 5000 machine (25 μm resolution). After image acquisition, the hybridization signals were quantified using Arraygauge software as described.[7]

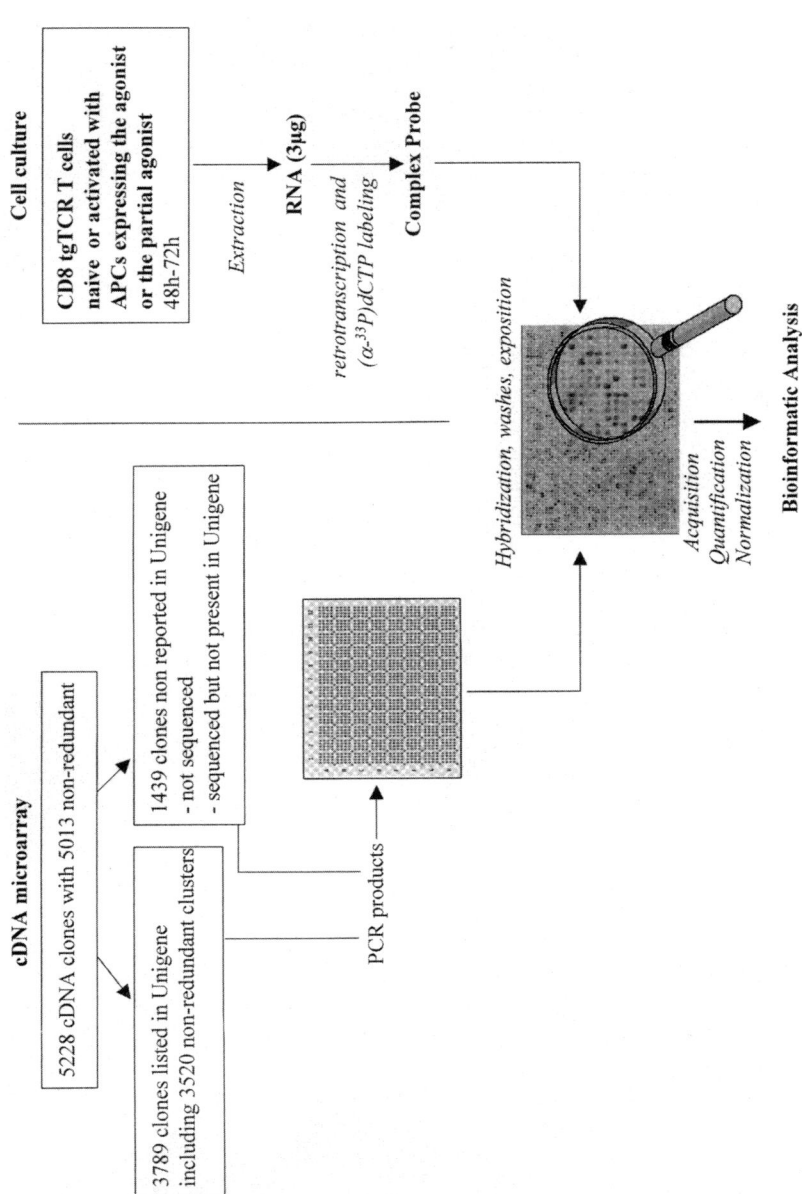

FIGURE 1. Schematic view of our design of custom-made cDNA microarrays and complex probe preparations.

cDNA Microarray Analysis

Data obtained both after vector and complex probes hybridizations were normalized. For vector analysis, mean background was calculated on blanks, the 30% lowest values were excluded and background was subtracted. For data obtained with complex probes, mean background was calculated on blanks and subtracted. Then, the complex probe value was divided by its vector counterpart. The median value of each microchip was calculated and used to normalize the complex probe value. Hierarchical clustering was applied using the Cluster program developed by Eisen et al.[8] (80% filter, Log transform, median center genes). Figures were displayed with the Tree View program.

RESULTS AND DISCUSSION

Common Gene Expression Profiles Associated with T Cell Activation

Custom made cDNA microarrays allowed us to screen for the expression level of around 5,000 different genes. Around 18% were differentially induced between naïve CD8 T cells and activated cells independent of whether the stimulating APC harbored the full or the partial agonist. Indeed, we observed genes that were upregulated after T cell activation (see FIGURE 2A) that are involved in cell metabolism (aldolase1, ATP synthase), in proteolysis (caspase 6, proteasome subunit beta type 2), in signaling (rlk/itk binding protein), and in cell cycle (cdc2a). We also identified genes that were downregulated in activated CD8 T cells as compared to naïve T cells (FIG. 2B): some of them are direct or indirect regulators of transcription (klf3, IkB beta). Altogether these clusters defined common gene expression profiles that signed for CD8 T cell activation whatever the nature of the initial TCR engagement was; that is, triggering by a low or a high avidity ligand.

Different Patterns of Gene Expression in the Response of Naive CD8 T Cells to a Full or a Partial Agonist

We also detected distinct gene expression profiles in differentially activated T cell populations. The first and most common pattern involved genes that were expressed at a low level in naïve CD8 T cells, being stably upregulated (at 48h and 72h) after activation by the full agonist, whereas only a transient increase (at 48h) was observed following encounter with the partial agonist (see FIGURE 3A). Among these genes, we found genes coding for cytolytic components, for chemokines, for signaling molecules and for cell cycle regulators, as well as unknown cDNA clones and ESTs that are presently being sequenced.

The reverse profile of stable versus transient downregulation of gene expression was also observed (FIG. 3B).

Another representative cluster included genes expressed at a low level in naïve CD8 T cells, that were weakly versus strongly induced after stimulation by a partial or a full agonist, respectively. Genes encoding surface receptors (FIG. 3C) are representative of this cluster, as well as genes coding for RNA binding proteins.

Altogether, it appeared that activation of naïve CD8 T cells by a partial agonist failed to durably regulate gene expression. Downregulation of mRNA expression levels can result from inefficient gene transactivation and/or from increased mRNA instability. The first level of regulation is complex and includes chromatin remodeling that is the consequence of DNA accessibility to transcription factors, together with hyperacetylation of associated histones and demethylation of CpG dinucleotides (reviewed in Orphanides and Reinberg[9]). The second level of regulation acting on mRNA instability has been less investigated. However, it is known that expression of cytokines is usually transient because their mRNAs are intrinsically unstable.[10] In our model, we have previously identified a correlation between the lack of IL-2 production and defective transactivation of AP-1.[4] Activation of transcription factors is a dynamic process that relies on nuclear import of cytoplasmic units. Indeed, there is a continuous shuttling of transcriptional factors between the cytoplasm and nucleus

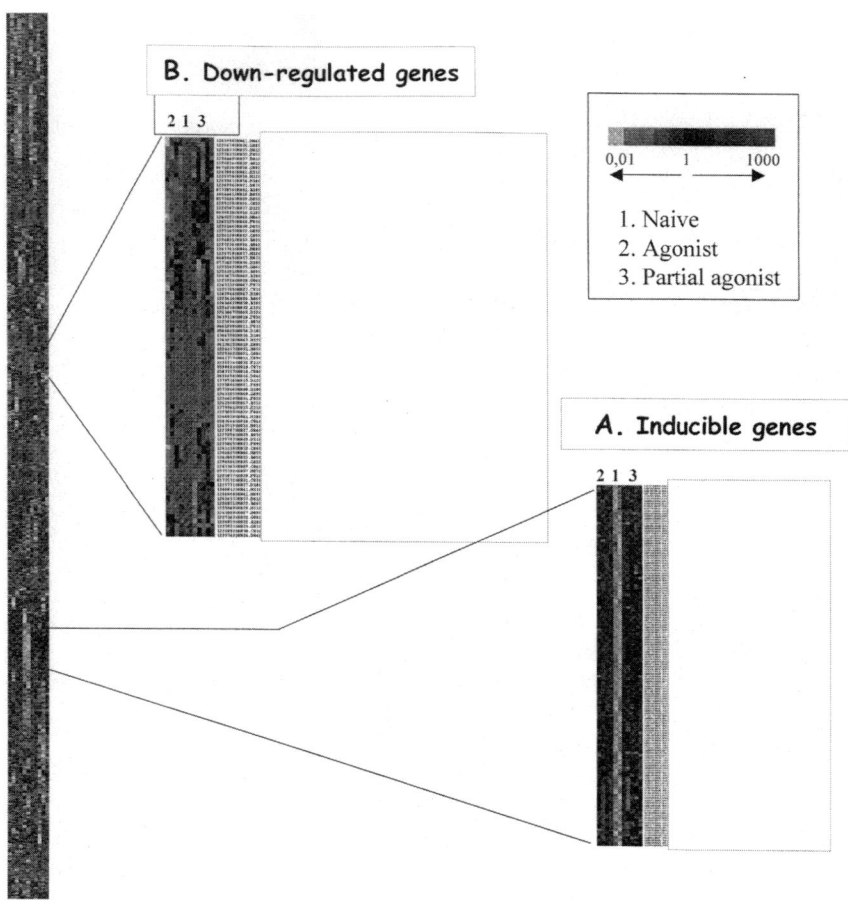

FIGURE 2. Hierarchical gene clustering defined common gene expression profiles in differentially activated CD8 T cell populations. Genes upregulated (**A**) or downregulated (**B**) in fully (2) or partially (3) activated CD8 T cells as compared to naïve cells (1). This figure appears in color on the web (www.annalsnyas.org).

and molecular regulation exists, controlling it in both directions.[11] Also, many transcription factors are unstable proteins that are destroyed by ubiquitin-mediated proteolysis.[12] Altogether, the combination of several mechanisms may be involved in the transient transcriptional pattern that we observed upon partial T cell activation.

Our results also showed that differential expression of mRNAs coding for surface receptors was correlated to a differential level of the corresponding protein at the cell surface (Auphan-Anezin *et al.*, submitted). This defective induction of co-stimulatory molecules by the partial agonist may affect (i) the extent of gene transcription by lowering activation of transcription factors[13] and/or (ii) the stability of mRNAs, as it was previously reported that signaling by CD28 regulated the stability of mRNAs coding for IL-2, IFNγ, TNFα and GM-CSF.[10] Indeed, we have previously observed that stimulation of naïve tgTCR CD8 by LPS-activated splenocytes expressing the partial agonist that had upregulated CD28 ligands, partially restored their proliferative response as well as transactivation of AP-1.[4] The observation that

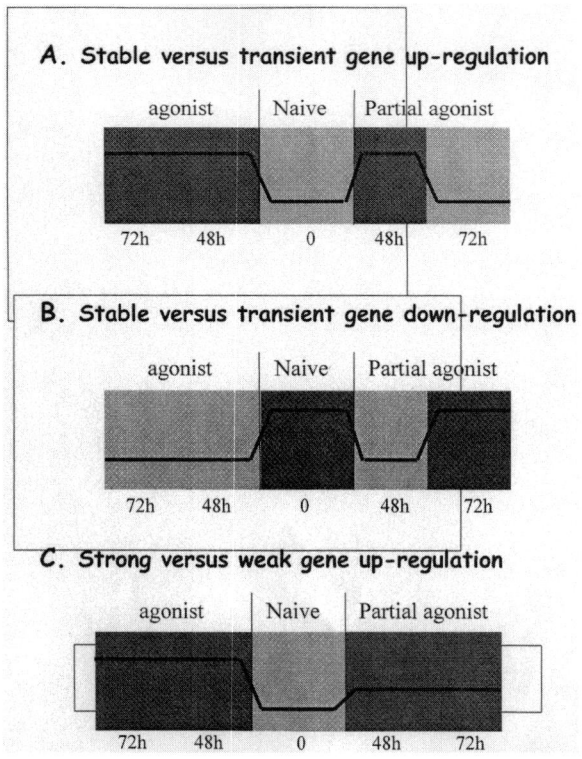

FIGURE 3. Hierarchical gene clustering defined distinct gene expression profiles in differentially activated CD8 T cell populations. Schematic view of (**A**) genes stably versus transiently upregulated in fully versus partially activated CD8 T cells as compared to naïve cells; the same representation applied to downregulated genes (**B**). Genes strongly versus weakly induced in fully versus partially activated CD8 T cells as compared to naïve cells (**C**). This figure appears in color on the web (www.annalsnyas.org).

naïve CD8 T cells failed to produce IL-2 in response to the partial agonist also raises the question of whether IL-2 is involved in the regulation of other genes stably induced by the full agonist such as genes coding for chemokines and cytolytic components. This line will be further explored.

Recently, cDNA or oligonucleotide microarrays have been used to monitor both CD4 and CD8 T cell responses. Therefore, the distinct effector functions of CD4$^+$ Th1/Th2 and CD8$^+$ Tc1/Tc2 cells have been correlated with distinct gene expression profiles and have enlarged the picture of markers associated with T cell polarization.[14] Also, molecular mechanisms associated (i) with enhanced cellular response of memory as compared to naïve CD4 T cells[15] and (ii) with decreased response of anergic as compared to activated CD4$^+$ T cells[16,17] have been documented. Here, we described that transient gene regulation is a hallmark of partial activation of CD8 T cells, rather than the induction of a specific set of genes. In fact, very few genes (10) were induced in naïve tgTCR CD8 cells by the altered ligand only. These genes correspond to ESTs or nonreferenced sequences for which no functional information is yet available.

CONCLUSION

Altogether, we observed (Auphan-Anezin *et al.*, manuscript in preparation) that partial T cell activation upon suboptimal stimulation of naïve CD8 T cells was regulated at the transcriptional level and mainly involved transient mRNA expression. Understanding the mechanisms underlying this observation will help to adapt vaccination protocols to avoid such incomplete immune responses or to manipulate existing defective CD8 T cells found in pathological situations in the context of immunotherapeutic approaches.

REFERENCES

1. WELSH, R.M. 2001. Assessing CD8 T cell number and dysfunction in the presence of antigen. J. Exp. Med. **193:** F19–F22.
2. CAO, W., S.S. TYKODI, M.T. ESSER, *et al.* 1995. Partial activation of CD8$^+$ T cells by a self-derived peptide. Nature **378:** 295–298.
3. SLOAN-LANCASTER, J. & P.M. ALLEN. 1996. Altered peptide ligand-induced partial T cell activation: molecular mechanisms and role in T cell biology. Annu. Rev. Immunol. **14:** 1–27.
4. AUPHAN, N., S. GHOSH, R.A. FLAVELL & A.-M. SCHMITT-VERHULST. 1999. Differential requirements for NF-κB and AP-1 transactivation in response to minimal TCR engagement by a partial agonist in naïve CD8 T cells. J. Immunol. **163:** 5219–5227.
5. AUPHAN, N., J. CURNOW, A. GUIMEZANES, *et al.* 1994. The degree of CD8 dependence of cytolytic T cell precursors is determined by the nature of the TCR and influences negative selection in TCR-transgenic mice. Eur. J. Immunol. **24:** 1572–1577.
6. BERNARD, K., N. AUPHAN, S. GRANJEAUD, *et al.* 1996. Multiplex messenger assay: simultaneous, quantitative measurement of expression of many genes in the context of T cell activation. Nucleic Acids Res. **24:** 1435–1442.
7. BERTUCCI, F., K. BERNARD, B. LORIOD, *et al.* 1999. Sensitivity issues in DNA array-based expression measurements and performance of nylon microarrays for small samples. Hum. Mol. Genet. **8:** 1715–1722.

8. EISEN, M.B., P.T. SPELLMAN, P.O. BROWN & D. BOTSTEIN. 1998. Cluster analysis and display of genome-wide expression patterns. Proc. Natl. Acad. Sci. USA **95:** 14863–14868.
9. ORPHANIDES, G. & D. REINBERG. 2002. A unified theory of gene expression. Cell **108:** 439–451.
10. LINDSTEN, T., C.H. JUNE, J.A. LEDBETTER, et al. 1989. Regulation of lymphokine messenger RNA stability by a surface-mediated T cell activation pathway. Science **244:** 339–343.
11. CHEN, L., W. FISCHLE, E. VERDIN & W.C. GREENE. 2001. Duration of nuclear NF-κB action regulated by reversible acetylation. Science **293:** 1653–1657.
12. THOMAS, D. & M. TYERS. 2000. Transcriptional regulation: kamikaze activators. Curr. Biol. **10:** R341–R343.
13. SU, B., E. JACINTO, M. HIBI, et al. 1994. JNK is involved in signal integration during costimulation of T lymphocytes. Cell **77:** 727–736.
14. CHTANOVA, T., R.A. KEMP, A.P. SUTHERLAND, et al. 2001. Gene microarrays reveal extensive differential gene expression in both CD4(+) and CD8(+) type 1 and type 2 T cells. J. Immunol. **167:** 3057–3063.
15. LIU, K., Y. LI, V. PRABHU, et al. 2001. Augmentation in expression of activation-induced genes differentiates memory from naïve CD4$^+$ T cells and is a molecular mechanism for enhanced cellular response of memory CD4$^+$ T cells. J. Immunol. **166:** 7335–7344.
16. LECHNER, O., J. LAUBER, A. FRANZKE, et al. 2001. Fingerprints of anergic T cells. Curr. Biol. **11:** 587–595.
17. MACIAN, F., F. GARCIA-COZAR, I. SIN-HYEOG, et al. 2002. Transcriptional mechanisms underlying lymphocyte tolerance. Cell **109:** 719–731.

Complexity of Inflammatory Responses in Endothelial Cells and Vascular Smooth Muscle Cells Determined by Microarray Analysis

OLGA BANDMAN, ROGER T. COLEMAN, JEANNE F. LORING,[a] JEFFREY J. SEILHAMER, AND BENJAMIN G. COCKS

Incyte Genomics, Palo Alto, California 94304, USA

ABSTRACT: To better understand the molecular basis of vascular cell system behavior in inflammation, we used gene expression microarrays to analyze the expression of 7,075 genes and their response to IL-1β and TNFα in cultures of coronary artery endothelium and smooth muscle derived from a single coronary artery. The most noticeable difference between the cell types was the considerably greater magnitude and complexity of the transcriptional response in the endothelial cells. Two hundred and nine genes were regulated in the endothelium and only 39 in vascular smooth muscle. Among the 209 regulated genes in the endothelium, 99 have not been previously associated with endothelial cell activation and many implicate the endothelium in unconventional roles. For example, the induced genes include several that have only been associated with leukocyte function (e.g., IL-7 receptor, EBI-3 receptor) and others related to antiviral and antibacterial defense (e.g., oligoadenylate synthetase, LMP7, toll-like receptor 4, complement component 3). In addition, 43 genes likely to participate in signal transduction (eg. IL-18 receptor, STK2 kinase, STAF50, ANP receptor, VIP receptor, RAC3, IFP35) were regulated providing evidence that a major effect of TNFα and IL-1β is to alter the potential of the endothelial cell to respond to various other external stimuli.

KEYWORDS: TNF-α; Interleukin-1 beta; gene expression profiling; inflammation; gene expression regulation

INTRODUCTION

TNFα and IL-1β are key regulators of inflammation. Sequelae of their effect on blood vessels are the alteration of the surface molecule repertoire of endothelial cells, attachment and transmigration of mononuclear cells, secretion of cytokines by the invading cells, and responding changes in gene expression by smooth muscle and endothelium.[1]

In order to understand better the nature of the inflammatory response and the gene products that mediate the ultimate effects of TNFα and IL-1β, we surveyed the gene expression pattern of 7050 individual genes in endothelium and vascular smooth muscle using cDNA microarrays. Consistent with the biological role of endothelium,

Address for correspondence: Benjamin G. Cocks, Incyte Genomics Inc., 3160 Porter Drive, Palo Alto, CA 94304. Voice: 650-845-4263; fax: 650-621-8514.
ben@incyte.com
[a]Present address: Arcos Inc., San Diego, CA.

the overall complexity and magnitude of the transcriptional response was considerably greater in endothelial cells than in smooth muscle cells. Many of the genes are well documented in the literature as TNFα/IL-1β–inducible genes, but we also identified a group of genes that have not been previously associated with the inflammatory response in the vascular system and provide new insights into the action of inflammatory cytokines.

MATERIAL AND METHODS

Cell Culture

Human coronary artery endothelial cells (HAEC) and human coronary artery smooth muscle cells (CASmMC) from the same donor were obtained from BioWhittaker, Inc. (San Diego, CA). Both cell types were cultured in Costar tissue-culture flasks in the media provided by BioWhittaker. Experiments were performed using cell cultures at 85% confluency. The smooth muscle cells and endothelial cells described in the paper were similar to those from other donors by a number of criteria we have examined. This includes morphology, expression of cell specific markers, and the ability to upregulate chemokine or cell surface marker expression with inflammatory mediators.

Recombinant human TNFα and IL-1β were purchased from R&D Systems (Minneapolis, MN). Both cytokines were used at a concentration of 10 ng/mL. After 24 hours both control and treated cells were collected and mRNA was extracted using Trizol (Life Technologies, Inc.) lysis followed by oligo dT selection (Qiagen).

Microarray Preparation

UniGEM V microarrays were used in all experiments. Sequences used for microarray fabrication were generated by PCR. Plasmids used as templates for generating PCR products are all available from Incyte Genomics, Inc. (Palo Alto, CA). PCR products were purified by gel filtration with Sephacryl-400 (Amersham Pharmacia Biotech, Inc., Piscataway, NJ) equilibrated in 0.2X SSC. The filtrate was dried and rehydrated in one-tenth-volume dH_2O for arraying. The DNA solutions were arrayed by robotics on modified glass slides essentially as described elsewhere.[2] All PCR products were re-sequenced to confirm gene identity prior to arraying. After arraying, slides were processed to fix the DNA to the prepared glass surface and washed three times in dH_2O at room temperature. Slides were then treated with 0.2% I-Block (Tropix, Bedford, MA) dissolved in 1X Dulbecco's phosphate buffered saline (Life Technologies, Gaithersburg, MD) at 60°C for 30 minutes. GEM microarrays were then rinsed in 0.2% SDS for two minutes followed by three one-minute washes in dH_2O.

Fluorescent Labeling of Probe

Isolated mRNA was reverse transcribed with 5' Cy3 or Cy5 labeled random 9-mers (Operon Technologies, Inc., Alameda, CA). Reactions were incubated for 2h at 37°C with 200ng polyA RNA, 200 Units M-MLV reverse transcriptase (Life Technologies, Gaithersburg, MD), 4mM DTT, 1 unit RNase Inhibitor (Ambion,

Austin, TX), 0.5 mM dNTPs, and 2 µg labeled 9-mers in 25 µL volume with enzyme buffer supplied by the manufacturer. The reactions were terminated by incubation at 85°C for 5 min. The paired reactions were combined and purified with a TE-30 column (Clontech, Palo Alto, CA), brought to 90 µL with dH_2O, and precipitated with 2 µL 1 mg/mL glycogen, 60 µL 5M NH_4OAc, and 300 µL EtOH. After centrifugation the supernatant was decanted and the pellet was resuspended in 24 µL of hybridization buffer: 5X SSC, 0.2% SDS, 1 mM DTT.

Hybridization

Probe solutions were thoroughly resuspended by incubating at 65°C for 5 min with mixing. The probe was applied to the array, covered with a 22 mm^2 glass coverslip, and placed in a sealed chamber to prevent evaporation. After hybridization at 60°C for 6.5 h, slides were washed in three consecutive washes of decreasing ionic strength.

Scanning

Microarrays were scanned in both Cy3 and Cy5 channels with Axon GenePixä scanners (Foster City, CA) with a 10-µm resolution. The signal was converted into 16-bits-per-pixel resolution, yielding a 65,536-count dynamic range.

Normalization and Ratio Determination

Incyte GEMtools™ software (Incyte Genomics, Inc., Palo Alto, CA) was used for image analysis. The elements were determined by a gridding and region-detection algorithm. The area surrounding each element image was used to calculate a local background, which was subtracted from the total element signal. Background-subtracted element signals were used to calculate Cy3:Cy5 ratios.

RESULTS

Endothelial and Smooth Muscle Cell Gene-Expression Patterns

Endothelial cell cultures were treated with a combination of the inflammatory mediators TNFα and IL-1β. The microarray analysis was performed using a competitive hybridization method described in detail previously[3]. The results are shown in FIGURE 1. The GenBank IDs of the sequences represented on the UniGEM V used in the experiment are available from Incyte Genomics, Inc. As FIGURE 1B shows, the endothelial cells responded to inflammatory stimuli by increasing expression levels of 137 sequences by twofold or more, and downregulating 72 sequences. The smooth muscle cells responded to inflammatory mediators with induced expression of 20 genes by twofold or more and downregulation of 19 (FIG. 1A). Comparing untreated samples in both Cy3 and Cy5 as a control for system variability yielded no false positives.

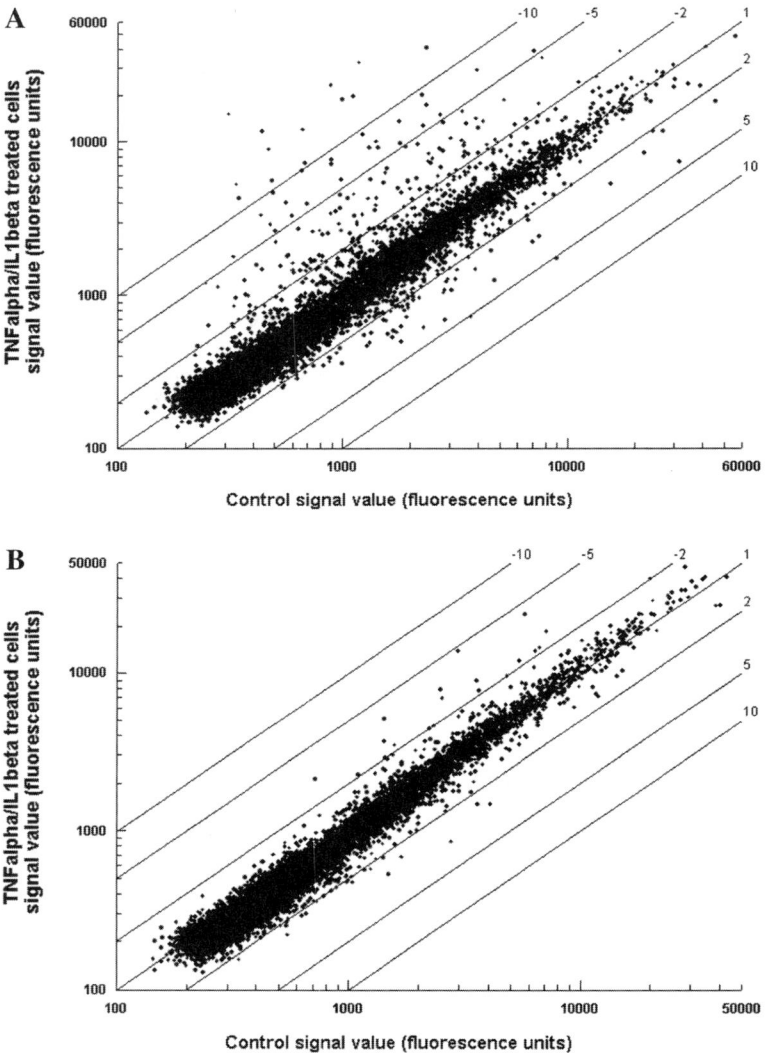

FIGURE 1. A. Endothelial cell gene expression. Scatter plot of the signals from a microarray analysis comparing activated to resting coronary artery endothelial cells. Cy5 labeled cDNA from activated cells is on the Y axis and Cy3 labeled cDNA from resting cells is on the X axis. The diagonal lines indicate the boundaries of a 2-, 5- and 10-fold change. Each point represents an individual element of the microarray. **B.** Vascular smooth muscle gene expression. Scatter plot of the signals from a microarray analysis comparing activated to resting coronary artery smooth muscle cells. Cy5 labeled cDNA from activated cells on the Y axis and Cy3 labeled cDNA from resting cells is on the X axis. The diagonal lines indicate the boundaries of a 2-, 5- and 10-fold change. Each point represents an individual element of the microarray.

Comparison of the in Vitro Inflammatory Response of Endothelium and Smooth Muscle

The complexity of the endothelial response to TNFα and IL-1β was much greater than that of the vascular smooth muscle. The fraction of regulated genes in endothelial cells represented 3.0% of the genes assayed, while 0.6% were regulated in smooth muscle cells. Interestingly, the gene sets induced by TNFα were largely different.

However, there was overlap in the induction response of the two cell types. TABLE 1 shows genes that were regulated by TNFα and IL-1β in both cell types. Comparison of the magnitude of induction of these genes indicates that in general the response was greater in endothelial cells. The induction levels for each gene varied, but they were consistently higher in endothelial cells; the average induction level for genes in endothelial cells was 9.9-fold compared to 2.5-fold in smooth muscle cells.

Identity of Regulated Genes

The regulated genes were grouped into functional categories, as summarized in TABLE 2. One of the most abundant categories was associated with leukocyte endothelial-cell interactions. In this category we placed genes with confirmed roles in

TABLE 1. Common set of regulated genes in endothelial cells and vascular smooth muscle cells

Gene name	GenBank ID	Magnitude of induction (induced/resting level)	
		Endothelial cells	Smooth muscle cells
GM-CSF	g31689	27.4	4.6
Serine/threonine kinase 2	g348244	26.1	2.7
ENA-78	g471242	18.9	3.1
SOD-2	g34710	18.8	2.5
MCP-1	g187434	7.0	2.2
IkBα	g187290	5.5	2.2
Interleukin 6	g32673	5.5	2.6
NK cell transcript 4	g189225	4.8	2.6
Metallothionein 1L	g435764	3.2	2.1
Metallothionein IB	g188709	3.1	2
PAI- I	g189541	2.2	2
Metallothionein 1E	g187538	2.1	2
Integrin a6	g33943	0.4	0.5
Thrombomodulin	g220126	0.3	0.5

TABLE 2. Categorization of regulated genes by function

Biological Process	Number of genes regulated
Cytoskeletal and ECM	15
Immunity	11
Leukocyte-endothelial interaction	41
Metabolism	27
Signal transduction and regulation of transcription	43
Vascular physiology	21
Not known: annotated	20
Cytokine-regulated of unknown function	10
Unannotated	12
Total	200

mediating chemoattraction, adhesion and activation of various leukocyte subsets. Other genes without a defined role in a particular cellular process could be identified as participating in signal transduction/transcriptional regulation and were categorized as such. Another category consists of genes for which only limited information about function is available and which have not previously been reported to be associated with the inflammatory response of endothelial/vascular smooth muscle cells.

TABLE 3 summarizes information about all of the regulated genes detected in this study. Microarray analysis confirmed many previous reports of gene regulation in endothelial cells. For example, E-selectin, mitochondrial superoxide dismutase, GM-CSF, and IL-8 have been previously identified as being regulated by inflammatory stimuli; and these genes were also observed to be modulated in the current microarray analysis. The regulation of these genes has been described in separate studies incorporating various endothelial cell systems and different detection technologies,[4–6] but here their regulation has been quantified simultaneously in one endothelial cell system. We have profiled other donors for the same response in other large artery endothelial cells and have confirmed that all the genes listed in TABLE 3 are also regulated in these other experiments.

DISCUSSION

Microarray analysis of aortic endothelial cells treated with TNFα and IL-1β reveals a complex inflammatory response comprised of mRNAs connected with several cellular processes. Predominant cellular functions represented by the regulated genes are leukocyte interaction, immunity, and vascular physiology. Among the highly upregulated genes are those that have been previously reported in separate studies to be induced during endothelial cell activation. Well-validated examples include COX-2, IL-8, MCP-1, eotaxin, gro-beta, MIP3a, G-CSF, GM-CSF, CSF-1, IL-6, E-selectin, VCAM-1, and ICAM-1, among others (TABLE 3).[5,7–11] We also observe prominent upregulation of several secreted and cell-surface molecules that are usually associated with leukocyte function, but have not been previously reported

TABLE 3. Genes regulated by TNFα/IL-1β in endothelial cells (continues next 4 pages)

Gene Name	GenBank ID	Fold-induction
Leukocyte-endothelial interaction		
Interleukin 8	g186367	22.8
GRO-beta	g183628	19.8
ENA-78	g471242	18.9
IP-10 chemokine	g33917	12.2
Fractalkine	g1888522	7.6
MCP-1	g187434	7
MIP-3 alpha	g1778716	4.2
MCP-2	g1905800	3.4
Eotaxin	g1280140	3.2
MIP-5	g1296608	0.4
G-CSF	g31689	27.4
M-CSF (CSF-1)	g181134	7.5
Interleukin 6	g32673	5.5
Interleukin 1 alpha	g33794	2.4
LIF	g34361	1.6
E-selectin	g537523	48.1
ICAM-1 (CD54)	g184532	8.8
Properdin	g452937	7.1
Sialyltransferase	g29433	4.8
VCAM-1	g3327169	4.2
Lactate dehydrogenase	g34328	3.3
Interleukin 15 receptor	g2661028	3.2
CD44	g29800	2.8
Galectin 9	g2385455	2.8
Beta-1,4-galactosyltransferase	g474986	2.5
CD51	g340306	2.5
Mac-2 binding protein	g307152	2.2
Cadherin 11	g575577	2.1
TNFα-inducible protein 6 (TSG-6)	g339994	2.1
Galectin 3	g179530	2
Neurexin 4	g1857707	2
PAPS synthetase	g2673861	0.5
CL-20 epithelial membrane protein	g1684789	0.5
Glypican 1	g31846	0.5
BH-protocadherin	g2979417	0.4
Integrin alpha 6	g33943	0.4
Epithelial V-like antigen	g3169829	0.4
ICAM-2	g32623	0.3
CD34	g180108	0.2

TABLE 3/continued 1.

Gene Name	GenBank ID	Fold-induction
Immunity		
Complement component 3	g1162925	10.7
EBI3 cytokine receptor	g632973	9
MxA	g5410450	8.5
2'-5'oligoadenylate synthetase 3	g338651	6.9
LMP7 proteasome subunit	g596139	5.6
Interleukin 7 receptor	g186365	5.4
MHC class I HLA BW62	g1620014	5.4
MxB	g188902	5.2
MECL-1 proteasome subunit	g2765347	2.8
Toll-like receptor 4	g3132527	2.7
MHC class II gamma chain	g188469	2
Signal transduction and transcriptional regulation		
Serine/threonine kinase 2	g348244	26.1
SOD-2	g34710	18.8
A20 TNF alpha-inducible protein	g177865	15.6
FIP2	g3127082	7.3
IKBA	g187290	5.5
Rac3	g2326205	5.5
Interferon-inducible guanilate binding protein 1	g183001	5.4
Interferon regulatory factor 1	g580208	3.8
Staf50	g899299	3.4
IAP-1	g3978243	3.3
Interleukin 18 receptor	g1206008	3
Interferon-inducible guanilate binding protein 2	g829176	2.6
P2X4 purinoreceptor	g4099120	2.6
Phosphatase PAP2-beta	g4105138	2.4
Interferon regulatory factor 7	g2098580	2.3
Caspase 1 or ICE	g717039	2.2
TAFII130	g1732072	2.2
FLN29	g2463530	2.2
RELB	g186549	2.1
CD47	g396704	2
Hypoxia-inducible factor 1 alpha	g1144012	2
RNA polymerase II elongation factor ELL2	g1946346	2
Serine/threonine protein kinase PK428	g1695872	2
Myosin light chain kinase (MLCK)	g1377819	2
Down syndrome candidate region 1	g2612867	1.2
Sodium channel beta-1 subunit	g307414	0.7
Chloride channel protein 4	g4760532	0.5
G-protein-coupled receptor (GPR39)	g2654160	0.5
Coxsackie virus and adenovirus receptor	g6690789	0.5

TABLE 3/continued 2.

Gene Name	GenBank ID	Fold-induction
Fatty acid binding protein	g182353	0.5
Guanin nucleotide binding protein G(I), alpha subunit	g3005736	0.5
Regulator of G-protein signalling 5	g2598186	0.5
Arg/Abl-interacting protein ARGBP2 B	g2952332	0.5
Cellular oncogene C-MER	g505664	0.5
cGMP inhibited phosphodiesterase A	g1039473	0.5
Orphan nuclear receptor NR5A2	g3810966	0.5
Cytoplasmic tyrosine protein kinase BMX	g951234	0.4
beta-Catalytic subunit of cAMP-dependent protein kinase	g189982	0.4
Extracellular protein S1-5	g458227	0.4
Cyclin A1	g1753108	0.4
Pirin	g1907075	0.3
Regulator of G-protein signaling 5	g1216372	0.3
Metabolism		
Diubiquitin	g2546963	26.6
Cationic amino acid transporter 2	g484049	17.9
Inducible 6-phosphofructo-2-kinase	g3676496	7.6
Golgi auto-antigen golgin-95	g306781	7.3
Spermidine/spermine N1-acetyltransferase	g1103903	4.6
Ferritin H chain	g182504	4.5
Apo-L	g2425057	4
Proteasome activator HPA28 subunit beta	g1008914	3.5
Metallothionein 1L	g435764	3.2
Interferon-gamma upregulated I-5111 protein	g186512	3
Butyrophilin BTF5	g2062705	2.4
Butyrophilin BTF1	g2062687	2.3
Carboxypeptidase D	g2462776	2.2
Tryptophanyl tRNA synthetase	g184656	2.2
Ubiquitin-conjugating enzyme RIG-B	g4335936	2.2
Cytochrome b-5	g181391	2.1
Metallothionein 1E	g187538	2.1
Butyrophilin BTF5	g2062705	2
Cysteine protease PRSC1	g1890049	2
Heme oxygenase 2	g248957	2
Estrogen sulfotransferase	g488282	0.5
Lysosomal hyaluronidase	g3702076	0.5
Metallothionein 1L	g435764	0.5
Sortilin	g1834494	0.5
Monoamine oxidase A	g34458	0.4
HSP40 homologue	g6031211	0.3
Alpha-2-macroglobulin	g177869	0.3

TABLE 3/continued 3.

Gene Name	GenBank ID	Fold-induction
Cytoskeletal and ECM		
Nef-associated factor 1	g3758820	5.8
TGFbeta-induced protein	g339567	3.1
Adducin-like protein ADDL	g2696053	2.9
Laminin 5 beta 3	g2429078	2.7
Collagen, type IV, alpha 1	g29548	2.2
Lysyl hydroxylase isoform 2 (PLOD2)	g2138313	2.2
Collagen, type VIII, alpha 1	g30081	2.1
Podocalyxin-like protein	g2213812	2
Lysyl oxidase	g733134	0.5
Keratin 15	g34074	0.5
Vimentin	g37851	0.5
Cytokeratin 2E	g181401	0.4
Serine protease OMI	g5870864	0.4
Cytokeratin 18	g34036	0.4
Keratin 7	g34067	0.2
Vascular physiology		
ANP-C receptor	g178651	17.2
VIP receptor	g1617516	11.5
TNFalpha-induced protein 2	g306463	9.7
Endoperoxide synthase type II (COX-2)	g291987	4.2
GTP cyclohydrolase 1	g5058996	3.3
VEGF-C	g1150988	2.7
Plasminogen activator inhibitor I	g189541	2.2
Platelet-derived growth factor	g338207	2.1
Endothelin-converting enzyme 1	g535181	2
Insulin-like growth factor binding protein 3	g398163	0.5
Thrombospondin 2	g307505	0.5
TIE1 receptor tyrosine kinase	g396814	0.5
NOS 3	g189211	0.5
Transglutaminase 2	g339520	0.4
Angiotensin I converting enzyme	g338666	0.4
Thrombomodulin	g220126	0.3
von Willebrand factor	g37946	0.3
Connexin 47	g6093424	0.3
Angiopoietin-2	g2257932	0.3
Pre-pro-multimerin	g927595	0.2
Bone morphogenetic protein 2b	g179503	0.2
Not known: cytokine-regulated of unknown function		
Interferon-induced protein 56	g32644	9.4
Interferon-induced protein 35	g2224902	4.6
Interferon-induced protein with tetratricopeptide repeats 4	g3719293	3.8

TABLE 3/continued 4.

Gene Name	GenBank ID	Fold-induction
Interferon induced protein 9-27	g177801	3.7
Interferon-inducible protein p27	g35183	3.6
Pentaxin PTX3	g35796	3.5
Hepatitis-associated microtubular aggregates protein	g218575	3.1
Homo sapiens cig5 mRNA	g2512970	2.9
Interferon-induced 17-kDa/15-kDa protein	g184570	2.9
Interferon induced transmembrane protein 3	g311374	2.3
Not known: annotated		
Hypothetical protein, expressed in osteoblast	g2564034	6.3
Natural killer cell transcript 4	g189225	4.8
Homo sapiens mRNA; cDNA DKFZp434F053	g5817205	3.4
KIAA0202	g1503987	3.1
Natural killer cell group 7 sequence (NKG7)	g487808	3
Activated B-cell factor-1 (ABF-1)	g3089604	2.4
Follistatin	g182718	2.3
Homo sapiens clone 25071 and 25177 mRNA sequences	g4406554	2.3
Homo sapiens polyA site DNA	g505034	2.1
LRR FLI-I interacting protein 1	g5257203	0.5
DKFZP586B0621 protein	g5817222	0.5
Homo sapiens clone 23860 mRNA sequence	g2795902	0.5
KIAA0758 protein	g3882236	0.5
KIAA1036 protein	g5689408	0.5
KIAK0002 gene	g285990	0.5
BRCA2 region, mRNA sequence CG003	g1685103	0.4
KIAA0680 gene product	g3327173	0.4
KIAA0836 protein	g4240160	0.4
KIAA0393 protein	g6683696	0.4
Homo sapiens clone 24432 mRNA sequence	g3387892	0.4
Not known: unannotated		
EST 1	g7019970	4
EST 2	g1031343	3.8
EST 3	g4508126	2.9
EST 4	g4003380	2.7
EST 5	g7020610	2.6
EST 6	g7106793	2.6
EST 7	g5262385	2.5
Homo sapiens PTD010 mRNA	g5531840	2.4
EST 8	g3927856	2.1
EST 9	g4165269	2
Nidogen	g1015511	0.5
Neuron-specific protein	g190258	0.3
EST 10	g4001608	4.8

to be regulated in activated endothelial cells. These structural classes include the EBI-3 (IL-12 related protein), NKG-7, TSG-6, CD44, CD51, cadherin-11, galectin-9, galectin-3, and MCP-2.[12,13] It is not yet clear what roles these molecules might play in endothelial cell function, and their involvement in mutual interactions between endothelial cells cannot be excluded.

The dramatic increase in transcription of over 200 genes induced by TNFα and IL-1β would be predicted to increase the ATP demands for the cell. Interestingly, we see that mRNA levels of phosphofructokinase are increased by the inflammatory stimuli. As the rate-limiting enzyme for glycolysis, phosphofructokinase is a target of allosteric regulation at the protein level; and it is intuitive that longer-term increases in the basal level of energy consumption would require an adjustment at the transcriptional level (and presumably the protein level) of this enzyme. Consistent with this idea, the level of lactate dehydrogenase mRNA level is also increased. The upregulation of superoxide dismutase, metallothionein, heme oxygenase, and ferritin may be associated with protection from oxidative damage, the potential of which is increased upon TNFα and IL-1β treatment due to the synthesis of reactive intermediates such as NO and as a by-product of increased metabolic activity.[14]

Consistent with the role of endothelium in regulating vascular tone, we found several genes associated with this function. Cationic amino acid transporter and GTP cyclohydrolase are critical for supply of arginine and tetrahydrobiopterin, two substrates required for NO synthesis.[15,16] In addition, COX-2, angiotensin I converting enzyme, ANP-C receptor, endothelin converting enzyme 1, and the VIP receptor were regulated by inflammatory cytokines.

In this study we report the regulation in endothelium of molecules that are considered to be important for cell function in cells of the immune system. The presence of these genes, IL-7 receptor, IL-18 receptor, IL-15 receptor, and CD34 may be indicative of the common lineage of hematopoietic cells and endothelial cells.[17–19] In addition, activated endothelial cells express several genes that can have anti-infective functions. Such genes include those known to be associated with anti-viral or anti-bacterial activity: toll receptor 4, Class I MHC, Class II MHC, 2′–5′ oligoadenylate synthetase, and complement components.[20–22] In addition to the anti-viral genes MxB and MxA, several other genes known to be IFNγ-responsive are induced in endothelial cells, some of which may be associated with anti-viral action, such as guanylate binding protein 2.[23,24] This may mean that endothelial cells participate directly in host defense more extensively than has previously been appreciated and the observed induction of many IFN-regulated genes is evidence that TNFα and IL-1β can, to some extent, trigger the IFNγ signal transduction pathway.

Several intracellular molecules known or likely to be involved in signal transduction are modulated by inflammatory stimuli. Many genes that participate in directly mediating TNFα and IL-1β signal transduction were regulated themselves at the mRNA level in this study.[25,26] These include IkBα, RelB, caspase 1, A20, cIAP, and the kinase STK2. Altering the levels of these components would be predicted to modulate the outcome of TNFα and IL-1β signal transduction in the cell. A20 and cIAP are likely to obviate apoptotic effects. It is possible that other genes in the signal transduction and transcription regulation category (TABLE 3) may also be directly involved in TNFα and IL-1β signal transduction. Interesting candidates include adducin (a known PKC substrate), and IFP35 (an AP-1 family member).[27]

It is noteworthy that among the induced genes there are many molecules including receptors that are known or likely to be involved in some type of signal transduction or transcriptional regulation. The large number of genes in this category indicates that a major effect of TNFα and IL-1β is to reset the signaling wiring and hence alter the potential of the endothelial cell to respond to various other external stimuli.

Microarray expression analysis is a valuable tool for examining complex cellular responses. In this simple *in vitro* model of inflammation, we were able to show that endothelial cells respond with a remarkably large repertory of genes that reflect changes in their physiology. The comparative simplicity of the response of smooth muscle cells supports the central regulatory role of the endothelial cell in the early stages of inflammation in the vasculature.

The simultaneous assessment of the activities of thousands of genes allowed some insight into a higher level of organization. The most interesting example of this difference in perspective was our parallel observation of the regulation of at least 43 signal transduction pathway components. This is indicative of interactions among many separate signal transduction pathways that form a "response network." Knowledge of the response network provides the basis for further understanding of the ways in which cells respond to inflammation, and help in designing therapeutic approaches for inflammatory diseases. This is particularly important given our observation that activation of the same pathway induces largely distinct genes and responses in different cell types.

REFERENCES

1. WENZEL, R.P. *et al.* 1996. Current understanding of sepsis. Clin. Infect. Dis. **22**(3): 407–412.
2. WEINSTEIN, J. *et al.* 1999. A cDNA microarray gene expression database for cancer drug discovery. Nature Genet. **23**: 81.
3. IYER, V. *et al.* 1999. The transcriptional program in the response of human fibroblasts to serum [see comments]. Science **283**(5398): 83–88.
4. MANTOVANI, A., S. SOZZANI & M. INTRONA. 1997. Endothelial activation by cytokines. Ann. N.Y. Acad. Sci. **832**: 93–116.
5. MANTOVANI, A. *et al.* 1998. Regulation of endothelial cell function by pro- and anti-inflammatory cytokines. Transplant. Proc. **30**(8): 4239–4243.
6. INTRONA, M. *et al.* 1993. IL-1 inducible genes in human umbilical vein endothelial cells. Eur. Heart J. **14**: 78–81.
7. SCHMEDTJE, J.J. *et al.* 1997. Hypoxia induces cyclooxygenase-2 via the NF-κB p65 transcription factor in human vascular endothelial cells. J. Biol. Chem. **272**(1): 601–608.
8. IMAIZUMI, T. *et al.* 1997. Human endothelial cells synthesize ENA-78: relationship to IL-8 and to signaling of PMN adhesion. Am. J. Respir. Cell Mol. Biol. **17**(2): 181–192.
9. LENHOFF, S. & T. OLOFSSON. 1996. Cytokine regulation of GM-CSF and G-CSF secretion by human umbilical cord vein endothelial cells (HUVEC). Cytokine **8**(9): 702–709.
10. KO, Y. *et al.* 1999. Cytokine-inducible growth factor gene expression in human umbilical endothelial cells. Mol. Cell Probes **13**(3): 203–211.
11. BOEHME, M.W. 2000. Interaction of endothelial cells and neutrophils in vitro: kinetics of thrombomodulin, intercellular adhesion molecule-1 (ICAM-1), E-selectin, and vascular cell adhesion molecule-1 (VCAM-1): implications for the relevance as serological disease activity markers in vasculitides. [Record Supplied By Publisher]. Clin. Exp. Immunol. **119**(1): 250–254.

12. WISNIEWSKI, H.G. & J. Vilcek. 1997. TSG-6: an IL-1/TNF-inducible protein with antiinflammatory activity. Cytokine Growth Factor Rev. **8**(2): 143–156.
13. DEVERGNE, O., M. BIRKENBACH & E. KIEFF. 1997. Epstein-Barr virus-induced gene 3 and the p35 subunit of interleukin 12 form a novel heterodimeric hematopoietin. Proc. Natl. Acad. Sci. USA **94**(22): 12041–12046.
14. LAZO, J.S. et al. 1998, The protein thiol metallothionein as an antioxidant and protectant against antineoplastic drugs. Chem. Biol. Interact. **112**: 255–262.
15. IRIE, K. et al. 1997. Cationic amino acid transporter-2 mRNA induction by tumor necrosis factor-alpha in vascular endothelial cells. Eur. J. Pharmacol. **339**(2-3): 289–293.
16. HATTORI, Y. et al. 1997. GTP cyclohydrolase I mRNA induction and tetrahydrobiopterin synthesis in human endothelial cells. Biochim. Biophys. Acta **1358**(1): 61–66.
17. HOFMEISTER, R. et al. 1999. Interleukin-7: physiological roles and mechanisms of action. Cytokine Growth Factor Rev. **10**(1): 41–60.
18. WALDMANN, T., Y. TAGAYA & R. BAMFORD. 1998. Interleukin-2, interleukin-15, and their receptors. Int. Rev. Immunol. **16**(3-4): 205–226.
19. DELIA, D. et al. 1993. CD34 expression is regulated reciprocally with adhesion molecules in vascular endothelial cells in vitro. Blood **81**(4): 1001–1008.
20. YU, F. 1999. Transcriptional induction of p69 2′-5′-oligoadenylate synthetase by interferon-alpha is stimulated by 12-O-tetradecanoyl phorbol-13-acetate through IRF/ISRE binding motifs. [In Process Citation]. Gene **237**(1): 177–184.
21. ZHANG, F. et al. 1999. Bacterial lipopolysaccharide activates nuclear factor-kappaB through interleukin-1 signaling mediators in cultured human dermal endothelial cells and mononuclear phagocytes. J. Biol. Chem. **274**(12): 7611–7614.
22. FAURE, E. et al. 2000. Bacterial lipopolysaccharide activates NF-kappaB through toll-like receptor 4 (TLR-4) in cultured human dermal endothelial cells. Differential expression of TLR-4 and TLR-2 in endothelial cells. J. Biol. Chem. **275**(15): 11058–11063.
23. HALLER, O., M. FRESE & G. KOCHS. 1998. Mx proteins: mediators of innate resistance to RNA viruses. Rev. Sci. Tech. **17**(1): 220–230.
24. MELEN, K. et al. 1996. Human MxB protein, an interferon-alpha-inducible GTPase, contains a nuclear targeting signal and is localized in the heterochromatin region beneath the nuclear envelope. J. Biol. Chem. **271**(38): 23478–23486.
25. NATOLI, G. et al. 1998. Apoptotic, non-apoptotic, and anti-apoptotic pathways of tumor necrosis factor signalling. Biochem. Pharmacol. **56**(8): 915–920.
26. LEDGERWOOD, E., J. POBER & J. BRADLEY. 1999. Recent advances in the molecular basis of TNF signal transduction. Lab. Invest. **79**(9): 1041–1050.
27. MATSUOKA, Y., X. LI & V. BENNETT. 1998. Adducin is an in vivo substrate for protein kinase C: phosphorylation in the MARCKS-related domain inhibits activity in promoting spectrin-actin complexes and occurs in many cells, including dendritic spines of neurons. J. Cell Biol. **142**(2): 485–497.

Integrated Genomic and Proteomic Analysis of Signaling Pathways in Dendritic Cell Differentiation and Maturation

JOHN RICHARDS,[a] FRANÇOIS LE NAOUR,[a] SAMIR HANASH,[b] AND LAURA BERETTA[a]

[a]*Department of Microbiology and Immunology,* [b]*Department of Pediatrics, University of Michigan, Ann Arbor, Michigan 48109, USA*

ABSTRACT: Dendritic cells (DCs) are antigen-presenting cells that play a major role in initiating primary immune responses. Their phenotypic and functional characteristics are intimately linked to their stage of maturation. The specific biochemical pathways and genes whose expression mediates differentiation of progenitors to DCs and their maturation are largely undefined. We recently utilized two approaches, DNA microarrays and proteomics, to analyze the expression profile of human $CD14^+$ blood monocytes and their derived DCs. Approximately 4% of the genes or proteins expressed were found to be regulated during DC differentiation. Most of these genes were not previously associated with DCs and included genes highly relevant to DC functions (genes involved in antigen presentation, cell adhesion and motility, lipid metabolism). Genes involved in specific signaling pathways, including IκBα, PPAR-γ and C/EBPα as well as two members of the family of transcription factors, interferon regulatory factors (IRFs), were also modified. Modulation of IRF gene expression is of particular interest because of their functional roles in innate and adaptive immune responses. IRF-family members control the expression of proteins that include type-1 interferons, interleukin-12, interleukin-15, MHC molecules and adhesion molecules. They have also been found to play an important role in lymphocyte development. In contrast to DC differentiation, very few genes were modified at the transcript level during DC maturation as determined by microarray experiments. Further analysis suggested that DC maturation is largely controlled by posttranscriptional and posttranslational modifications. The use of proteomics is therefore necessary for a full comprehension of DC maturation process.

KEYWORDS: genomic analysis; proteomic analysis; signaling pathways; dendritic cell differentiation; dendritic cell maturation

DENDRITIC CELL DIFFERENTIATION AND MATURATION

Dendritic cells (DCs) are potent antigen-presenting cells derived from bone marrow that have an integral role in regulating the immune response.[1,2] The function of DCs correlates directly with their degree of differentiation and maturation.[2]

Address for correspondence: Laura Beretta, Department of Microbiology and Immunology, University of Michigan, 6744 MSII, 1150 West Medical Center Drive, Ann Arbor, Michigan 48109-0620. Voice: 734 615 5964; fax: 734 615 6150.
berettal@umich.edu

Immature DCs are not potent antigen-presenting cells, but continually uptake material from their surroundings by phagocytosis, macropinocytosis, and receptor-mediated endocytosis.[2] DC maturation leads to the cessation of antigen uptake for antigen presentation. Mature DCs have greater surface levels of MHC, costimulatory, and adhesion molecules making them potent activators of T cells.[2] Furthermore, mature DCs secrete chemokines such as SLC and MIP-3β, which promote the recruitment of naïve and memory T cells.[3] In vivo, the location of DCs is highly concordant with their function. Immature DCs are located in body tissues were they act as sentinels.[4] Upon encounter with a pathogen or at a site of inflammation, DCs undergo maturation and migrate through the afferent lymphatics to secondary lymphoid organs where they interact and activate antigen-specific T cells.[5] Activated T cells leave the secondary lymphoid organs, migrate to the inflammation site, and perform effector functions leading to the clearance of the pathogen.[1,2]

DCs were initially known for their ability to activate T cells.[4] More recently, the ability of DCs to regulate T cells has become of great interest. A striking example of DC-induced T cell tolerance was observed when influenza matrix peptide (MP)–pulsed immature DCs were injected into healthy individuals.[6] Evaluation of the immune response pre- and post-DC injection demonstrated a decrease in T cell reactivity against MP. Injection of MP-loaded, mature DCs showed the opposite effect, as T cells had a more robust response towards MP.[6,7] Determination of whether DCs will be tolerogenic or immunogenic may be related to DC subsets or DC plasticity. An example of how different human DC populations can give different immune responses is demonstrated by comparing human myeloid DCs with human plasmacytoid DCs.[8] Allogeneic T cell stimulation with myeloid DCs and plasmacytoid DCs results in T cell secretion of IFN-γ and IL-4, IL-5, or IL-10, respectively. Closer analysis of the DCs showed that myeloid DCs secreted IL-12 while plasmacytoid DCs did not. These data along with data obtained in murine models helped develop the idea that tolerance and activation might be induced by different DC subsets.[9] However, to complicate matters, DC subsets have plasticity in that they exhibit the ability to both activate and tolerize T cells.[10] The plasticity is associated with the microenvironment where the DC resides.[10] For example, myeloid DCs cultured in the presence of IL-10 induce T cell tolerance, whereas DCs cultured in the presence of inflammatory stimuli will augment T cell activation and dsRNA will augment T cell activation as well as polarize T cells towards a type 1 response.[11,12]

The ability of DCs to stimulate different immune responses is associated with different states of maturation.[2] Several microbial products such as dsRNA, LPS, peptidoglycan, and bacterial CpG islands all seem to stimulate DC maturation.[13] The capacity of these molecules to stimulate DC maturation is associated with their binding to specific Toll-like receptors present on the DC surface.[10] Toll-like receptors send signals that result in the activation in NF-κB. NF-κB has been associated with the transcriptional regulation of many genes that are detected during DC maturation, including the cytokine IL-12p40 and costimulatory molecules CD80 and CD86.[14] The common activation of NF-κB by toll-like receptors and cytokines does not explain the diversity in DC maturation. For example, DCs matured with peptidoglycans secrete high levels of TNF-α, low levels of IL-6 and IL-12, and no IFN-α, while poly I:C induces the secretion of IL-12p70, low levels of IFN-α, and no TNF-α or IL-6 after 24 hours incubation.[13] Individual inflammatory mediators such as TNF-α, IL-1β, IL-6, and prostaglandin E2 (PGE2) have the ability to induce DC maturation.[15] However, the combinations of inflammatory mediators are synergistic in their ability to induce DC maturation. NF-κB is definitely involved in these responses but what other biochemical pathways and transcription factors are involved in the generation of diversity found in the immune response?

DCs have become accessible for detailed molecular and cell biological analysis and for clinical applications. Microarrays and proteomics are emerging and potentially complementary technologies for identifying the mRNA and protein constituents of living organisms and determining their pattern of expression.[16–18] Few studies have been undertaken that simultaneously analyzed cell populations at both RNA and protein levels. Potential sources of discordance between RNA and protein levels include translational control and altered protein stability. Additionally, proteomic analysis may uncover posttranslational modifications that are not predictable at the RNA level. Using both oligonucleotide microarrays and proteomics, we performed a global analysis of gene expression during DC differentiation and maturation.[19]

GENOMICS APPLIED TO DENDRITIC CELL DIFFERENTIATION AND MATURATION

The identification of expressed sequences in a number of species has ushered in the post-genome era. In this era, technologies are becoming available that allow the profiling of tissues and cell populations at the RNA and protein levels. Microarray technology is a promising approach to comparatively analyze genome-wide patterns of mRNA expression,[20–27] the ultimate goal being to develop arrays that contain every gene in a genome, or selected subsets, against which mRNA expression levels can be quantitatively assessed. DNA microarrays provide an important new tool for the characterization of tissues and cell lines. Large sets of genes involved in signal transduction, differentiation, apoptosis, cell cycle progression, etc., all could be analyzed simultaneously with respect to their expression. Microarray analysis exemplifies the type of comprehensive, large throughput technologies that could yield a molecular based understanding of physiological processes and disease states. There are at present a substantial variety of arrays that may be utilized as well as choices of hardware, software, and multiple sources of DNA for arraying and a variety of protocols for implementation. One technology for cDNA-based microarrays is based on an approach in which cDNA clone inserts are robotically printed onto glass slides and subsequently hybridized to two differentially fluorescently labeled probes to compare the expression patterns of the cells from which they were derived. Another leading technology relies on the use of oligonucleotides. One concept that has been implemented involves the synthesis of tens of thousands of oligonucleotides onto chips using photolithography, as developed by Affymetrix.

Differentiation of CD14$^+$ blood monocytes into mature DCs can be induced *in vitro* by treatment with a combination of GM-CSF, IL-4 and TNF-α.[10,16] Using oligonucleotide arrays, RNA transcript levels for different genes expressed during DC differentiation were determined at day 1 (CD14$^+$ monocytes) and after seven days of GM-CSF/IL-4 treatment (immature DCs) and 14 days of GM-CSF/IL-4 plus TNF-α treatment (mature DCs). Transcripts for approximately 40% of the 6,300 unique genes assessed were detected in all the cell populations tested. We identified a subset of genes which differed in their expression levels during DC differentiation and maturation, by 2.5-fold or greater.

We identified close to 4% of the genes and proteins analyzed as regulated during DC differentiation. The regulated genes were in major part related to cell adhesion and motility, growth control, regulation of the immune response and antigen presentation, transcription and signal transduction, and lipid metabolism. Genes known to be differentially expressed during DC differentiation changed their expression accordingly in our analysis. This group included the monocytic marker CD14, CD163 and C5a anaphylatoxin receptor (CD88), which were strongly downregulated, and the cell surface proteins MHC class II, CD1a, CD1b, CD1c, CD36, CD59, CD83, CD86, and CCR7 which were upregregulated with DC differentiation and maturation. The secretion of proteins TARC (CCR4 ligand), MCP-4 and the macrophage-derived chemokine (MDC) was also observed. Most of the 255 regulated genes we uncovered were not previously known to be differentially expressed in DCs.

Interestingly, we identified a large number of genes encoding for proteins involved in cell adhesion and motility which are regulated during DC differentiation. Expression of galectin 2, CD11a/LFA-1 alpha, ninjurin 1, macmarcks, syndecan 2, CD44E, and presenilin 1 was downregulated. Expression of secreted proteins involved in cell motility, autotaxin-t and semaphorin E, reported to play a role in axon guidance in the nervous system,[28] was upregulated. Therefore, the concomitant decrease in expression of integrins and cell adhesion molecules, the increase in expression of genes involved in cell motility, and regulated expression of enzymes such as alpha 1 antitrypsin and macrophage metalloelastase (HME), likely have an effect on the enhanced migration properties of DCs compared to their precursors.

Differentiation of DCs was accompanied by differential expression of genes involved in the immune response. Noticeable was the upregulation of genes encoding antiinflammatory proteins such as cyclophilin C and TSG-6 [29,30] with a concomitant decrease in the production of proinflammatory cytokines. Several genes encoding proinflammatory cytokines and their receptors, such as prointerleukin-1-β, TNF-α, CD163, C5a anaphylatoxin receptor, IL-6 receptor, and TNF receptor were downregulated. A noticeable change was the downregulation of a set of chemokines belonging to the IL-8 superfamily such as CTAPIII, MIP2-α, MIP2-β, ENA78, PF4, and IL-8. It has been reported that these chemokines are proinflammatory cytokines that act as potent neutrophil chemoattractants and activators.[31] Interestingly, these chemokines which were coordinately downregulated have been co-localized to the same genomic region.[32] Osteopontin, a key cytokine involved in T-lymphocyte activation[33] was upregulated. The maturation of DCs was accompanied by the upregulation of Mac-2 binding protein. Mac-2 binding protein is an adhesion molecule with a potent immune stimulatory activity. Indeed, it has been demonstrated that Mac-2 binding protein stimulates host defense systems, such as NK and LAK cell activities, and induces the secretion of IL-2.[34] Upregulation of TGF-α was also observed during DC maturation.

Expression of mRNAs encoding for proteins localized in the nuclear compartment or involved in signaling has been poorly described in DCs. Expression of the interferon regulatory factor 4 (IRF-4), C/EBPa, mrg1, PPARg, TRIP7, SLA,

Rap1GAP, cAMP-dependent protein kinase, IP3 protein kinase B, cyclophilin C and cyclins A1, D2, G2 and H genes, was increased. Expression of IRF-7A, TAL2, NAP-2, EGF-response factor 2, CtBP, IEX-1, SAP49, HRH1, I-κB alpha, Fyb, Net and cyclophilin F genes was decreased. Of these genes, IRF-4 and IRF-7 are of particular interest. In IRF-4$^{-/-}$ mice, there are severe immunological defects in T and B cell function.[35] Antigen-presenting cells appeared normal as T cell lines recognized processed antigen. However, these mice were unable to mount a primary immune response against an allogeneic tumor, suggesting a defect in DC function. The role of IRF-7 has been traditionally involved in the activation of type 1 interferons.[36,37] More recently, IRF-7 was shown to be involved in the differentiation of monocytes into macrophages.[38] The decrease in IRF-7 during DC differentiation versus increased expression in macrophage differentiation may suggest a critical role for IRF-7 at the crossroad between macrophage and DC differentiation from monocytes.

Finally, the regulation of a large group of genes encoding for lipid-binding proteins or enzymes involved in lipid metabolism was observed in DC differentiation. Several genes encoding enzymes or proteins involved in the production, uptake, transport, and solubilization of cholesterol and fatty acids were upregulated in DCs. This group includes apolipoprotein E, apolipoprotein C-I, ABCG1, lysosomal acid lipase, and lipoprotein lipase. The fatty acids are translocated from the extracellular environment to the cytoplasm by the fatty acid translocase (FAT/CD36) and then solubilized and transported by fatty acid binding proteins (FABPs) to the site where they are metabolized.[39] We reported marked upregulation of CD36 as well as of the lipid binding proteins FABP3, FABP4, FABP5, CRABPII, and ACBP. Upregulation of FABPs was concomitant with a strong downregulation of the S100 proteins, MRP8 and MRP14. Interestingly, MRP8 and MRP14 are expressed by myeloid cells during inflammatory reactions, and it has been reported that MRP-8/MRP-14 heterodimer (FA-p34) has a fatty acid binding activity and specifically binds (poly)unsaturated fatty acids.[40–42] In contrast, FABP4 and FABP5 bind saturated or (mono)unsaturated fatty acids with a high affinity. Long-chain fatty acids and acyl-CoA esters affect a large number of cell functions during cell growth and differentiation, including signal transduction, gene regulation, ion channel activities, and membrane fusion.[39,43] In this context, we observed an upregulation of 15-lipoxygenase which promotes the formation of lipoxins that are modulators of leukocyte recruitment.[44–46]

PROTEOMICS APPLIED TO DENDRITIC CELL DIFFERENTIATION AND MATURATION

Proteins are the most functional component encoded for in the genome. The large-scale profiling of gene expression at the protein level has a long history that predates profiling at the RNA level.[47] In the past decade, mass spectrometry has provided the means for the identification, through sequence database searching, of proteins separated by two-dimensional electrophoresis or other means, at an unprecedented level of sensitivity and speed.[48] The availability of a full set of human and other mammalian sequences of expressed genes and the emergence of mass spectrometry as an important tool for protein identification have led to a resurgence of interest in protein analysis. Critical to protein investigations has been the availability of suitable technology for the large-scale analysis of complex protein mixtures that provides high speed and automation as well as high sensitivity. A number of technologies have been investigated or are under development. However it is generally agreed that at the present time, 2D-PAGE remains the "gold standard" for resolving large protein mixtures.

To identify protein changes during the differentiation and maturation of the monocyte-derived DCs, total proteins were extracted as described for the microarray analysis. Following protein separation by two-dimensional gel electrophoresis, gels were silver stained and digitized. 2-D protein patterns were matched by computer analysis; 900 protein spots were matched and quantitated. Whereas the overall 2-D patterns of $CD14^+$ monocytes, immature and mature DCs were largely similar, numerous protein changes were reproducibly detected. As for the microarray analysis, we selected protein spots whose intensities changed in all experiments by 2.5-fold or greater during DC differentiation or maturation. A set of 37 proteins was identified.

Of the 37 spots excised from the gels, 18 were identified without ambiguity, by mass spectrometry. Specific antibodies confirmed the identification based on mass spectrometry for all proteins analyzed by Western-blotting. The proteins identified were members of specific families including chaperones, Ca^{2+}-binding proteins, fatty acid binding proteins and structural proteins. Expression of three members of the fatty acid binding protein (FABP) family, FABP4, FABP5 and Acyl-CoA-binding protein, (ACBP) was highly increased after seven days of culture. The increased protein and RNA levels for these genes were concordant. Concomitant with the upregulation of FABP4 and FABP5, we observed a strong downregulation of two members of the S100 family, the myeloid-related proteins MRP14 and MRP8. Interestingly, it has been recently shown that the heterodimer MRP8/MRP14, designated fatty-acid p34 (FA-p34), exerts a fatty-acid binding activity.[40–42] MRP14 and MRP8 downregulation was progressive upon DC differentiation and maturation, leading to a 9- and 12-fold decrease in spot intensities, respectively. Again, the results obtained for these two genes at both the RNA and protein levels were highly concordant.

Several proteins known for their chaperone activity including hsp73, hsp27, and calreticulin were also regulated during DC differentiation. An emerging hypothesis is that heat shock proteins participate in antigen processing and presentation and play a central role in the activation of T lymphocytes by DCs.[49–51] Hsp70 targets immature DC precursors to enhance antigen uptake.[52] We observed an upregulation of hsp73 protein, related to the hsp70 family,[53] during DC differentiation. Hsp73 has been recently reported to bind specifically to the cell surface of monocytic and dendritic cell lines and to be internalized spontaneously by receptor-mediated endocytosis.[50] In addition, the murine hsp73 has been recently reported to accumulate in exosomes from immatures DCs.[54] The role of hsp27 upregulation during DC differentiation is less clear. It has been reported that an increase in cellular levels of hsp27 promotes a resistance of monocytes to apoptotic cell death.[55,56] Increased hsp27 expression in DCs may therefore have a protective role against cytotoxicity. In contrast to hsp27 and hsp73, the cognate chaperone protein calreticulin was downregulated during DC differentiation owing to posttranslational modification. In addition, whereas the expression of hsp27 and hsp73 was maximal in immature DCs, calreticulin was mostly downregulated during DC maturation. Calreticulin participates in the assembly of MHC class I with peptide and beta 2-microglobulin in the endoplasmic reticulum, a process required for the presentation of antigenic peptides to CTLs at the cell surface.[57,58] In addition, it has been recently reported that calreticulin elicits tumor- and peptide-specific immunity.[59] Calreticulin displays *in vivo* peptide-binding activity and can elicit CTL responses against bound peptides.[60]

There were discrepancies between the protein and gene expression data for vimentin, hsp27, and calreticulin. Close analysis of the microarray hybridization data showed saturation level intensities for vimentin and hsp resulting from their high-level expression. Therefore, the discordance between mRNA and protein levels observed in our data for these genes most likely reflects their high expression level, reaching saturation at the RNA hybridization level using microarrays, but not at the protein level using 2-D gels. The calreticulin protein was found to be downregulated with DC differentiation in our 2-D gel analysis, whereas the corresponding transcript was unchanged at the RNA level by microarray analysis. Hybridization data for calreticulin transcript did not show any saturation. Interestingly, a protein with an estimated MW of 32 kDa and PI of 4.1, was found to be induced in immature DCs. After enzymatic digestions using trypsin or endoproteinase Lys-C and analysis of the resulting peptides by MALDI-TOF mass spectrometry, the peptide masses were consistent with those of peptides derived from calreticulin, a protein with a MW of 48 kDa and a PI of 4.3. Altogether, proteomic analysis allowed us to identify a truncated form of calreticulin, present only in DCs. We designated this novel form of calreticulin as Crt32. This form contains the P-domain, a site of chaperone activity, and the C-domain, which contains the endoplasmic reticulum retrieval sequence, but lacks the N-domain. A calreticulin fragment corresponding to the N-domain has been recently purified from the supernatant of an EBV-immortalized cell line. This fragment, named vasostatin, is an angiogenesis inhibitor that exerts antitumor effects *in vivo*.[61,62] Therefore, even though the C-terminal end of vasostatin has not been precisely characterized, Crt32 most likely corresponds to the complementary part of vasostatin, following cleavage of calreticulin. A decrease in levels of the cognate form of calreticulin and an increase in Crt32 levels may be relevant to DC function and the precise function(s) of Crt32 in mature DCs is currently under investigation. Therefore, whereas microarray analysis did not show any changes involving calreticulin, proteomic analysis allowed the detection of a posttranslational modification of calreticulin occurring during DC differentiation.

FINAL COMMENTS

DCs acquire their function with differentiation and maturation, which occurs through a programmed expression of specific proteins. The combination of both genomics relying on the quantitative analysis of mRNAs, and proteomics, relying on quantitative analysis and identification of proteins, demonstrated a good correlation between transcripts and proteins during DC differentiation, but not during DC maturation. Therefore complete understanding of the mechanisms underlying DC maturation would necessitate further proteomic analysis of specific subcellular fractions of the cell. Indeed, proteins represent the most functional compartment of a cell, and the information obtained at the protein level cannot simply be predicted from examining expression at the RNA level. The proteomics approach is also appropriate to identify posttranslational modifications, which may regulate protein function. An example is that during DC differentiation MHC class II molecules are synthesized but are not stably expressed on the cell surface.[63] However, fully mature DCs stably express MHC class II molecules on the cell surface while biosynthetic and endocytic traffic ceases.[63]

The oligonucleotide array and proteomics analyses have uncovered novel genes and proteins with potential roles in DC function, differentiation and/or maturation. Microarray analysis has identified important changes in genes involved in cell adhesion and motility, immune response, and growth control as well as in lipid metabolism. Following the simultaneous analysis of several thousand genes at the mRNA level, the challenge is to efficiently utilize this information to develop a better understanding of DC function. This study also demonstrates that a proteomics approach may provide information that could not be obtained at the RNA level, owing either to poor correlation between mRNA and protein levels or to posttranslational modifications that may result in several isoforms generated from one mRNA, as in the case of calreticulin in our study. Genes and proteins identified to be selectively expressed in DCs, may provide further understanding of the biological function of DCs in host defense systems and of the mechanisms of antigen processing and presentation.

REFERENCES

1. BANCHEREAU, J. et al. 2000. Immunobiology of dendritic cells. Annu. Rev. Immunol. **18:** 767–811.
2. BANCHEREAU, J. & R.M. STEINMAN. 1998. Dendritic cells and the control of immunity. Nature **392:** 245–252.
3. CYSTER, J.G. 1999. Chemokines and cell migration in secondary lymphoid organs. Science **286:** 2098–2102.
4. STEINMAN, R.M. 1991. The dendritic cell system and its role in immunogenicity. Annu. Rev. Immunol. **9:** 271–296.
5. STEINMAN, R.M. 2001. Dendritic cells and the control of immunity: enhancing the efficiency of antigen presentation. Mt. Sinai J. Med. **68:** 106–166.
6. DHODAPKAR, M.V. et al. 2001. Antigen-specific inhibition of effector T cell function in humans after injection of immature dendritic cells. J. Exp. Med. **193:** 233–238.
7. DHODAPKAR, M.V. et al. 1999. Rapid generation of broad T-cell immunity in humans after a single injection of mature dendritic cells. J. Clin. Invest. **104:** 173–180.
8. RISSOAN, M.C. et al. 1999. Reciprocal control of T helper cell and dendritic cell differentiation [see comments]. Science **283:** 1183–1186.
9. MALDONADO-LOPEZ, R. & M. MOSER. 2001. Dendritic cell subsets and the regulation of Th1/Th2 responses. Semin. Immunol. **13:** 275–282.
10. LANZAVECCHIA, A. & F. SALLUSTO. 2001. The instructive role of dendritic cells on T cell responses: lineages, plasticity and kinetics. Curr. Opin. Immunol. **13:** 291–298.
11. STEINBRINK, K. et al. 1997. Induction of tolerance by IL-10-treated dendritic cells. J. Immunol. **159:** 4772–4780.
12. CELLA, M. et al. 1999. Maturation, activation, and protection of dendritic cells induced by double-stranded RNA. J. Exp. Med. **189:** 821–829.
13. KADOWAKI, N. et al. 2001. Subsets of human dendritic cell precursors express different toll-like receptors and respond to different microbial antigens. J. Exp. Med. **194:** 863–869.
14. HOFFMANN, J.A. et al. 1999. Phylogenetic perspectives in innate immunity. Science **284:** 1313–1318.

15. JONULEIT, H. *et al.* 1997. Pro-inflammatory cytokines and prostaglandins induce maturation of potent immunostimulatory dendritic cells under fetal calf serum-free conditions. Eur. J. Immunol. **27:** 3135–3142.
16. LOCKHART, D.J. & E.A. WINZELER. 2000. Genomics, gene expression and DNA arrays. Nature **405:** 827–836.
17. HANASH, S.M. 1998. Two-dimensional Gel Electrophoresis. *In* Gel Electrophoresis of Proteins: A Practical Approach. B.D. Hames & D. Rickwood, Eds.: 189–211. Oxford University Press. Oxford.
18. PANDEY, A. & M. MANN. 2000. Proteomics to study genes and genomes. Nature **405:** 837–846.
19. LE NAOUR, F. *et al.* 2001. Profiling changes in gene expression during differentiation and maturation of monocyte-derived dendritic cells using both oligonucleotide microarrays and proteomics. J. Biol. Chem. **276:** 17920–17931.
20. CHEN, Y., E. DOUGHERTY & M. BITTNER. 1997. Ratio-based decisions and the quantitative analysis of cDNA micro-array images. J. Biomed. Optics **2:** 365.
21. BROWN, P.O. & D. BOTSTEIN. 1999. Exploring the new world of the genome with DNA microarrays. Nat. Genet. **21:** 33–37.
22. DERISI, J. *et al.* 1996. Use of a cDNA microarray to analyse gene expression patterns in human cancer. Nat. Genet. **14:** 457–460.
23. KHAN, J. *et al.* 1998. Gene expression profiling of alveolar rhabdomyosarcoma with cDNA microarrays. Cancer Res. **58:** 5009–5013.
24. SCHENA, M. 1996. Genome analysis with gene expression microarrays. Bioessays **18:** 427–431.
25. SCHENA, M. *et al.* 1995. Quantitative monitoring of gene expression patterns with a complementary DNA microarray. Science **270:** 467–470.
26. SCHENA, M. *et al.* 1996. Parallel human genome analysis: microarray-based expression monitoring of 1000 genes. Proc. Natl. Acad. Sci. USA **93:** 10614–10619.
27. TRENT, J.M. *et al.* 1997. Use of microgenomic technology for analysis of alterations in DNA copy number and gene expression in malignant melanoma. Clin. Exp. Immunol. **107**(Suppl. 1): 33–40.
28. BAGNARD, D. *et al.* 1998. Semaphorins act as attractive and repulsive guidance signals during the development of cortical projections. Development **125:** 5043–5053.
29. TRAHEY, M. & I.L. WEISSMAN. 1999. Cyclophilin C-associated protein: a normal secreted glycoprotein that down-modulates endotoxin and proinflammatory responses in vivo. Proc. Natl. Acad. Sci. USA **96:** 3006–3011.
30. WISNIEWSKI, H.G. & J. VILCEK. 1997. TSG-6: an IL-1/TNF-inducible protein with anti-inflammatory activity. Cytokine Growth Factor Rev. **8:** 143–156.
31. BAGGIOLINI, M., P. LOETSCHER & B. MOSER. 1995. Interleukin-8 and the chemokine family. Int. J. Immunopharmacol. **17:** 103–108.
32. O'DONOVAN, N., M. GALVIN & J.G. MORGAN. 1999. Physical mapping of the CXC chemokine locus on human chromosome 4. Cytogenet. Cell Genet. **84:** 39–42.
33. ASHKAR, S. *et al.* 2000. Eta-1 (osteopontin): an early component of type-1 (cell-mediated) immunity. Science **287:** 860–864.
34. ULLRICH, A. *et al.* 1994. The secreted tumor-associated antigen 90K is a potent immune stimulator. J. Biol. Chem. **269:** 18401–18407.
35. MITTRUCKER, H.W. *et al.* 1997. Requirement for the transcription factor LSIRF/IRF4 for mature B and T lymphocyte function. Science **275:** 540–543.
36. TANIGUCHI, T. *et al.* 2001. IRF family of transcription factors as regulators of host defense. Annu. Rev. Immunol. **19:** 623–655.
37. MAMANE, Y. *et al.* 1999. Interferon regulatory factors: the next generation. Gene **237:** 1–14.
38. LU, R. & P.M. PITHA. 2001. Monocyte differentiation to macrophage requires interferon regulatory factor 7. J. Biol. Chem. **276:** 45491–45496.
39. GLATZ, J.F. & G.J. VAN DER VUSSE. 1996. Cellular fatty acid-binding proteins: their function and physiological significance. Prog. Lipid Res. **35:** 243–282.
40. KLEMPT, M. *et al.* 1997. The heterodimer of the Ca2+-binding proteins MRP8 and MRP14 binds to arachidonic acid. FEBS Lett. **408:** 81–84.

41. KERKHOFF, C. et al. 1999. The two calcium-binding proteins, S100A8 and S100A9, are involved in the metabolism of arachidonic acid in human neutrophils. J. Biol. Chem. **274:** 32672–32679.
42. SIEGENTHALER, G. et al. 1997. A heterocomplex formed by the calcium-binding proteins MRP8 (S100A8) and MRP14 (S100A9) binds unsaturated fatty acids with high affinity. J. Biol. Chem. **272:** 9371–9377.
43. FAERGEMAN, N.J. & J. KNUDSEN. 1997. Role of long-chain fatty acyl-CoA esters in the regulation of metabolism and in cell signalling. Biochem. J. **323**(Pt. 1): 1–12.
44. CLARKSON, M.R. et al. 1998. Leukotrienes and lipoxins: lipoxygenase-derived modulators of leukocyte recruitment and vascular tone in glomerulonephritis. Nephrol. Dial. Transplant. **13:** 3043–3051.
45. KUHN, H. & B.J. THIELE. 1995. Arachidonate 15-lipoxygenase. J. Lipid Mediat. Cell Signal. **12:** 157–170.
46. SIGAL, E. & D.J. CONRAD. 1994. Human 15-lipoxygenase: a potential effector molecule for interleukin-4. Adv. Prostaglandin Thromboxane Leukotriene Res. **22:** 309–316.
47. HANASH, S.M. 2000. Biomedical applications of two-dimensional electrophoresis using immobilized pH gradients: current status. Electrophoresis **21:** 1202–1209.
48. PATTERSON, S.D. 2000. Mass spectrometry and proteomics. Physiol. Genomics **2:** 59–65.
49. COLACO, C.A. 1998. Towards a unified theory of immunity: dendritic cells, stress proteins and antigen capture. Cell. Mol. Biol. (Noisy-le-grand) **44:** 883–890.
50. ARNOLD-SCHILD, D. et al. 1999. Cutting edge: receptor-mediated endocytosis of heat shock proteins by professional antigen-presenting cells. J. Immunol. **162:** 3757–3760.
51. MANARA, G.C. et al. 1993. New insights suggesting a possible role of a heat shock protein 70-kD family-related protein in antigen processing/presentation phenomenon in humans. Blood **82:** 2865–2871.
52. TODRYK, S. et al. 1999. Heat shock protein 70 induced during tumor cell killing induces Th1 cytokines and targets immature dendritic cell precursors to enhance antigen uptake. J. Immunol. **163:** 1398–1408.
53. DWORNICZAK, B. & M.E. MIRAULT. 1987. Structure and expression of a human gene coding for a 71 kd heat shock 'cognate' protein. Nucleic Acids Res. **15:** 5181–5197.
54. THERY, C. et al. 1999. Molecular characterization of dendritic cell-derived exosomes. Selective accumulation of the heat shock protein hsc73. J. Cell Biol. **147:** 599–610.
55. JAATTELA, M. & D. WISSING. 1993. Heat-shock proteins protect cells from monocyte cytotoxicity: possible mechanism of self-protection. J. Exp. Med. **177:** 231–236.
56. SAMALI, A. & T.G. COTTER. 1996. Heat shock proteins increase resistance to apoptosis. Exp. Cell Res. **223:** 163–170.
57. MICHALAK, M. et al. 1999. Calreticulin: one protein, one gene, many functions. Biochem. J. 344 (Pt. 2): 281–292.
58. KRAUSE, K.H. & M. MICHALAK. 1997. Calreticulin. Cell **88:** 439–443.
59. BASU, S. & P.K. SRIVASTAVA. 1999. Calreticulin, a peptide-binding chaperone of the endoplasmic reticulum, elicits tumor- and peptide-specific immunity. J. Exp. Med. **189:** 797–802.
60. NAIR, S. et al. 1999. Calreticulin displays in vivo peptide-binding activity and can elicit CTL responses against bound peptides. J. Immunol. **162:** 6426–6432.
61. PIKE, S.E. et al. 1998. Vasostatin, a calreticulin fragment, inhibits angiogenesis and suppresses tumor growth. J. Exp. Med. **188:** 2349–2356.
62. PIKE, S.E. et al. 1999. Calreticulin and calreticulin fragments are endothelial cell inhibitors that suppress tumor growth. Blood **94:** 2461–2468.
63. WATTS, C. 1997. Immunology. Inside the gearbox of the dendritic cell. Nature **388:** 724–725.

CD30—Governor of Memory T Cells?

ECKHARD R. PODACK, NATASA STRBO,
VLATKA SOTOSEC, AND HIROMI MUTA

*Department of Microbiology and Immunology,
University of Miami School of Medicine, Miami, Florida 33136, USA*

ABSTRACT: CD30 is well recognized as a marker expressed by a heterogeneous group of lymphomas and in several immune and autoimmune disorders. However, the function of CD30 in theses diseases or in the normal immune response has remained unclear. Studying gene expression patterns induced by stimulating CD30 signals on a large granular lymphoma cell line, YT, with an agonistic anti-CD30 antibody, we found that CD30 signals affected proapoptotic and antiapoptotic genes, regulated cytotoxicity, and controlled molecules regulating T cell traffic. Creating CD30-L deficient mice and studying CD8 CTL activation and memory responses, it was observed that the absence of CD30-L resulted in diminished primary clonal expansion of CD8 cells. In addition the absence of CD30-L abolished clonal contraction after primary expansion and interfered with secondary expansion upon boosting. The studies suggest that CD30 regulates CD8 CTL function and survival during memory responses and is important for clonal contraction.

KEYWORDS: CD30; memory T-cells; T regulatory cells

INTRODUCTION

CD30, member of the TNF-receptor family,[14] is expressed on many lymphomas of B, T, and NK-cell origin.[1] CD30 is found on anaplastic large cell lymphoma, Hodgkin's and non-Hodgkin's lymphoma, skin-associated lymphomas, and germ cell tumors. CD30 is also expressed on multiple myeloma (our own unpublished data) and virally associated lymphomas. CD30 is over expressed on T cells in rheumatoid arthritis, atopic dermatitis, and in immunodeficiency syndromes Increased CD30 expression in lymphomas is associated with disease progression and unfavorable prognosis, suggesting that it contributes to the oncogenic process. Despite this obvious clinical importance,[2–6] very little is known about the function of CD30 in lymphomagenesis and in normal T cell responses.

CD30 can be expressed by activated B and T cells.[7–9] CD30 expression on normal B cells can inhibit isotype switching upon CD30-L (CD153) binding.[10–12] CD30 expression on T cells is transient and late following activation, and CD30 signals have been shown to induce IL-5 and IFN-γ production.[13] The intracellular domain of CD30 binds several members of the TRAF family and signals via the MAP-kinases c-Jun N-terminal (JNK) and p38, via NFκB and via FADD.[15–23] CD30's functions are pleiotropic, capable of mediating apoptosis, cell activation, and effec-

---

Address for correspondence: Eckhard R. Podack, Department of Microbiology and Immunology, University of Miami School of Medicine, P.O. Box 016960, Miami, FL 33101, USA. Voice: 305-243-6655; fax: 305-243-4623.

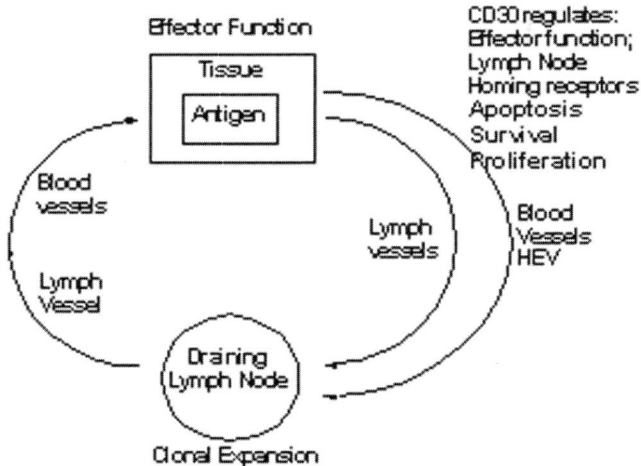

FIGURE 1.

tor function, respectively.[24] The ligand for CD30 is the CD30-Ligand (CD153). CD30-L is expressed constitutively on polymorphonuclear granulocytes and can be induced on monocytes and on activated B and T cells and, as we recently found, on immature dendritic cells.

Why is there comparatively little known about CD30 despite its clinical role? The answer probably lies in a lack of good models for investigation. CD30 knock-out (k.o.) mice have been generated and have only a minimal phenotype characterized by a partial defect in negative selection of thymocytes,[25] although this has been disputed.[26] The majority of antibodies to CD30 have no effect on CD30 signaling. Few anti-CD30 antibodies, including our own named C10, have agonistic effects and are suitable for *in vivo* and *in vitro* studies. An additional obstacle is the fact that CD30 is expressed only very transiently and at a low level on activated T cells. It is known that CD30 is constitutively expressed on a very small fraction of human PBL (about 2%), positive for CD45RO and secreting IFN-γ and IL-5.[27] The function of these cells is unclear.

CD30 signals via TRAF2-dependent and -independent pathways to JNK, p38, NFκB and FADD. CD30 can induce proliferation, inflammation, modulate effector function, regulate trafficking molecules, and induce apoptosis (see FIGURE 1). This complex signaling and functional modulation places CD30 into an ideal position to govern T cell memory function in the context of other signals. The studies described below support such a model.

RESULTS

Naïve T cells are activated in draining lymph nodes entering from the blood through CCR7 expression on the T cell and SLC on the high endothelial venules.[28–30]

Encountering antigen presented by dendritic cells in the lymph node, T cells undergo rapid clonal expansion and leave the lymph node via the lymphatic vessels (see FIGURE 1). At this point, the naïve cell has been activated to an effector cell and has lost the expression of both the CD45RA marker and CCR7. The CD45RO T cells recirculate in the blood stream and enter tissues at sites of inflammation, attracted through chemokines and other inflammatory signals. Upon reencountering antigen via the T cell receptor the effector cell upregulates CD30 and executes its effector function. CD45-RO T cells upon reactivation express high levels of CD30 and sustain CD30 expression longer than naïve CD45-RA T cells (see FIGURE 2). This observation suggests that CD30 function may be more critical for the regulation of CD45-RO positive T cells (memory T cells) than for naïve T cells.

Memory T cells (CD45-RO$^+$) have been categorized into two groups according to their CCR7 expression.[31] Memory effector cells that are able to express effector function upon TCR engagement are CCR7 negative. In contrast, central memory cells that express CCR7 do not execute effector function upon TCR engagement. CCR7 positive effector cells are able to reenter lymph nodes via SLC expressed in HEV. Presumably prior to entering lymph nodes it is necessary to suppress effector function so that antigen encounter does not cause effector function within the lymph node environment, which could be disruptive.

To gain further insight into the function of CD30 we studied gene expression profiles induced by CD30 signals. For this purpose the human large granular, NK like lymphoma line YT which expresses very high levels of CD30 was used. We have previously generated an antibody to CD30 (named C10) that has agonistic activity upon CD30 binding.[32] The YT lymphoma is a useful model cell line for cytotoxic cells. In addition to CD30 YT cells express CD56 but not TCR and CD16. YT kill Raji cells via B7/CD28, ICAM-1/LFA-1 interaction. YT cells express granules which contain perforin and granzyme B and which express Fas-Ligand. They are thus endowed with the two primary cytotoxic pathways used by NK and cytotoxic lymphocytes (CTL). YT therefore can serve as model effector cells for NK and possibly CTL.

YT cells were incubated with the agonistic C10 antibody or a control antibody for up to 72 hours. cDNA microarrays (Incyte) for approximately 8,000 genes were

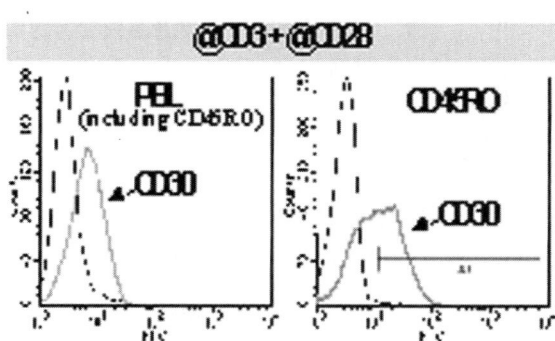

FIGURE 2. CD45RO cells express CD30 upon activation. Human PBL and purified CD45RO T cells were activated with anti-CD3 and anti-CD28 for three days and then analyzed for CD30 expression by flow cytometry.

hybridized and the effects of CD30 signaling evaluated by measuring differential regulation of message levels in C10 treated and control antibody-treated cells. Levels of mRNA upregulated or downregulated 1.5-fold or more were considered potentially significant. Genes of particular interest were validated in their regulation by RT-PCR, by RNA-protection assay, by FACS analysis, by Western blot, and by functional assays.[33]

A global analysis revealed that CD30 induced about 750 genes two or more fold and repressed about 90 genes two or more fold. Grouping genes by function the following patterns were observed.

Members of the TNF-Receptor and Ligand Superfamilies and Their Signaling/Adaptor Molecules

The strongest upregulation is seen for TRAF6, HVEM, TRAIL; Fas upregulation is also seen and was verified by FACS; TRAIL upregulation was verified by RNA protection assays. In addition we observed complete downregulation of Fas-L and upregulation of death receptor 3 (DR3) (see FIGURE 3).

The downregulation of Fas-Ligand by CD30 indicates that CD30 signals disable killing via induction of Fas-mediated apoptosis, which was verified. The upregulation of Fas, DR3 and Trail may suggests that CD30 signals increase the susceptibility of the cells to apoptotic signals by other cells.

Metalloproteinases

An unexpected finding of CD30 signaling was the strong upregulation of metalloproteinases (MP) by CD30. Using enzymatic assays we found MP9 and MP2

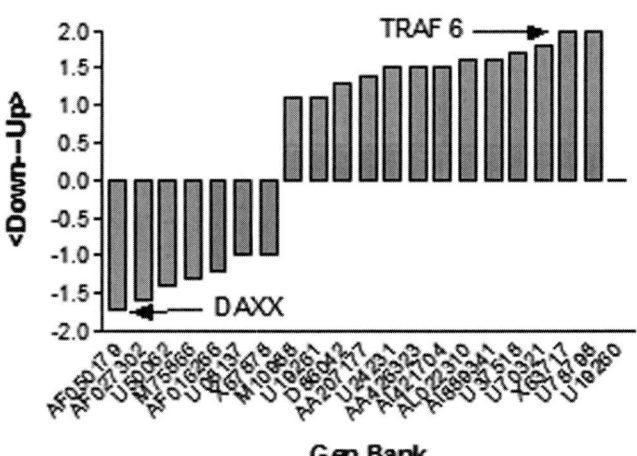

FIGURE 3. Down- and upregulation of members of the TNF-receptor and -ligand superfamilies by CD30. Expression at level 1 or −1 fold indicates no change. Expression at level 0 indicates that the gene is not expressed by YT. Negative numbers indicate fold downregulation, positive numbers upregulation.

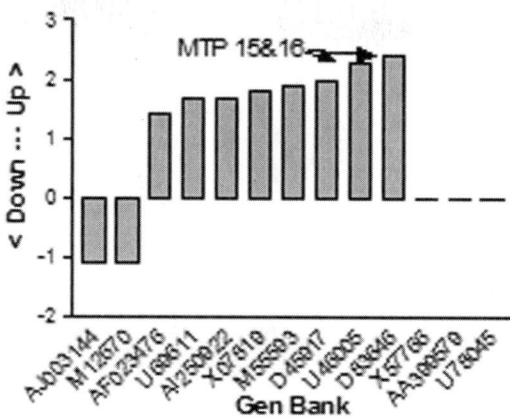

FIGURE 4. Induction of metalloproteinases by CD30 signals.

gelatinases also strongly upregulated (Owen et al., unpublished). Metalloproteinases are required for digestion of matrix proteins (collagen, laminin, etc.) to allow for migration of cells through tissues. In this context the expression of MPs may represent the ability of cytotoxic cells to travel through tissues or the ability of the LGL lymphoma to metastasize (see FIGURE 4).

Survival and Antiapoptotic Genes

CD30 strongly upregulated c-IAP 2 and xIAP. In addition CD30 strongly upregulated Bfl-1/A1. Bfl-1 is associated with cell survival and over expression in myeloid tumors and its induction indicates that CD30 can have prosurvival function. Under appropriate conditions CD30 may act as a costimulus for cell expansion and survival. Interestingly, the prosurvival gene Mcl-1 is downregulated by CD30 signals in YT (see FIGURE 5).

Granule-Associated Genes

The granule exocytosis mechanism is the most effective cytotoxic pathway for the removal of infectious agents and tumor rejection. Cytolytic granules contain perforin and granzymes as their major constituents. CD30 signals suppress perforin and granulysin expression and induce granzyme A and TIA1 message levels (see FIGURE 6). Independently, RNA protection assays confirmed perforin suppression and revealed that granzyme B was also downregulated (not detected on the gene chip). Since perforin is suppressed, CD30 signals would appear to reduce cytotoxic activity by the two major pathways, Fas-L and perforin (granule exocytosis). The inability of killing by perforin is accompanied by the inability to deliver granzymes to the target cell.

Chemokines and Chemokine Receptors

CD30 strongly upregulates CCR7 as measured with the gene chip. Upregulation was verified by RT-PCR (see FIGURE 7). This finding was unexpected and suggested

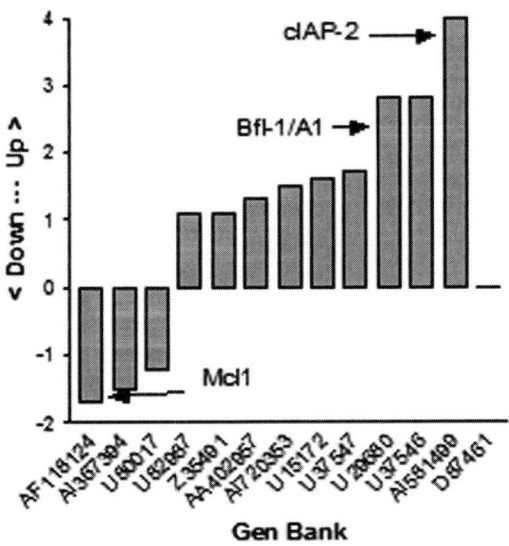

FIGURE 5. Bcl/IAP prosurvival genes induced and repressed by CD30.

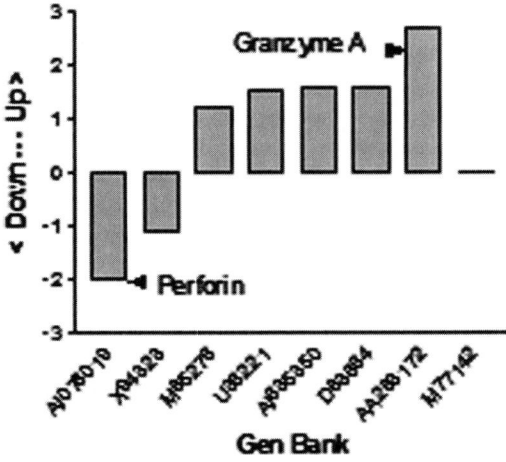

FIGURE 6. Induction and suppression of granule-associated proteins by CD30.

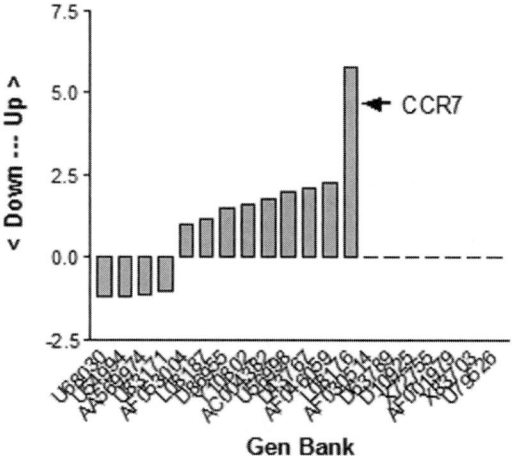

FIGURE 7. Regulation of chemokines and chemokine receptors by CD30.

that CD30 may regulate trafficking of CTL by regulating homing receptors. CCR7 is the receptor for SLC and directs cells to enter lymph nodes. As mentioned above, CCR7 expression is associated with a lack of effector function in CD45-RO$^+$ memory T cells. Therefore CD30 may be associated with the coordinated regulation of effector function and lymphocyte homing to lymph nodes.

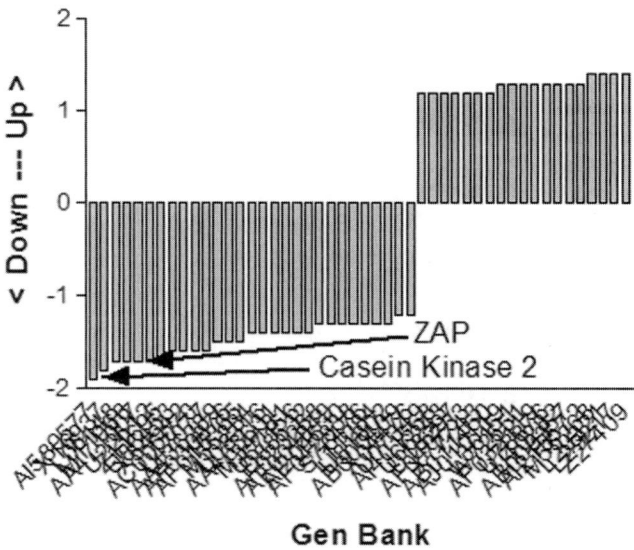

FIGURE 8. Regulation of kinases by CD30.

Kinases

A large number of kinases are affected by CD 30 signaling. Interestingly, the majority of kinases are downregulated, including the TCR zeta chain associated ZAP kinase. It is not clear at this time how to interpret and group the observed regulation of kinases by CD30 (see FIGURE 8). It also not clear how the regulation of kinases relates to the functions of CD30 schematized in FIGURE 1.

Interleukins, Interleukin Receptors and Caspases

The results are shown in FIGURES 9 and 10. The most highly induced gene is the interleukin 1 receptor antagonist, while Il-10 expression is suppressed. Caspase 1 and caspase 4 are fairly strongly upregulated by CD30 signals.

The gene expression data can be summarized as follows. CD30 can regulate T cell homing molecules, and this regulation is coordinated with regulation of effector function. Thus, the upregulation of lymph node homing molecules (CCR7) is coordinated with downregulation of cytotoxicity by perforin and Fas-Ligand. CD30 apparently can convert effector memory cells to central memory cells—and it appears to be the first molecule to which this function can be attributed. This regulatory action is accompanied by increased expression of proapoptotic molecules rendering the cells more susceptible to apoptosis. Simultaneously, however, a number of antiapoptotic molecules are also upregulated protecting the cells from apoptosis. Most notable among these is Bfl-1/A1, which has prominent survival function. The CD30 gene chip data were obtained with a CD30 expressing lymphoma line and extrapolation to normal T or NK cells has to be done with care. It is likely that the oncogenic transformation of YT has led to the dysregulation of survival pathways. It will therefore be necessary to measure gene expression patterns induced by CD30 in normal cells. This work is in progress.

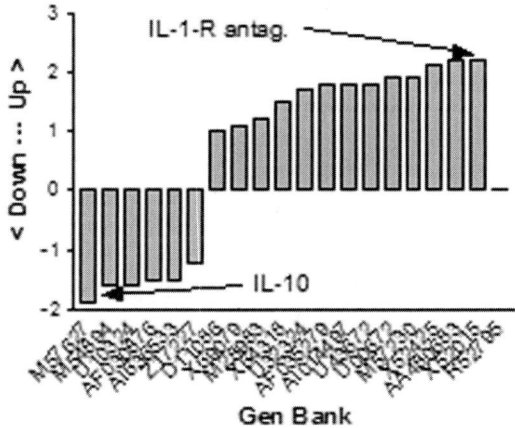

FIGURE 9. Regulation of interleukins and their receptors by CD30 signals.

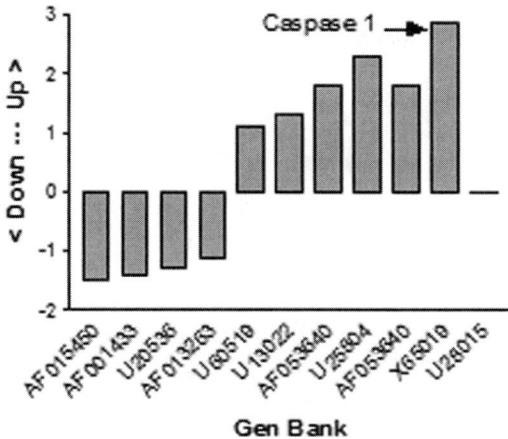

FIGURE 10. Regulation of caspases by CD30.

Defect of Homeostasis of CD8 CTL in CD30-L Knockout Mice

In order to better understand the role of CD30 in CTL responses, we generated CD30-L k.o. mice. These mice will not be able to deliver signals to CD30 on activated T cells owing to the absence of the CD30-Ligand (CD153). In order to determine the role of CD30 in CTL homeostasis, we devised a system by which CD8 CTL expansion, contraction, and secondary expansion could be precisely quantitated.

OT-1 are TCR transgenic CD8 cells specific for Kb-ova (SIINFEKL).[34] OT-1 cells can be detected specifically with Kb-ova tetramers or with the TCR variable region specific antibodies anti-va2 and -vb5.1-2 by flow cytometry. EG7 is a lymphoma syngeneic with C57Bl/6 derived from the EL4 cell line by ovalbumin transfection. GP96-Ig is a fusion protein generated from the ER resident heat shock protein gp96 by deletion of the ER retention signal KDEL and fusion to the Fc portion of mouse IgG1. Owing to the KDEL deletion, gp96-Ig is secreted upon transfection and expression in EG7 cells. EG7-gp96Ig immunization of B6 mice renders them immune to challenge with EG7, EL4, and ovalbumin-transfected LLC. Immunity is mediated by CD8 cells even in the absence of CD4 help.[35]

Mechanistically, immunity is generated by the activation of dendritic cells (DC) by secreted gp96-Ig, recognized by CD91 on DC. Endocytosis of gp96-Ig with associated tumor peptides results in re-presentation of tumor peptides by MHC I of the DC. Endocytosis also results in activation and maturation of DC enabling the activation of specific CD8 cells without CD4 help.[35] Since EG7-gp96Ig express ovalbumin, it is expected that secreted gp96-Ig will be associated with ovalbumin-derived peptides. After uptake of gp96-Ig by DC, processing and presentation of the ova-peptide SIINFEKL by Kb, Kb-ova specific OT-1 T cells therefore respond with clonal expansion to EG7-gp96Ig immunization (see FIGURE 11). One million OT-1 adoptively transferred to mice establish a frequency of 0.5% within the CD8 population. One week after immunization with one million EG7-gp96Ig i.p., the OT-1

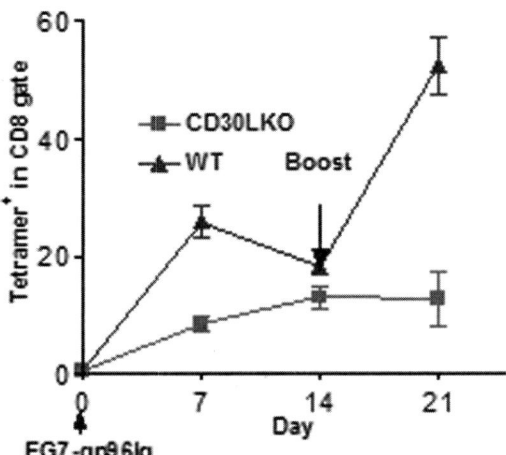

FIGURE 11. Diminished OT-1 expansion in CD30-L. CD30-LKO and three wild-type mice received 1 million OT-1 i.v. on day 2 and were immunized on day 0 and day 14 with 1 million EG7-gp96Ig i.p. (*arrows*). OT-1 expansion was measured in PBL with Kb-ova-tetramers by FACS.

cells expand to a frequency of 25% of all CD8 cells in wild-type (w.t.) mice, but to only 8% in CD30-LKO. During the second week, OT-1 undergo clonal contraction in w.t. mice, but continue to expand in CD30-LKO (FIG. 11). After the second immunization with one million EG7-gp96Ig on day 14, OT-1 respond with boosted, secondary expansion in w.t. mice to a frequency of almost 50% of all CD8 cells. In CD30-LKO the secondary immunization is not followed by secondary, boosted expansion of OT-1 cells suggesting an important role for CD30 signals both for clonal contraction and secondary (memory) response. Since the OT-1 cells used in this experiment are not CD30-L deficient, it is evident that CD30-L must be provided by other cells for OT-1 expansion in w.t. mice. Initial experiments suggest that w.t. DC are able to partially correct the defect of OT-1 expansion in CD30-LKO. This experiment demonstrates that CD30 has important functions in CTL homeostasis. The most notable defect is the inability of CTL generated in the absence of CD30 signals to clonally contract after primary (although diminished) activation. Taking this observation together with the gene expression studies, the failure of CD30 to upregulate proapoptotic genes (Fas, DR3, Trail) may be responsible for the inability of CD8 CTL to clonally contract in CD30-LKO mice. Another interesting finding is the inability of CD8 CTL to respond with boosted expansion to secondary immunization. This observation in the context of the gene expression studies allows two interpretations. First, clonal contraction may be coupled in some way to secondary expansion. Only those cells surviving clonal contraction have been licensed for memory responses. The second, and possibly more attractive hypothesis holds that absence of CD30 signals results in a failure of the upregulation of CCR7 (accompanied by the downregulation of cytotoxicity), and hence the inability of CD8 CTL to return home to the draining lymph node. It is at this site were secondary expansion may have to occur and the inability of CTL in CD30-LKO to migrate there would explain their failure to undergo secondary, boosted expansion.

This study seems to throw light on the mystery of CD30 function, greatly facilitated by the combination of gene expression studies with *in vivo* studies in mice. However the study opens also a number of new questions that need to be addressed —which are the cells expressing CD30-Ligand? How are CD30 signals interpreted over time and how are decisions made between pro- and antiapoptotic signaling? Are the signaling pathways via MAP-kinases, via NF-κB and via FADD separately regulated—and what kind of genes are addressed by these pathways? How do they relate to the governing function of CD30 for CD8 CTL? Precisely because CD30 signaling is so complex, it is ideally suited to regulate multiple functions, apoptosis, survival, effector function, migration and homing and proliferation. CD30 is in a pivotal position for effector cell regulation.

ACKNOWLEDGMENT

This work was supported by NIH grants CA80228 and AI/DK49829

REFERENCES

1. GERDES, J., R. SCHWARTING & H. STEIN. 1986. High proliferative activity of Reed Sternberg associated antigen Ki-1 positive cells in normal lymphoid tissue. J. Clin. Pathol. **39:** 993.
2. LIU, V. & P.H. MCKEE. 2002. Cutaneous T-cell lymphoproliferative disorders: approach for the surgical pathologist: recent advances and clarification of confused issues. Adv. Anat. Pathol. **9:** 79.
3. HWONG, H., D. JONES, V.G. PRIETO, *et al.* 2001. Persistent atypical lymphocytic hyperplasia following tick bite in a child: report of a case and review of the literature. Pediatr. Dermatol. **18:** 481.
4. WEITZMAN, S., K. SURYANARAYAN & H.J. WEINSTEIN. 2002. Pediatric non-Hodgkin's lymphoma: clinical and biologic prognostic factors and risk allocation. Curr. Oncol. Rep. **4:** 107.
5. FIORANI, C., G. VINCI, S. SACCHI, *et al.* 2001. Primary systemic anaplastic large-cell lymphoma (CD30$^+$): advances in biology and current therapeutic approaches. Clin. Lymphoma **2:** 29.
6. KAWAMURA, T., T. INAMURA, K. IKEZAKI, *et al.* 2001. Primary Ki-1 lymphoma in the central nervous system. J. Clin. Neurosci. **8:** 574.
7. GILFILLAN, M.C., P.J. NOEL, E.R. PODACK, *et al.* 1998. Expression of the costimulatory receptor CD30 is regulated by both CD28 and cytokines. J. Immunol. **160:** 2180.
8. NAKAMURA, T., R.K. LEE, S.Y. NAM, *et al.* 1997. Roles of IL-4 and IFN-gamma in stabilizing the T helper cell type 1 and 2 phenotype. J. Immunol. **158:** 2648.
9. NAKAMURA, T., R.K. LEE, S.Y. NAM, *et al.* 1997. Reciprocal regulation of CD30 expression on CD4$^+$ T cells by IL-4 and IFN-gamma. J. Immunol. **158:** 2090.
10. CERUTTI, A., E.C. KIM, S. SHAH, *et al.* 2001. Dysregulation of CD30+ T cells by leukemia impairs isotype switching in normal B cells. Nat. Immunol. **2:** 150.
11. CERUTTI, A., A. SCHAFFER, R.G. GOODWIN, *et al.* 2000. Engagement of CD153 (CD30 ligand) by CD30+ T cells inhibits class switch DNA recombination and antibody production in human IgD+ IgM+ B cells. J. Immunol. **165:** 786.
12. CERUTTI, A., A. SCHAFFER, S. SHAH, *et al.* 1998. CD30 is a CD40-inducible molecule that negatively regulates CD40-mediated immunoglobulin class switching in non-antigen-selected human B cells. Immunity **9:** 247.

13. BOWEN, M.A., R.K. LEE, G. MIRAGLIOTTA, *et al.* 1996. Structure and expression of murine CD30 and its role in cytokine production. J. Immunol. **156:** 442.
14. SMITH, C.A., H.J. GRUSS, T. DAVIS, *et al.* 1993. CD30 antigen, a marker for Hodgkin's lymphoma, is a receptor whose ligand defines an emerging family of cytokines with homology to TNF. Cell **73:** 1349.
15. DUCKETT, C.S., R.W. GEDRICH, M.C. GILFILLAN & C.B. THOMPSON. 1997. Induction of nuclear factor kappaB by the CD30 receptor is mediated by TRAF1 and TRAF2. Mol. Cell Biol. **17:** 1535.
16. DEVERGNE, O., E. HATZIVASSILIOU, K.M. IZUMI, *et al.* 1996. Association of TRAF1, TRAF2, and TRAF3 with an Epstein-Barr virus LMP1 domain important for B-lymphocyte transformation: role in NF-kappaB activation. Mol. Cell Biol. **16:** 7098.
17. ANSIEAU, S., I. SCHEFFRAHN, G. MOSIALOS, *et al.* 1996. Tumor necrosis factor receptor-associated factor (TRAF)-1, TRAF-2, and TRAF-3 interact in vivo with the CD30 cytoplasmic domain; TRAF-2 mediates CD30-induced nuclear factor kappa B activation. Proc. Natl. Acad. Sci. USA **93:** 14053.
18. ISHIDA, T., S. MIZUSHIMA, S. AZUMA, *et al.* 1996. Identification of TRAF6, a novel tumor necrosis factor receptor-associated factor protein that mediates signaling from an amino-terminal domain of the CD40 cytoplasmic region. J. Biol. Chem. **271:** 28745.
19. LEE, S.Y., G. KANDALA, M.L. LIOU, *et al.* 1996. CD30/TNF receptor-associated factor interaction: NF-kappa B activation and binding specificity. Proc. Natl. Acad. Sci. USA **93:** 9699.
20. GEDRICH, R.W., M.C. GILFILLAN, C.S. DUCKETT, *et al.* 1996. CD30 contains two binding sites with different specificities for members of the tumor necrosis factor receptor-associated factor family of signal transducing proteins. J. Biol. Chem. **271:** 12852.
21. LEE, S.Y., C.G. PARK & Y. CHOI. 1996. T cell receptor-dependent cell death of T cell hybridomas mediated by the CD30 cytoplasmic domain in association with tumor necrosis factor receptor-associated factors. J. Exp. Med. **183:** 669.
22. HORIE, R., T. WATANABE, Y. MORISHITA, *et al.* 2002. Ligand-independent signaling by overexpressed CD30 drives NF-kappaB activation in Hodgkin-Reed-Sternberg cells. Oncogene **21:** 2493.
23. ARCH, R.H., R.W. GEDRICH & C.B. THOMPSON. 2000. Translocation of TRAF proteins regulates apoptotic threshold of cells. Biochem. Biophys. Res. Commun. **272:** 936.
24. GRUSS, H.J., N. BOIANI, D.E. WILLIAMS, *et al.* 1994. Pleiotropic effects of the CD30 ligand on CD30-expressing cells and lymphoma cell lines. Blood **83:** 2045.
25. AMAKAWA, R., A. HAKEM, T.M. KUNDIG, *et al.* 1996. Impaired negative selection of T cells in Hodgkin's disease antigen CD30-deficient mice. Cell **84:** 551.
26. DEYOUNG, A.L., O. DURAMAD & A. WINOTO. 2000. The TNF receptor family member CD30 is not essential for negative selection. J. Immunol. **165:** 6170.
27. ALZONA, M., H.M. JACK, R.I. FISHER & T.M. ELLIS. 1994. CD30 defines a subset of activated human T cells that produce IFN-gamma and IL-5 and exhibit enhanced B cell helper activity. J. Immunol. **153:** 2861.
28. SAEKI, H., A.M. MOORE, M.J. BROWN & S.T. HWANG. 1999. Cutting edge: secondary lymphoid-tissue chemokine (SLC) and CC chemokine receptor 7 (CCR7) participate in the emigration pathway of mature dendritic cells from the skin to regional lymph nodes. J. Immunol. **162:** 2472.
29. YOSHIDA, R., M. NAGIRA, M. KITAURA, *et al.* 1998. Secondary lymphoid-tissue chemokine is a functional ligand for the CC chemokine receptor CCR7. J. Biol. Chem. **273:** 7118.
30. BAEKKEVOLD, E.S., T. YAMANAKA, R.T. PALFRAMAN, *et al.* 2001. The CCR7 ligand elc (CCL19) is transcytosed in high endothelial venules and mediates T cell recruitment. J. Exp. Med. **193:** 1105.
31. SALLUSTO, F., D. LENIG, R. FORSTER, *et al.* 1999. Two subsets of memory T lymphocytes with distinct homing potentials and effector functions [see comments]. Nature **401:** 708.
32. BOWEN, M.A., K.J. OLSEN, L. CHENG, *et al.* 1993. Functional effects of CD30 on a large granular lymphoma cell line, YT. Inhibition of cytotoxicity, regulation of CD28 and IL-2R, and induction of homotypic aggregation. J. Immunol. **151:** 5896.

33. MUTA, H., L.H. BOISE, L. FANG & E.R. PODACK. 2000. CD30 signals integrate expression of cytotoxic effector molecules, lymphocyte trafficking signals, and signals for proliferation and apoptosis [In Process Citation]. J. Immunol. **165:** 5105.
34. HOGQUIST, K.A., S.C. JAMESON, W.R. HEATH, *et al.* 1994. T cell receptor antagonist peptides induce positive selection. Cell **76:** 17.
35. YAMAZAKI, K., T. NGUYEN & E.R. PODACK. 1999. Cutting edge: tumor secreted heat shock-fusion protein elicits CD8 cells for rejection. J. Immunol. **163:** 5178.

Stronger Correlation of bcl-3 than bcl-2, bcl-x_L, Costimulation, or Antioxidants with Adjuvant-Induced T Cell Survival

THOMAS C. MITCHELL,[a] T. KENT TEAGUE,[b] DAVID A. HILDEMAN,[c] JEREMY BENDER,[d] WILLIAM A. REES,[e] ROSS M. KEDL,[f] BRAD SWANSON,[g] JOHN W. KAPPLER,[g–j] AND PHILIPPA MARRACK[g–i]

[a]*Institute for Cellular Therapeutics, University of Louisville School of Medicine, Louisville, Kentucky 40202, USA*

[b]*Department of Surgery, University of Oklahoma College of Medicine, Tulsa, Oklahoma, USA*

[c]*Immunobiology, Children's Hospital Medical Center, Cincinnati, Ohio, USA*

[d]*Ancora Pharmaceuticals, Cambridge Massachusetts, USA*

[e]*Corixa Corporation, Seattle Washington, USA*

[f]*3M Corp, St. Paul, Minnesota, USA*

[g]*Howard Hughes Medical Institute, Department of Medicine, National Jewish Medical and Research Center;* [h]*Departments of Biochemistry and Molecular Genetics,* [i]*Integrated Immunology, and* [j]*Pharmacology, University of Colorado Health Sciences Center, Denver, Colorado 80206, USA*

ABSTRACT: A set of signals separate from those needed for T cell activation and clonal expansion acts to sustain a T cell response once it has begun. Immunologic adjuvants can initiate these signals in a process we designate adjuvant-induced survival (AIS). Here, the natural adjuvant LPS was used in a superantigen model of AIS to understand which factors are needed to sustain T cell survival after activation. Flow cytometric stains for antiapoptotic Bcl-2 and Bcl-xL showed that neither factor was well correlated with AIS, although both were increased transiently upon T cell activation. T cells protected via AIS showed no increased ability to resist death caused by reactive oxygen species, and cellular division was not accelerated as might be expected if AIS were to operate through co-stimulatory pathways. Finally, microarray analyses were performed that showed increased expression of Bcl-3, an NFκB/IκB factor, was correlated with AIS. It is proposed that T cell survival during productive immune responses occurs by successive activities of Bcl-2, Bcl-xL and Bcl-3, with Bcl-3 requiring innate immune responses to adjuvants for its expression.

KEYWORDS: bcl-3; bcl-2; bcl-x_L; T cell survival; adjuvants

Addresses for correspondence: Thomas C. Mitchell, 570 S. Preston St., Baxter Building, Suite 404, Louisville, KY 40202. Voice: 502-852-2073; fax: 502-852-2085.
tom.mitchell@louisville.edu
Philippa Marrack, 1400 Jackson St., Goodman Building, 5th floor, Denver, CO 80206.
marrackp@njc.org

INTRODUCTION

The clonal expansion of T cells reacting to antigen is well-known to be a critical event in the generation of immunity. It is somewhat less well-known that a set of signals separate from those needed for activation and clonal expansion are needed to sustain the T cell response once it has begun. If sustaining signals are not given, a T cell population's clonal expansion can ultimately cause its removal, because the reacting cells proliferate and then go on to die. This abortive activation of mature T cells was initially shown by Kawabe and Ochi[1] and Webb et al.,[2] who found that antigenic stimulation of T cells in mice caused proliferation and then death of the responding cells. The extent to which clonal deletion of mature cells, as opposed to thymic deletion of developing cells,[3] regulates immunologic tolerance of T cells to self has not been resolved. It is obvious, however, that the most effective vaccinations are those in which clonal deletion of pathogen-specific T cells is prevented.

Many research groups have now shown that clonal deletion of T cells can be prevented by coadministration of immunological adjuvants and protein antigens.[4–13] The first visualization of the effect of adjuvants on T cell numbers was reported by Kearney et al.,[7] who tracked T cells from TCR-transgenic mice in nontransgenic recipients after T cell responses were stimulated with protein antigen in the presence or absence of complete Freund's adjuvant. Vella et al.[12] showed this was true for nontransgenic T cells in reporting that a natural adjuvant, lipopolysaccharide (LPS), prevented superantigen-induced clonal deletion in mice. Natural adjuvants are materials associated with invading organisms that trigger innate immune responses by conserved receptors. LPS for example is bound by Toll-like receptor 4 (Tlr4) and its coreceptor CD14 on antigen-presenting cells.[14] Even with effective immune responses, most T cells that are mobilized die via antigen withdrawal or activation-induced death, but adjuvant effects nevertheless prevent the responses from being abortive by supporting the survival of a sufficient number of cells for long-lasting immunity to be established.

In spite of the critical role played by adjuvants in making productive T cell responses possible, the mechanisms supporting that role remain to be fully elucidated. It is by now well established that T cell stimulation initially requires two signals: engagement of T cell receptor (TCR) by major histocompatibility complexes (MHC) that are loaded with peptide antigen (signal 1), and costimulation via cross-linking of CD28 on T cells by antigen-presenting cell (APC)–derived B7 molecules (signal 2).[15] Adjuvant-induced survival (AIS) of stimulated T cells is most commonly assumed to result from costimulatory signals that help drive proliferation. However, the notion that costimulation is present only when an adjuvant is present is belied by the fact that T cells in mice proliferate extensively after exposure to antigen alone, whether injected or expressed in uninfected tissue.[1,2,4,7,16–22] The proliferation that is seen, moreover, is already CD28-dependent,[23,24] indicating that signal 2 was available without coadministration of adjuvant. Therefore, the signals transmitted to T cells to keep them alive after they have proliferated appear to result from an as yet unknown "signal 3."[25] A striking example of the distinct nature of this signal (or signals) can be found in Vella's observation that survival signals can be initiated well after T cell activation has begun.[12] Because costimulation of T cells is associated with Bcl-x_L,[26,27] we tested for its expression in order to confirm or refute the idea that co-stimulation is dependent on the presence of adjuvants.

Another possible mechanism of AIS is via induction of prosurvival cytokines. This idea is supported by observations that several members of the IL-2 family of cytokines (IL-2, IL-4, IL-7, and IL-15) increase T cell survival when added to activated T cells in culture.[28,29] Because cytokine treatment of T cells is associated with expression of the antiapoptotic molecule Bcl-2,[8] we tested here for its expression in a mouse model of abortive vs. productive T cell responses. Neither it nor Bcl-x_L expression in T cells was found to be correlated with AIS. Further analysis showed that neither the extent of T cell proliferation nor the reactive oxygen content of T cells was affected in a way that could explain AIS. Finally, microarray analyses were performed in an effort to identify new candidate molecules. These analyses pointed toward an NFκB/IκB protein, Bcl-3, as an important mediator of AIS in T cells.[13]

THE SUPERANTIGEN+LPS MODEL OF AIS IN MICE

Because relatively large numbers of activated cells were needed for the flow cytometric and the microarray analyses described here, superantigens were used to stimulate T cells in normal mice. A superantigen (Sag) is capable of binding simultaneously to an MHCII molecule on an APC and to the variable portion of the β chain (Vβ) of a TCR.[30] This binding event thereby makes available to the T cell all of the APC-derived stimulation signals normally given during presentation of a conventional peptide antigen. Different Sags have binding preferences for different Vβ segments and stimulate different proportions of the circulating T cell population, based on the frequency with which a given Vβ was used for TCR rearrangement during T cell development. For example, a Sag designated SEA (staphylococcal enterotoxin A) stimulates T cells bearing Vβ3 segments as part of their TCR, while the Sag SEB stimulates T cells bearing Vβ8. Because Vβ3 is present on about 5% of CD4$^+$ T cells in B10.BR mice, that proportion of cells will initially become activated upon injection of SEA. As with normal antigens, the affected T cells proliferate for 2–3 days, but then begin to die rapidly.

Vella et al.[12] developed the B10.BR/SEA/LPS model in 1995 and reported that the injection of LPS at the same time or 24 h after SEA was sufficient to transform an abortive immune response into one that was productive. It is important to note that LPS almost certainly acted on T cells indirectly, via an accessory cell, because exposure of purified T cells to LPS had no effect.[12] A typical time course of the CD4$^+$Vβ3$^+$ T cell response using this model is shown in FIGURE 1, in which injection of LPS 20h after SEA greatly increased both the peak of expansion and the long-term retention of CD4$^+$Vβ3$^+$ T cells. The protected cells are not anergic when tested for proliferation upon *in vitro* exposure to SEA[25] and show all of the surface phenotypes typical of memory T cells (data not shown). Using the same model, VV-infection was shown to drive the same pattern of AIS.[8] This model system therefore permits the effect of adjuvants on T cells to be isolated and examined because an identical antigenic stimulus can be given under varying conditions of adjuvant exposure.

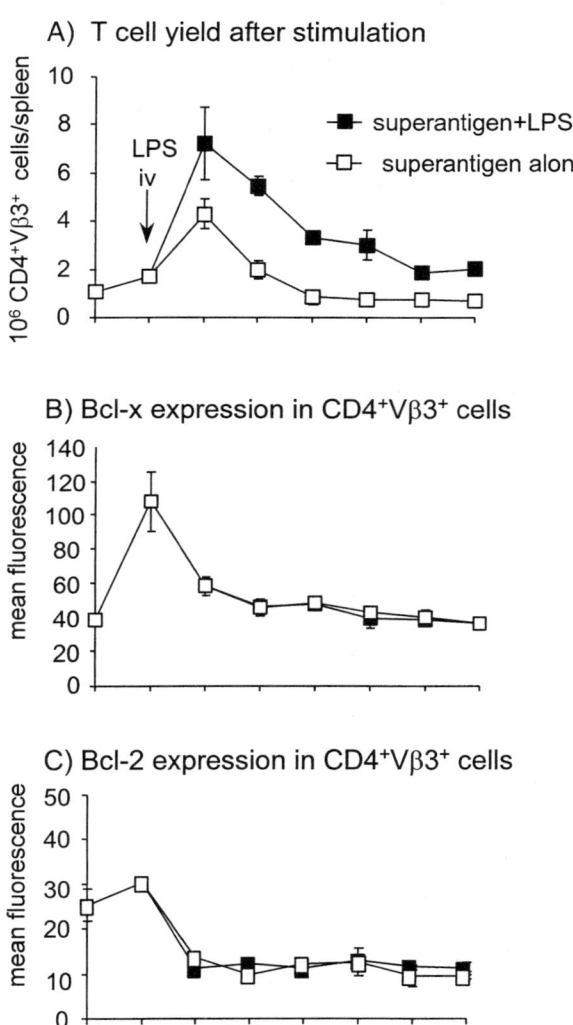

FIGURE 1. Adjuvant treatment of mice does not change Bcl-2 or Bcl-x_L expression in superantigen-stimulated CD4+ cells. B10.BR mice were given the superantigen (Sag) SEA, which stimulates all T cells bearing Vβ3 as part of their TCR. Some of the mice were given the adjuvant LPS 20h later. On each day for seven days thereafter, replicate mice were sacrificed to determine (**A**) the total number of CD4+Vβ3+ cells per spleen, (**B**) the level of Bcl-x_L expression per CD4+Vβ3+ cell, or (**C**) the level of Bcl-2 expression per CD4+Vβ3+ cell. Bcl-x_L and Bcl-2 expression was measured in arbitrary units of fluorescence, ± S.E.M, after staining saponin-permeabilized cells with anti-Bcl-x_L and anti-Bcl-2 antibodies as described previously.[8]

AIS IS NOT CORRELATED WITH BCL-x_L EXPRESSION

Vella et al.[24] found that the prolonged survival of SEB-activated T cells from mice given LPS as adjuvant was not dependent on signaling via the costimulatory receptor CD28 because prolonged survival was observed in CD28$^{-/-}$ mice. Further analysis of a downstream target of CD28 signaling, Bcl-x_L, showed that expression of this antiapoptotic factor was not altered in activated T cells from VV-infected mice.[8] In order to learn whether the same was true of LPS, flow cytometric stains for Bcl-x_L were performed with activated T cells from B10.BR mice. A cohort of B10.BR mice was given SEA on d0, one-half of these mice were given LPS on d1, and at daily intervals for a week three mice from each group were sacrificed for analysis. As shown in FIGURE 1B, the pattern of Bcl-x_L expression observed in mice that had been treated with Sag plus LPS was indistinguishable from the pattern seen in mice that had been given Sag alone. Bcl-x_L was observed to increase over two days to exactly the same extent in cells from both groups, and to decrease at exactly the same rate thereafter, even though the addition of LPS treatment markedly increased T cell yield (FIG. 1A). Hence, Bcl-x_L was correlated with costimulation, because its expression increased as cells began to proliferate, but not with adjuvant exposure because Bcl-x_L expression was not increased further nor was its level of expression sustained or extended as a result of adjuvant treatment.

AIS IS NOT CORRELATED WITH INCREASED PROLIFERATION

Because CD28 is not the only T cell molecule capable of costimulation, it was possible that adjuvants influenced costimulation via another pathway. In order to evaluate adjuvant-induced costimulatory effects on T cells by some means other than measuring Bcl-x_L expression, proliferation *in vivo* was visualized using cells loaded with the dye 5-(and-6)-carboxyfluorescein diacetate, succinimidyl ester (CFSE). The fluorescence of CFSE-loaded cells decreases 50% with each successive cellular division, which both allows for enumeration of the number of cell cycles undergone by a population of cells,[31] and requires that cells be tracked independently of the CFSE label (which becomes undetectable after 7–8 rounds of division). Thy1.1$^+$ B6.PL mice were therefore used as the source of T cells to be loaded with CFSE and transferred to Thy1.2$^+$ C57BL/6 mice, permitting use of an anti-Thy1.1 antibody to track transferred T cells. After loading and transferring T cells, recipient mice were given 100µg SEB, which stimulates the 20–25% of CD4$^+$ T cells in B6 mice which bear Vβ8 as part of their TCR. Subsets of SEB-treated mice were given either 7 µg LPS as adjuvant, or 7µg LPS and 100µg of a monoclonal antibody, 1C10,[32] which potentiates the adjuvant effect of LPS by cross-linking CD40 molecules on the surface of APC.[33] After two or four days, spleens were harvested from replicate mice and cell division was assessed by plotting the CFSE fluorescence of Vβ8$^+$ CD4$^+$Thy1.1$^+$ cells (i.e., those that were transferred from B6.PL mice).

By d2 of Sag treatment, T cells stimulated by SEB in mice given adjuvants had proliferated somewhat less than their equivalents given SEB alone (see FIGURE 2A). Injection of SEB alone resulted in an average of 2.9 rounds of cellular division among the 74% of T cells that divided at least once. The addition of LPS decreased slightly the average number of divisions, to 2.6, and the addition of both LPS and anti-CD40mAb decreased that number still further to 2.4. The fact that adjuvants decreased rather than increased initial rates of division suggest that AIS was not the result of increased costimulation. The lack of correlation between adjuvant exposure and costimulatory proliferation was not specific to LPS, because the same pattern was seen with AIS mediated by VV infection.[8]

Tabulation of the total yield of Thy1.1$^+$CD4$^+$ T cells from these mice (FIG. 2B) showed that adjuvant treatment was associated with retention of the peak numbers of cells from d2 to d4, relative to treatment with SEB alone. Adjuvant effects on d2 were most evident in a culture test of AIS (FIG. 2B). Here, spleen cells harvested on d2 were cultured in normal culture medium, without added growth factors, and tested after 25h for the proportion that had survived. Treatment with Sag alone sensitized CD4$^+$Vβ8$^+$ to rapid death relative to no treatment controls, whereas treatment with LPS or LPS and anti-CD40 prevented this sensitization.

By d4 of Sag treatment, all populations of T cells continued to divide, but T cell accumulation was observed only if adjuvant had been given (FIG. 2). T cell populations that had expanded two days after treatment with Sag alone were lost and their propensity for rapid death upon culture remained (FIG. 2B), as expected in the absence of adjuvant. T cells from mice given Sag and LPS were as abundant on d4 as on d2, and had cycled more than cells from mice given Sag alone (4.7 vs. 3.5 average divisions, respectively), but this increase in proliferation was not correlated with prolonged survival in culture because the cells died rapidly upon culture (FIG. 2B). We concluded that costimulation was either inversely related to survival effects, or the appearance of increased costimulation was actually due to a relative enrichment of cells that had undergone cellular divisions in Sag plus LPS-treated mice, as compared to a loss of cells that had already divided in mice treated with Sag alone. Support for this latter interpretation comes from consideration of the percentage of cells that did not divide (FIG. 2A). From d2 to d4 in Sag-treated mice, the percentage of cells which had not divided increased from 26 to 48%, a result that could occur only by a relative loss of dividing cells. In Sag plus LPS-treated mice these values were essentially unchanged, 20 to 24%, over the same time period indicating more survival of cells that had divided.

With the addition of CD40 cross-linking antibody, these patterns were amplified. Robust expansion of the population of Thy1.1$^+$CD4$^+$Vβ8$^+$ cells was associated with slightly fewer cell cycles and substantially more *in vitro* survival than was seen with Sag alone (FIG. 2). By d4 many more cells had divided and the total number of cells was much greater. Interestingly, resistance to rapid death upon culture was retained on d4 by cells from mice given Sag plus LPS plus anti-CD40, whereas this property had been lost in mice that did not receive anti-CD40 mAb treatment. One explanation for this pattern is that anti-CD40 treatment amplifies adjuvant effects because it keeps APC alive longer,[34] an argument supported by the observation that anti-CD40 mAb treatment cannot replace LPS in promoting long-term T cell survival.[25]

AIS IS NOT CORRELATED WITH BCL-2 EXPRESSION

An alternative hypothesis to explain adjuvant effects is that cytokines with survival activity for activated T cells are induced by adjuvants. Cytokines known to

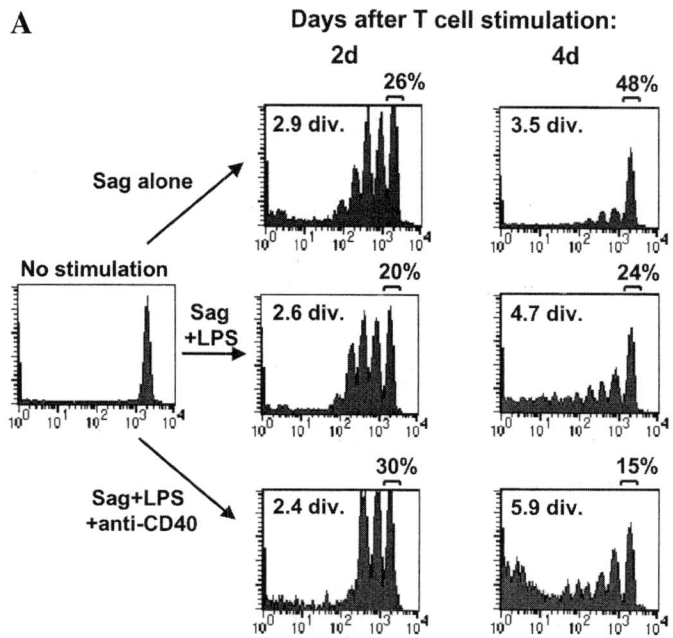
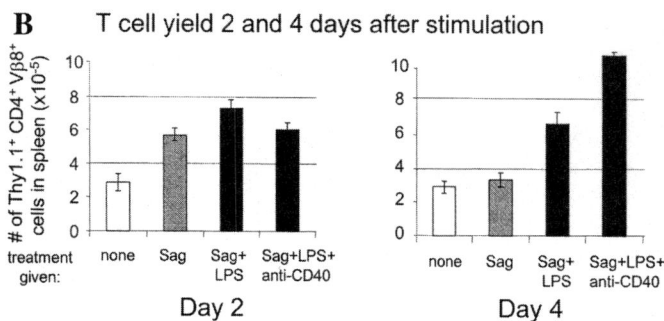
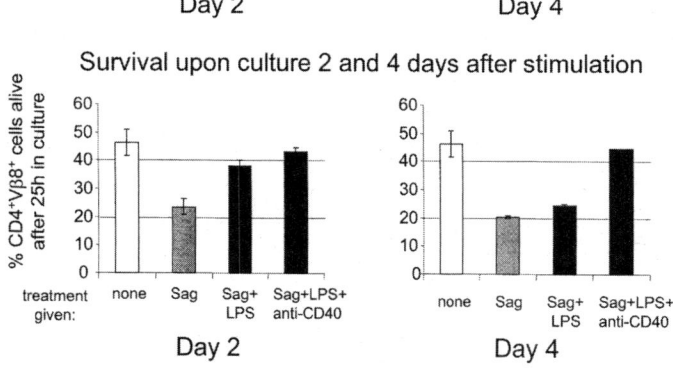

increase T cell survival when added to cultures include IL-2, IL-4, IL-7, and IL-15 (but not IL-9, the remaining member of this 'common γ chain' family).[28,29] It is reasonable to suppose that adjuvants cause increased levels of some or all of these factors, but simple tests of cytokine concentrations in serum do little to reveal the actual amounts of cytokines in lymphoid organs. We have shown previously that doses of IL-2, -4, -7, or -15 that are sufficient to increase T cell survival in culture also induce expression of the antiapoptotic protein, Bcl-2,[8] while doses too small to increase survival fail to induce Bcl-2. Therefore, a cell's expression of Bcl-2 can serve as a marker of its exposure to members of the IL-2-family of cytokines. We previously found that Sag-activated T cells from VV-infected mice did not have increased levels of Bcl-2, relative to Sag-activated cells from uninfected mice,[8] suggesting that the adjuvant properties of viral infection are not mediated by IL-2 related proteins.

In order to determine whether or not LPS treatment also failed to influence Bcl-2 expression by T cells, flow cytometric stains for intracellular Bcl-2 were performed on T cells from Sag plus LPS-treated mice (FIG. 1C). Using Bcl-2 as a marker, T cells from mice given SEA plus LPS did not show more exposure to IL-2 family of cytokines than cells from mice treated with SEA alone, even though an adjuvant effect was evident (FIG. 1A). The pattern of expression of Bcl-2 in mice given SEA alone or SEA plus LPS indicated instead that T cell exposure to Bcl-2–inducing cytokines occurred in the first 24 hours of activation. After that point, Bcl-2 content per cell decreased markedly as the cells divided. T cells from adjuvant-treated mice were not refractory to cytokine signaling because Bcl-2 expression increased as soon as IL-2 family members were added to cultures of explanted T cells.[8] As was true for Bcl-x_L, Bcl-2 was correlated with T cell activation, because its expression increased as the cells prepared to proliferate, but Bcl-2 was not detectably correlated with adjuvant exposure.

FIGURE 2. Adjuvant-induced survival of activated T cells is not necessarily associated with increased cellular proliferation. Female C57BL/6 (Thy1.2$^+$) mice were infused with CFSE dye-loaded cells from female B6.Pl (Thy1.1$^+$) mice. Several days after infusion, the recipient mice were given the Sag SEB to stimulate Vβ8$^+$ T cells, or Sag and LPS, or Sag and LPS and anti-CD40 mAb 1C10. Two and four days after stimulation with Sag, splenic cells were stained for Thy1.1, CD4 and Vβ8 and analyzed using flow cytometry to visualize cellular division by the method of Lyons and Parrish.[31] (**A**) The proportion of cells that had undergone one or more cellular divisions was measured and used to calculate the average number of cell doublings undergone by the population of Thy1.1$^+$ CD4$^+$ Vβ8$^+$ cells. The percentages shown at upper left of each histogram indicate the proportion of cells that did not divide, as judged by retention of CFSE. (**B**) The total yield and survival properties of Thy1.1$^+$CD4$^+$Vβ8$^+$ cells were measured on day 2 and day 4 after each of the treatments described above. Values for cell yield are shown as mean ± S.E.M. for cells found in spleen. Cell survival was assessed after 25 h culture in triplicate of 4×10^5 splenocytes/well of a 96-well plate in culture medium containing fetal bovine serum but no added growth factors. The percentage of cells ± S.E.M. alive after culture was determined from forward vs. side light scatter characteristics as in Mitchell et al.[8]

A TRANSIENT EFFECT OF LPS ON BCL-X_L AND BCL-2 EXPRESSION

Because it seemed implausible that LPS injection would have no effect whatsoever on expression of Bcl-x_L and Bcl-2, more timepoints within the first 48h of T cell stimulation were examined. As shown in FIGURE 3, injection of LPS induced slightly more Bcl-x_L and Bcl-2 expression by T cells at the 36h timepoint, but this increase was almost completely lost within the next 12 hours. Overall, LPS injection delayed decreases in levels of Bcl-x_L and Bcl-2, but did not prevent them, with kinetics that indicated the effects of LPS on these signaling pathways lasted no more than 24 hours. This timeframe is consistent with an earlier observation that injection of LPS 24 h before Sag generated little or no AIS.[12] While not ruling out a role for Bcl-2 or Bcl-x_L in AIS, the timing of these events suggests that these factors are not likely to play a role. For example, it is formally possible that increased Bcl-2 expression at 36h could promote survival of cells whose culture began at 48h and lasted 25h, even though increased Bcl-2 was not detected at the outset of the culture period. However, AIS is strong even if LPS and Sag are injected simultaneously,[12] showing that resistance to death upon culture can persist for up to 48 hours. While not formally disproving a role for Bcl-2 or Bcl-x_L, these considerations led us to conclude that other factors or events must be responsible for AIS.

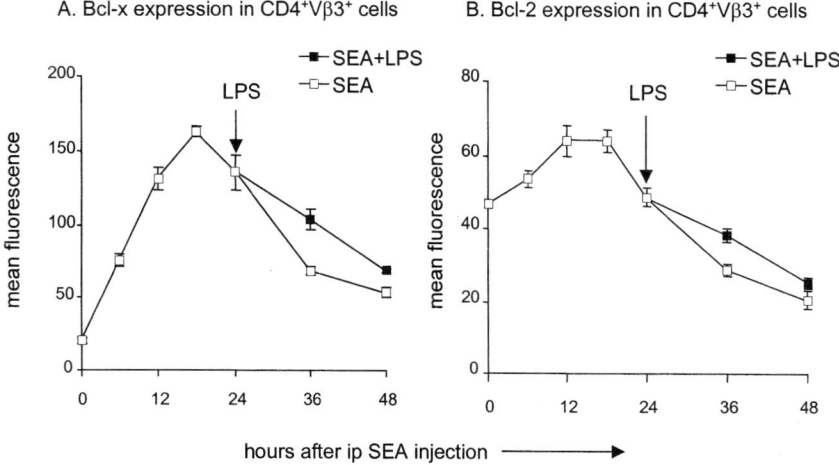

FIGURE 3. The LPS adjuvant effect lasts less than 24 h. Groups of B10.BR mice were given either SEA alone or SEA at time 0 and LPS at 24 h. Every 12 h for the next 24 h, splenic T cells from three mice in each group were harvested (**A**) the level of Bcl-x_L expression per CD4$^+$Vβ3$^+$ cell, or (**B**) the level of Bcl-2 expression per CD4$^+$Vβ3$^+$ cell. Bcl-x_L and Bcl-2 expression was measured in arbitrary units of fluorescence, ± S.E.M, after staining saponin-permeabilized cells with anti-Bcl-x_L and anti-Bcl-2 antibodies as described previously.[8]

ADJUVANTS DO NOT INDUCE ANTIOXIDANT ACTIVITY

A third possible explanation for AIS is that adjuvant treatment reduces the levels of damaging reactive oxygen species (ROS) in activated T cells. This possibility emerged when Hildeman et al. showed that a catalytic antioxidant, MnTBAP, protected activated T cells from apoptotic death.[35] The antioxidant ascorbic acid was reported to have the same effect,[36] and retroviral transduction of MnSOD or catalase inhibits death of activated T cells,[37] showing that intracellular scavengers of reactive oxygen species can promote T cell survival. These results led to the theory that adjuvants might function by inducing the expression or activity of detoxifying enzymes.

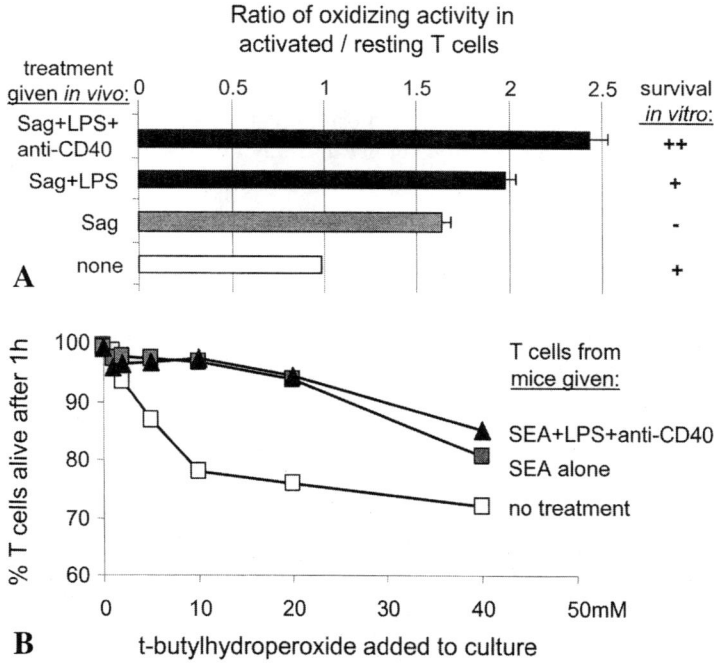

FIGURE 4. Adjuvant treatment does not reduce intracellular reactive oxygen levels or induce antioxidant activity in activated T cells. B10.BR mice were given no treatment, the Sag SEA to stimulate CD4$^+$Vβ3$^+$ T cells, Sag and LPS, or Sag and LPS and anti-CD40 mAb. (**A**) 48 h after Sag injection, T cells were harvested from spleen, stained with CD4- and Vβ3-specific antibodies and then with the oxidation-sensitive dye dihydroethidium as described previously.[35] The level of oxidation in activated T cells is presented as the ratio of ethidium fluorescence in activated cells over resting cells present in the same well (flow cytometric gating was on Vβ3$^+$ or Vβ3^{neg} CD4$^+$ T cells). Survival upon *in vitro* culture is shown as: + for survival similar to resting cells, – for rapid death in culture, and ++ for survival greater than resting T cells. (**B**) T cells were harvested from spleen, cultured for 1 h at 37°C at the indicated concentration of *t*-butylhydroperoxide, and analyzed flow cytometrically for the proportion of live vs. dead CD4$^+$Vβ3$^+$ cells. The proportion of cells alive was determined from forward versus side light scatter properties of the cells as described previously.[13]

However, measurement of intracellular reactive oxygen levels with dihydroethidium showed that they were higher, not lower, in T cells destined to live longer due to adjuvant effects (see FIGURE 4A). Upon oxidation, cell-permeable dihydroethidium (HE) is converted to ethidium, which is able to bind cellular DNA and fluoresce. Using HE staining, reactive oxygen levels were measured as the ratio of ethidium fluorescence in activated ($V\beta3^+$ in SEA-treated mice) versus 'resting' cells ($V\beta3^{neg}$ cells not targeted by SEA) in the same population. In $V\beta3^+$ cells from untreated mice, this ratio was 1.0 as expected, whereas in cells activated by Sag alone it had increased to 1.5. Addition of LPS, or LPS plus anti-CD40, produced ratios of 2.0 or greater, indicating that ROS levels were positively correlated with AIS, not inversely correlated as had been theorized.

To test T cells directly for their susceptibility to ROS-induced death, activated T cells were harvested from mice and cultured with t-butylhydroperoxide, which kills cells lacking antioxidant activity (FIG. 4B). T cells from Sag-treated mice were observed to be no more susceptible to ROS-induced death upon 1 h exposure to peroxide than cells from Sag plus LPS-treated mice. Interestingly, it was resting cells that were the most sensitive to ROS, indicating that T cell activation is associated with increased antioxidant activity, but not in a way that was correlated with adjuvant treatment. Put together, the experiments summarized in FIGURE 4 showed that regulation of ROS was not likely to be the basis for AIS.

AN NFκB/IκB PROTEIN, BCL-3, IS INDUCED BY ADJUVANTS

Affymetrix gene microarrays were used in an unbiased screen for genes whose expression in activated T cells was correlated with adjuvant treatment.[13] C57BL/10 mice were injected with SEB alone to stimulate $V\beta8^+$ T cells, or SEB plus bystander VV infection, or SEB plus LPS plus anti-CD40. Cells from the lymph nodes and spleens of treated mice were isolated at the peak of their expansion, just before they began to die. T cells from the three groups of mice were purified by high speed cell sorting to yield populations that were greater than 97% $V_\beta8^+$ and less than 0.5% MHC class II$^+$. RNA was prepared from these cells and analyzed using the mu6400 Affymetrix gene array system.[13] Of the genes and expressed sequence tags (ESTs) represented on the mu6400 genechip, 288 scored as increased in T cells after SEB plus VV treatment and 141 scored as increased after SEB plus LPS plus anti-CD40 treatment, as compared to T cells stimulated with SEB alone (see FIGURE 5). Of these, 23 previously described genes were increased both by the viral and by the bacterial adjuvants. Several of the 23 genes, such as those for the granzymes A and B, IL-7Rα, STAT-1, and ICAM-1, are relevant to T cell immune responses. The gene most increased in expression was Bcl-3, which showed 10- and 17-fold increases in hybridization intensity following treatment with VV and LPS, respectively.

Ohno and McKeithan[38] discovered Bcl-3 as the overexpressed gene product of a translocation event between human chromosomes 14 and 19 that is found in some cases of B cell chronic lymphocytic leukemia (B-CLL). Inspection of its secondary structure revealed that Bcl-3 had ankyrin repeats and it was therefore classified as an IκB protein.[39] However, Bcl-3 is expressed primarily in the nuclei of cells and is regulated at the level of *de novo* protein synthesis, distinguishing it from IκB proteins.[40]

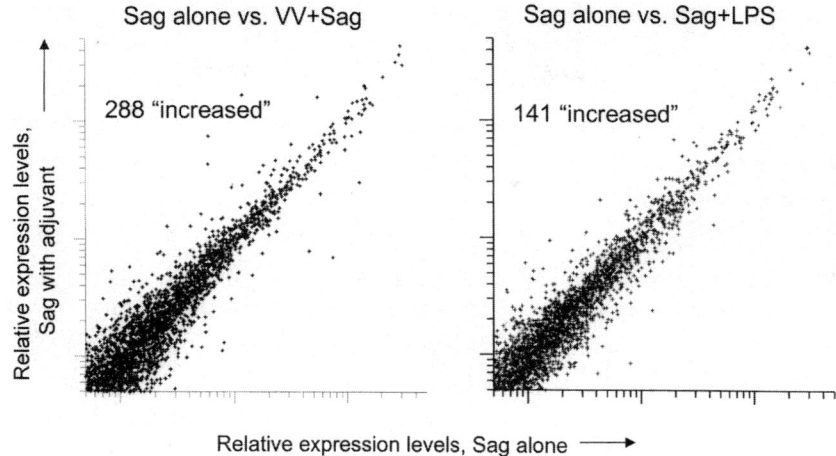

FIGURE 5. Pair-wise comparison of genes expressed by T cells after adjuvant treatment. Determination of gene expression in these cells was described previously.[13] Briefly, C57BL/10 mice were given SEB or SEB and LPS and anti-CD40 mAb, or were inoculated intravenously with Vaccinia Virus (VV) and then given SEB; 48 h after SEB treatment, T cells were harvested, purified by high-speed FACS and lysed to obtain poly(A)$^+$ RNA. Affymetrix mu6400 microarrays were probed with labeled cRNA prepared from these RNA populations, and the amounts of transcript of each gene represented were measured as hybridization intensity in arbitrary units using Affymetrix GeneChip software.[13]

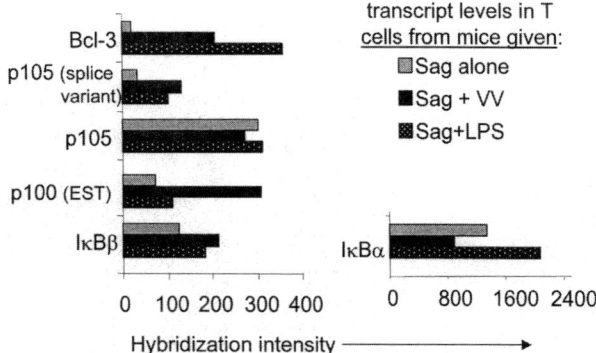

FIGURE 6. Adjuvant-correlated expression of NFκB/Rel/IκB transcription factors in activated mouse T cells. Hybridization intensities for each of the genes indicated were determined from the Affymetrix mu6400 analysis described in FIGURE 6. Some of these values were reported previously in Mitchell *et al.*[13] The Genbank identifiers for the shown were: Bcl-3, M90397; p105 splice variant, L28118; p105, L28117; p100, AA144430; IκB-β, U19799; IκB-α, U36277.

Subsequent analyses showed that Bcl-3 could drive transcription, rather than inhibit it, when partnered with selected DNA-binding proteins.[41–43] This transactivation function of Bcl-3 was mapped to non-ankyrin domains at the amino- and carboxyl-termini of the protein.[41] Effectively, Bcl-3 has attributes of both the transcriptionally transactivating and the inhibiting members of the NFκB/Rel/IκB superfamily of transcription factors. The normal function of Bcl-3 in lymphocytes has not yet been discovered, although our microarray results pointed to it as an adjuvant-induced survival factor for T cells.

Analysis of hybridization signals for other members of the NFκB/Rel/IκB superfamily showed a trend toward increased expression of IκB proteins (see FIGURE 6). IκBβ showed higher levels after either adjuvant treatment, VV or LPS adjuvant treatment. The precursor to NFκB p50, p105 showed no differences, but a splice variant of p105 showed adjuvant-associated increases. Interestingly, this splice variant expresses an ankyrin repeat protein that is primarily nuclear, much like Bcl-3.[44,45] The archetype of the family, IκBα, was increased by LPS but not VV infection while the reverse was true for NFκB p100. IκB proteins are commonly subject to transcriptional regulation by NFκB/Rel proteins,[46] and so these fluctuations may reflect increased activation of NFκBs in T cells from adjuvant treated animals.

BCL-3 SUPPORTS T CELL SURVIVAL WITHOUT DRIVING PROLIFERATION

As described elsewhere, Bcl-3 promotes survival of activated T cells when expressed via retroviral vectors,[13] and had earlier been ascribed an antiapoptotic role in cultured T lymphoid cell-lines.[47] Importantly, T cells transduced with Bcl-3 retroviruses did not show spontaneous proliferation, or heightened proliferation upon stimulation with antigen in culture, a result which is consistent with the idea that Bcl-3 acts via pathways not associated with co-stimulation and acts 'only' as a survival factor. (For further detail on Bcl-3, see Mitchell *et al.*, A Short Domain within Bcl-3 Is Responsible for Its Lymphocyte Survival Activity, in this volume.)

CONCLUSIONS

The hypothesis that Bcl-3 is an adjuvant-induced survival factor remains to be proved conclusively, but several observations argue that our microarray screen produced a valid candidate. First, independent quantitation of Bcl-3 expression by "real-time" polymerase chain reaction (PCR) confirmed that transcript levels were higher after adjuvant treatment.[13] An independent microarray analysis showed that Bcl-3 transcription was increased by about 5-fold in CD4 memory as compared to naïve T cell populations (see FIGURE 8). A demonstration of increased protein levels has been hampered by high background signals from the only commercially available antibody specific for mouse Bcl-3. Finally, *Bcl3*$^{-/-}$ mice were generated independently by two groups,[48,49] and both reported that the knock-out mice had defective immune responses. Although the mice developed normally and had normal numbers of B and T cells, immunization or infection revealed immune defects that are consistent with deficiencies in T cell-dependent responses. These defects included failure to form germinal centers and to produce immunogen-specific antibodies, high mortality following *T.gondii* and *S.pneumoniae* infection, failure to clear *L. monocytogenes*, and poor responses to infection by influenza virus.[48,49] Also, susceptibility to *T. gondii* was correlated with an abortive IFNγ response to *Toxoplasma* antigens,[49] which is reminiscent of the abortive response of T cells following proliferation in the absence of adjuvant treatment. The apparent role of Bcl-3 in adjuvant-induced survival of T cells makes our relatively primitive microarray analysis one of the early examples of successful use of the technology to find an unanticipated correlation between a gene product and an important biological phenomenon.

Altogether, the experiments described here and elsewhere indicate that several layers of signaling are needed to achieve productive T cell responses. Greatly simplified views of the processes involved are summarized in FIGURES 7 and 8. Because LPS does not appear to act directly on T cells, it is sensible to suppose that an APC with receptors for LPS must play a role (FIG. 7). Discovery of the precise molecular interactions that make APC 'aware' of lytic viral infections of nonlymphoid cells remains an important challenge. The operative APC is likely to be a non-B CD40+ cell because the effects of CD40 cross-linking in this model system are profound and AIS is fully operative in B-cell deficient mice.[50] Also, the APC must transmit much more than signals 1 (MHC-antigen-TCR) and 2 (B7-CD28 or other costimulatory pathways) in order to sustain a T cell response after it has begun. Induction of Bcl-3

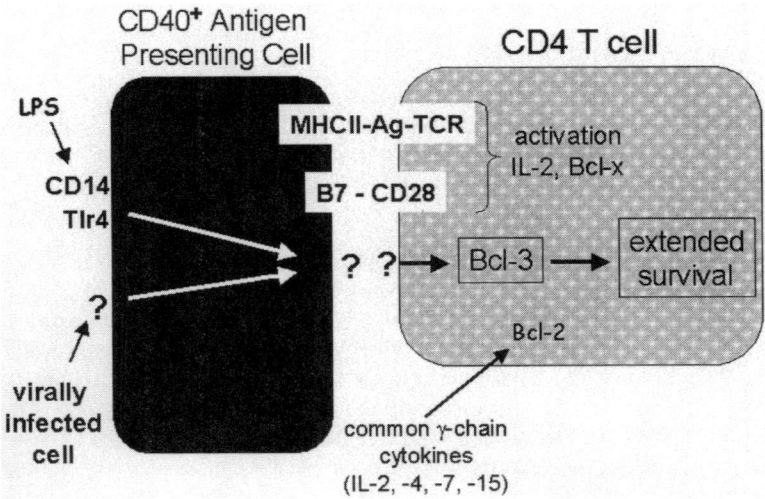

FIGURE 7. Model for the mechanism of adjuvant-induced T cell survival. Adjuvant-induced T cell survival is postulated to result from the actions of natural adjuvants on CD40+ antigen-presenting cells (APC). LPS is known to signal via CD14 and Tlr-4; the signals received by APC upon viral infection of non-lymphoid cells remain unknown. Substantial activation via signal 1 (MHCII-Ag-TCR) plus signal 2 (B7-CD28) does not require the presence of adjuvants, whereas adjuvant exposure is required for increased Bcl-3 expression and extended T cell survival.

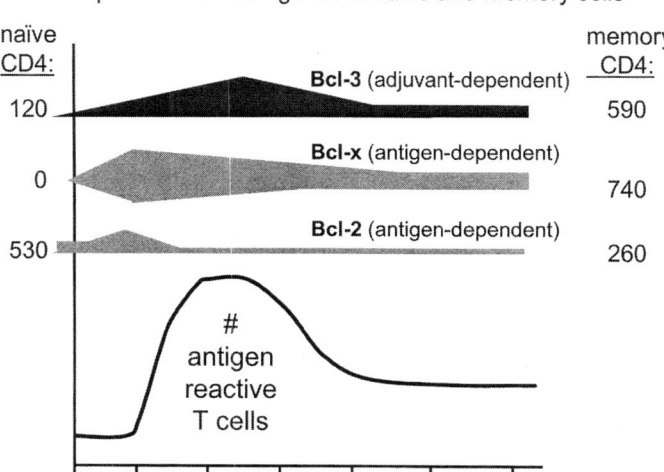

FIGURE 8. Idealized time course of Bcl-2, Bcl-xL and Bcl-3 expression after T cell activation. The roles of Bcl-2, Bcl-x_L, and Bcl-3 are proposed to comprise a series of transient effects. T cell yield during the course of an immune response to antigen in the presence of adjuvant is depicted as a solid line, with peak yield occurring 2–3 days postimmunization. Approximated levels of expression of Bcl-3 (*in black*), or Bcl-2 and Bcl-x_L (*both in gray*) are compiled from flow cytometric stains (Fig. 1 in ref. 8, and unpublished data), and Affymetrix mu6400 (FIG. 5, ref. 13) and 11K (Swanson *et al.*, in preparation) microarrays. Numbers shown indicate the expression levels for Bcl-2, Bcl-x_L, and Bcl-3, as determined from Affymetrix analyses of naive-phenotype (small, $CD44^{low}$, and $CD62L^{high}$) or memory phenotype (small, $CD44^{high}$, and $CD62L^{low}$) CD4+ cells sorted from C57BL/10 retired breeders as described previously (Swanson *et al.*, in preparation).

is appealing as a molecular lure with which to fish out the ill-defined upstream and downstream events involved in extending survival of T cells. As shown in FIGURE 8, the conventional anti-apoptotic factor Bcl-2 is likely to play its greatest role within the first 24 h following T cell activation. Bcl-x_L also shows most of its expression in the first 24 h, but its persistence in memory cells indicates it is likely to play a major role there, presumably in an adjuvant-independent fashion. Bcl-3 may be most important 2-3 days after activation, but given the transient nature of the LPS survival effect (FIG. 2) it seems unlikely to be sufficient for the maintenance of populations of CD4+ memory cells. Still, a short-term boost to survival may have a strongly beneficial effect on memory T cell generation, especially in light of the "rested effector" model of memory formation recently described by Swain and coworkers (Hu *et al.*[51]). In those experiments, the only event needed to convert activated effector cells to memory cells was survival of growth factor withdrawal. That is, activated T cells maintained in culture by a cocktail of cytokines were only able to enter the memory pool efficiently when injected into recipient mice if they first survived removal of the cytokines. Adjuvant-induced survival appears to play a critical role in generating long-lasting T cell populations, but it is clearly just one of a series of boosts needed to generate and maintain the right population of T cells for effective immunity.

ACKNOWLEDGMENTS

This work was made possible by USPHS AI5137, the Commonwealth of Kentucky Research Challenge Trust Fund, the Jewish Hospital Foundation (T.C.M) and USPHS AI17134, 18785, and 22295 (P.M.). The authors are grateful to Carolyn R. Casella and Bruce S. Thompson for comments on the manuscript, and to G.W.H. for help with the mice.

REFERENCES

1. KAWABE, Y. & A. OCHI. 1991. Programmed cell death and extrathymic reduction of Vbeta8+ CD4+ T cells in mice tolerant to *Staphylococcus aureus* enterotoxin B. Nature **349:** 245–248.
2. WEBB, S., C. MORRIS & J. SPRENT. 1990. Extrathymic tolerance of mature T cells: clonal elimination as a consequence of immunity. Cell **63:** 1249–1256.
3. KAPPLER, J.W., N. ROEHM & P. MARRACK. 1987. T cell tolerance by clonal elimination in the thymus. Cell **49:** 273–280.
4. AOKI, Y., K. HIROMATSU, J. USAMI, *et al.* 1994. Clonal expansion but lack of subsequent clonal deletion of bacterial superantigen-reactive T cells in murine retroviral infection. J. Immunol. **153:** 3611–3621.
5. CHILLER, J.M. & W.O.WEIGLE. 1973. Termination of tolerance to human gamma globulin in mice by antigen and bacterial lipopolysaccharide (endotoxin). J. Exp. Med. **137:** 740–750.
6. EHL, S., J. HOMBACH, P. AICHELE, *et al.* 1998. Viral and bacterial infections interfere with peripheral tolerance induction and activate CD8+ T cells to cause immunopathology. J. Exp. Med. **187:** 763–774.
7. KEARNEY, E.R., K.A. PAPE, D.Y. LOH & M.K. JENKINS. 1994. Visualization of peptide-specific T cell immunity and peripheral tolerance induction in vivo. Immunity **1:** 327–339.
8. MITCHELL, T., J. KAPPLER & P. MARRACK. 1999. Bystander virus infection prolongs activated T cell survival. J. Immunol. **162:** 4527–4535.
9. OHASHI, P.S., S. OEHEN, K. BUERKI, *et al.* 1991. Ablation of "tolerance" and induction of diabetes by virus infection in viral antigen transgenic mice. Cell **65:** 305–317.
10. OLDSTONE, M.B., M. NERENBERG, P. SOUTHERN, *et al.* 1991. Virus infection triggers insulin-dependent diabetes mellitus in a transgenic model: role of anti-self (virus) immune response. Cell **65:** 319–331.
11. ROCKEN, M., J.F. URBAN & E.M. SHEVACH. 1992. Infection breaks T-cell tolerance. Nature **359:** 79–82.
12. VELLA, A.T., J.E. MCCORMACK, P.S. LINSLEY, *et al.* 1995. Lipopolysaccharide interferes with the induction of peripheral T cell death. Immunity **2:** 261–270.
13. MITCHELL, T.C., D. HILDEMAN, R.M. KEDL, *et al.* 2001. Immunological adjuvants promote activated T cell survival via induction of Bcl-3. Nat. Immunol. **2:** 397–402.
14. POLTORAK, A., I. SMIRNOVA, X. HE, *et al.* 1998. Genetic and physical mapping of the Lps locus: identification of the toll-4 receptor as a candidate gene in the critical region. Blood Cells Mol. Dis. **24:** 340–355.
15. MUELLER, D.L., M.K. JENKINS & R.H. SCHWARTZ. 1989. Clonal expansion versus functional clonal inactivation: a costimulatory signalling pathway determines the outcome of T cell antigen receptor occupancy. Annu. Rev. Immunol. **7:** 445–480.

16. ADLER, A.J., C.T. HUANG, G.S. YOCHUM, *et al.* 2000. In vivo CD4$^+$ T cell tolerance induction versus priming is independent of the rate and number of cell divisions. J. Immunol. **164:** 649–655.
17. BERTOLINO, P., W.R. HEATH, C.L. HARDY, *et al.* 1995. Peripheral deletion of autoreactive CD8$^+$ T cells in transgenic mice expressing H-2Kb in the liver. Eur. J. Immunol. **25:** 1932–1942.
18. CARLOW, D.A., S.J. TEH, N.S. VAN OERS, *et al.* 1992. Peripheral tolerance through clonal deletion of mature CD4-CD8$^+$ T cells. Int. Immunol. **4:** 599–610.
19. JONES, L.A., L.T. CHIN, D.L. LONGO & A.M. KRUISBEEK. 1990. Peripheral clonal elimination of functional T cells. Science **250:** 1726–1729.
20. MCCORMACK, J.E., J.E. CALLAHAN, J. KAPPLER & P.C.MARRACK. 1993. Profound deletion of mature T cells in vivo by chronic exposure to exogenous superantigen. J. Immunol. **150:** 3785–3792.
21. ROCHA, B. & H.VON BOEHMER. 1991. Peripheral selection of the T cell repertoire. Science **251:** 1225–1228.
22. ZHANG, L.I., D.R. MARTIN, W.P. FUNG-LEUNG, *et al.* 1992. Peripheral deletion of mature CD8+ antigen-specific T cells after in vivo exposure to male antigen. J. Immunol. **148:** 3740–3745.
23. KHORUTS, A., A. MONDINO, K.A. PAPE, *et al.* 1998. A natural immunological adjuvant enhances T cell clonal expansion through a CD28-dependent, interleukin (IL)-2-independent mechanism. J. Exp. Med. **187:** 225–236.
24. VELLA, A.T., T. MITCHELL, B.GROTH, *et al.* 1997. CD28 engagement and proinflammatory cytokines contribute to T cell expansion and long-term survival in vivo. J. Immunol. **158:** 4714–4720.
25. MAXWELL, J.R., C. RUBY, N.I. KERKVLIET & A.T. VELLA. 2002. Contrasting the roles of costimulation and the natural adjuvant lipopolysaccharide during the induction of T cell immunity. J. Immunol. **168:** 4372–4381.
26. BOISE, L.H., M. GONZALEZ-GARCIA, C.E. POSTEMA, *et al.* 1993. Bcl-x, a bcl-2-related gene that functions as a dominant regulator of apoptotic cell death. Cell **74:** 597–608.
27. BOISE, L.H., A.J. MINN, P.J. NOEL, *et al.* 1995. CD28 costimulation can promote T cell survival by enhancing the expression of Bcl-XL. Immunity **3:** 87–98.
28. AKBAR, A.N., N.J. BORTHWICK, R.G. WICKREMASINGHE, *et al.* 1996. Interleukin-2 receptor common gamma-chain signaling cytokines regulate activated T cell apoptosis in response to growth factor withdrawal: selective induction of anti-apoptotic (bcl-2, bcl-xL) but not pro-apoptotic (bax, bcl-xS) gene expression. Eur. J. Immunol. **26:** 294–299.
29. VELLA, A.T., S. DOW, T.A. POTTER, *et al.* 1998. Cytokine-induced survival of activated T cells in vitro and in vivo. Proc. Natl. Acad. Sci. USA **95:** 3810–3815.
30. WHITE, J., A. HERMAN, A.M. PULLEN, *et al.* 1989. The V beta-specific superantigen staphylococcal enterotoxin B: stimulation of mature T cells and clonal deletion in neonatal mice. Cell **56:** 27–35.
31. LYONS, A.B. & C.R.PARISH. 1994. Determination of lymphocyte division by flow cytometry. J. Immunol. Methods 171: 131–137.
32. HEATH, A.W., W.W. WU & M.C.HOWARD. 1994. Monoclonal antibodies to murine CD40 define two distinct functional epitopes. Eur. J. Immunol. **24:** 1828–1834.
33. MAXWELL, J.R., J.D. CAMPBELL, C.H. KIM & A.T.VELLA. 1999. CD40 activation boosts T cell immunity in vivo by enhancing T cell clonal expansion and delaying peripheral T cell deletion. J. Immunol. **162:** 2024–2034.
34. VAN KOOTEN, C. & J. BANCHEREAU. 2000. CD40-CD40 ligand. J. Leukocyte Biol. **67:** 2–17.
35. HILDEMAN, D.A., T. MITCHELL, T.K. TEAGUE, *et al.* 1999. Reactive oxygen species regulate activation-induced T cell apoptosis. Immunity **10:** 735–744.
36. CAMPBELL, J.D., M. COLE, B. BUNDITRUTAVORN & A.T.VELLA. 1999. Ascorbic acid is a potent inhibitor of various forms of T cell apoptosis. Cell. Immunol. **194:** 1–5.
37. HILDEMAN, D.A., B. WHITLOCK, S. GARDAI, *et al.* 2002. Intracellular expression of free radical scavengers protects activated T cells from death. In preparation.

38. OHNO, H., G. TAKIMOTO & T.W. MCKEITHAN. 1990. The candidate proto-oncogene bcl-3 is related to genes implicated in cell lineage determination and cell cycle control. Cell **60:** 991–997.
39. KERR, L.D., C.S. DUCKETT, P. WAMSLEY, *et al.* 1992. The proto-oncogene bcl-3 encodes an I kappa B protein. Genes Dev. **6:** 2352–2363.
40. NOLAN, G.P., T. FUJITA, K. BHATIA, *et al.* 1993. The bcl-3 proto-oncogene encodes a nuclear I kappa B-like molecule that preferentially interacts with NF-kappa B p50 and p52 in a phosphorylation-dependent manner. Mol. Cell. Biol. **13:** 3557–3566.
41. BOURS, V., G. FRANZOSO, V. AZARENKO, *et al.* 1993. The oncoprotein Bcl-3 directly transactivates through kappa B motifs via association with DNA-binding p50B homodimers. Cell **72:** 729–739.
42. FRANZOSO, G., V. BOURS, S. PARK, *et al.* 1992. The candidate oncoprotein Bcl-3 is an antagonist of p50/NF-kappa B-mediated inhibition. Nature **359:** 339–342.
43. FUJITA, T., G.P. NOLAN, H.C. LIOU, *et al.* 1993. The candidate proto-oncogene bcl-3 encodes a transcriptional coactivator that activates through NF-kappa B p50 homodimers. Genes Dev. **7:** 1354–1363.
44. GRUMONT, R.J. & S. GERONDAKIS. 1994. Alternative splicing of RNA transcripts encoded by the murine p105 NF-kappa B gene generates I kappa B gamma isoforms with different inhibitory activities. Proc. Natl. Acad. Sci. USA **91:** 4367–4371.
45. GRUMONT, R.J., J. FECONDO & S. GERONDAKIS. 1994. Alternate RNA splicing of murine nfkb1 generates a nuclear isoform of the p50 precursor NF-kappa B1 that can function as a transactivator of NF-kappa B-regulated transcription. Mol. Cell. Biol. **14:** 8460–8470.
46. GILMORE, T.D. 1999. The Rel/NF-kappaB signal transduction pathway: introduction. Oncogene **18:** 6842–6844.
47. REBOLLO, A., L. DUMOUTIER, J.C. RENAULD, *et al.* 2000. Bcl-3 expression promotes cell survival following interleukin-4 deprivation and is controlled by AP1 and AP1-like transcription factors. Mol. Cell. Biol. **20:** 3407–3416.
48. SCHWARZ, E.M., P. KRIMPENFORT, A. BERNS & I.M. VERMA. 1997. Immunological defects in mice with a targeted disruption in Bcl-3. Genes Dev. **11:** 187–197.
49. FRANZOSO, G., L. CARLSON, T. SCHARTON-KERSTEN, *et al.* 1997. Critical roles for the Bcl-3 oncoprotein in T cell-mediated immunity, splenic microarchitecture, and germinal center reactions. Immunity **6:** 479–490.
50. VELLA, A.T., M.T. SCHERER, L. SCHULTZ, *et al.* 1996. B cells are not essential for peripheral T-cell tolerance. Proc. Natl. Acad. Sci. USA **93:** 951–955.
51. HU, H., G. HUSTON, D. DUSO, *et al.* 2001. CD4(+) T cell effectors can become memory cells with high efficiency and without further division. Nat. Immunol. **2:** 705–710.

A Short Domain within Bcl-3 Is Responsible for Its Lymphocyte Survival Activity

THOMAS C. MITCHELL,[a] BRUCE S. THOMPSON,[a] JOHN O. TRENT,[b] AND CAROLYN R. CASELLA[a]

[a]*Institute for Cellular Therapeutics,* [b]*J. Graham Brown Cancer Center, University of Louisville School of Medicine, Louisville, Kentucky 40202, USA*

ABSTRACT: The NFκB factor Bcl-3 influences the survival of T cells when they are activated to take part in immune responses. Because treatment of mice with adjuvant results in the increased expression of Bcl-3 in T cells, where it has survival-promoting effects, Bcl-3 may be an important, limiting factor that is supplied to T cells only when they are contributing to an appropriate immune response to infection, and not when spuriously activated by self-antigens. Although Bcl-3 is a member of the NFκB/Rel/IκB family of transcription factors, the means by which it promotes T cell survival is not obvious because Bcl-3 is unique in having an ankyrin repeat domain, like inhibitory IκB proteins, while also possessing domains capable of transcriptional activation, like Rel proteins. In order to understand the basis for the survival activity of Bcl-3, deletion mutants were engineered and tested in a retroviral gene transfer sytem. We report that most of Bcl-3 can be deleted without diminishing its ability to prolong the survival of activated T and B cells, and find that its lymphocyte survival domain maps to the vicinity of its first and second ankyrin repeats. This information sets the stage for experiments in which a focused search can be made for mediators of Bcl-3 survival effects.

KEYWORDS: Bcl-3; lymphocyte survival activity

INTRODUCTION

The NFκB factor Bcl-3 influences the survival of T cells during their mobilization to take part in a productive immune response.[1] Bcl-3 is an unusual but relatively little studied member of the NFκB family of transcription factors. It was discovered by Ohno and McKeithan in 1990[2] as the overexpressed gene product of a translocation event between human chromosomes 14 and 19 that is found in some cases of B cell chronic lymphocytic leukemia (B-CLL). Recently, expression of Bcl-3 was found to be increased in activated T cells only when adjuvants or an infectious state were present.[1] Moreover, enforced Bcl-3 expression was shown to prolong the survival of T lymphocytes and T lymphoid cell-lines.[1,3] From these findings one can conclude that Bcl-3 may be a limiting factor that is supplied to T cells only when they are taking part in an appropriate immune response from infection, and not when spuriously activated by self-antigens.

Addresss for correspondence: Thomas C. Mitchell, 570 S. Preston St., Baxter Building, Suite 404, Louisville, KY 40202. Voice: 502-852-2073; fax: 502-852-2085.
  tom.mitchell@louisville.edu

Bcl-3 is most likely to exert its effects via other members of the NFκB superfamily of transcription factors, which themselves have been ascribed important survival functions in a variety of cell-types.[4] NFκB/Rel/IκB factors in vertebrate animals consist of 5 DNA-binding proteins, 4 cytoplasmic inhibitors of the DNA-binding family members, and Bcl-3 (see TABLE 1). The 5 DNA-binding members are p50 (proteolytic product of NFκB1), p52 (proteolytic product of NFκB2), RelA (p65), RelB, and c-Rel.[5] Each of these can self-associate to form homodimers, or bind other members to form heterodimers. Each dimer has different binding specificities for DNA promoter elements, and accordingly drives (or represses) distinct patterns of gene expression. The heterodimer of p50 and RelA is the species to which most investigators refer when using the general term "NFκB," but virtually all possible combinations of heterodimers have been reported. The transcriptional activities of NFκB/rel transcription factors are held in check by the 4 inhibitors IκBα, IκBβ, IκBγ, and IκBε. These inhibitors bind to NFκB/Rel proteins and sequester them in the cytoplasm. Phosphorylation-induced proteolysis of these cytoplasmic IκB factors is usually required to remove them from NFκB/Rel complexes, which permits their translocation to the nucleus. Each inhibitor has distinct binding specificities for the various NFκB proteins. For example, IκBα primarily binds and inhibits heterodimers of p50/p65 and p50/c-Rel. IκB proteins are distinguished from other members of the NFκB superfamily by having ankyrin repeat domains (ARDs) that mediate protein-protein interactions.[6]

Bcl-3 is unique in that it has features of both the NFκB/Rel and the IκB proteins. Early inspection of its secondary structure revealed that Bcl-3 had ankyrin repeats and it was therefore classified as an IκB protein.[7] In agreement with this conclusion, initial studies found that NFκB-driven transcription was inhibited by Bcl-3 in transfection experiments and that purified Bcl-3 protein blocked DNA binding of some NFκB heterodimers in electrophoretic mobility shift assays.[7-9] However, Bcl-3 is often found in the nuclei of cells and is regulated at the level of *de novo* protein synthesis, distinguishing it from conventional IκB proteins.[10,11] Subsequently, Bcl-3 was found to function as a transcriptional transactivator when coexpressed with selected NFκB proteins. Transcriptional activation was dependent on its proline-rich amino- and serine-rich carboxyl-termini, and presumably on its ARD for protein–protein binding interactions.[10] The secondary structure of mouse Bcl-3 is shown

TABLE 1. Members of the NFκB/Rel/IκB family of transcription factors

Rel proteins (bind DNA, drive transcription)	RelA (p65), RelB, c-Rel
NFκB proteins (bind DNA but do not drive transcription by themselves)	p50, p52
IκB proteins (ankyrin repeats, inhibit NFKB/Rel complexes)	IκBα (MAD-3), IκBβ,γ,ε
NFκB/IκB precursor proteins (ankyrin repeats, precursors to p52, p50)	p100, p105
Bcl-3 (ankyrin repeats, binds homodimers of p50 or p52, no DNA binding)	

in FIGURE 1 with potential phosphorylation sites identified using NetPhos 2.0 software[12] and major structural motifs. A proline-glutamic acid-serine-threonine (PEST) sequence[13] that might signal degradation of Bcl-3 upon being phosphorylated was also identified (FIG. 1).

Within the NFκB/IκB family, Bcl-3 shows the most binding affinity for p50 or p52 proteins, which have DNA-binding domains but cannot drive transcription (TABLE 1).[9,10] Coexpression of Bcl-3 and p52 was sufficient to drive transcription from reporter plasmids, and it was postulated that Bcl-3 forms a higher order complex with p52,[10,14] which provides the DNA-binding specificity while Bcl-3 supplies transactivation functions (see FIGURE 4). Bcl-3 can cooperate with p50[15–18] in driving transcription as well, but in a fashion that may be strikingly different from that of p52. Bcl-3 can bind to and remove p50-p50 homodimers from DNA, thus derepressing transcription that would otherwise have been inhibited at that site.[15–18]

The mechanism by which Bcl-3 promotes T cell survival is currently unknown, but could involve one or both of the interactions with p50 and p52 described above. A third possible mechanism for Bcl-3's effects is for it to function as a shuttle that determines the nuclear vs. cytoplasmic residence of p50, thereby increasing[19] or decreasing,[20] respectively, its availability to form heterodimers with Rel proteins. In HepG2 cells, downregulation of Bcl-3 expression was correlated with increased NFκB-dependent expression from reporter plasmids,[20] indicating that Bcl-3 normally downregulates NFκB activity in this cell-type. If such an inhibitory function were responsible for the survival effects of Bcl-3 in activated T cells, some aspects of NFκB-driven transcription would have to be regarded as proapoptotic even though most reports in the literature focus on the compelling antiapoptotic effects of NFκB proteins in a variety of cell types.[4,21,22] However, some investigators do find that NFκB factors are associated with proapoptotic effects. For example, c-Rel expression is strongly correlated with apoptosis in embryonic avian tissues,[23] inhibitors of NFκB promote survival of T lymphoid cell-lines,[24] enforced c-Rel expression kills

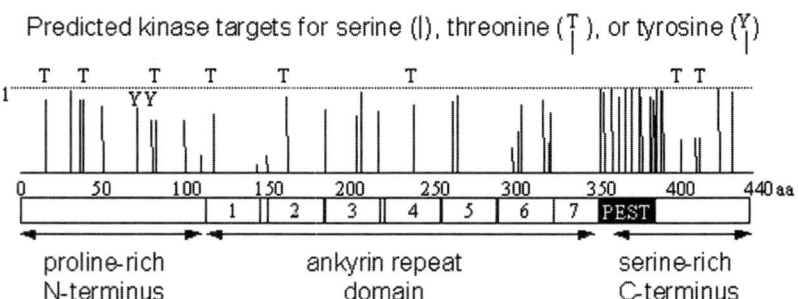

FIGURE 1. Protein motifs in Bcl-3. Mouse Bcl-3 has 440 amino acids, with seven ankyrin repeats flanked by proline-rich (N-terminus) and serine-rich (C-terminus) regions. Possible phosphorylation targets at serine, threonine, and tyrosine residues are indicated with lines. The length of the lines denotes 'phosphorylation potential' as determined by NetPhos 2.0 software[12] (www.cbs.dtu.dk/services/NetPhos/). Increased length of these lines indicates residues most likely to be phosphorylated. Seven previously identified ankyrin repeats are indicated as numbered boxes, and a possible PEST domain is shown in black, as predicted using PESTfind software[13] (http://emb1.bcc.univie.ac.at/embnet/tools/bio/PESTfind/).

primary T cells,[1] and NFκB activation can kill developing thymocytes and pro-B lymphoid cell-lines.[25,26]

In order to begin to understand how Bcl-3 supports T cell survival, we constructed deletion mutants of the protein and tested them for survival-enhancing activity. Our results show clearly that large sections of Bcl-3 can be removed without impairing its prosurvival activity, which probably means that Bcl-3 does not keep T cells alive

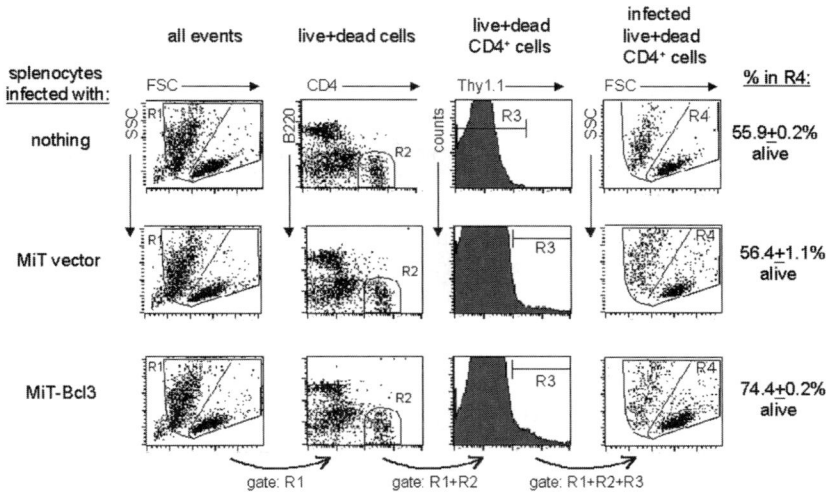

FIGURE 2. Flow cytometric gating method used to test Bcl-3 for survival activity in T cells. Activated T cells from VβDO transgenic mice were either left uninfected, infected with an 'empty' MiT retroviral vector, or infected with its derivative MiT-Bcl3[1] and cultured in triplicate wells. MiT expresses Thy1.1 alone as a marker of infection; MiT-Bcl3 expresses Bcl-3 and Thy1.1 from a bicistronic RNA transcript. After 20 h culture in medium containing no growth factors, the T cells were stained with antibodies specific for CD4, B220, and Thy1.1 and analyzed with a FACSCalibur flow cytometer. T cell survival was assessed by sequential gating of populations as follows. All cytometric events collected from uninfected T cell populations were plotted using forward vs. side light scatter (shown as FSC and SSC, respectively) to distinguish live and dead cells (R1) from debris. Live+dead cells were plotted next by B220 vs. CD4 staining to distinguish B from T_h cells, which were gated with region R2. Live and dead CD4$^+$ cells were then plotted in a histogram showing cell count vs. Thy1.1 staining. For uninfected samples, live+dead CD4$^+$ Thy1.1-negative cells (R3) were assessed for survival using forward vs. side light scatter; region R4 was drawn to distinguish live from dead cells. Next, samples of MiT-infected cells were gated to plot live+dead CD4$^+$ cells in a histogram showing Thy1.1 expression (live+dead CD4$^+$ cells). R3 was moved to include all Thy1.1$^+$ cells, with its left-hand boundary set so that the percentage of cells in R4 from this population matched that of CD4$^+$ cells from uninfected treatment groups. Finally, Bcl-3 survival activity was measured in cells infected with MiT-Bcl3 and gated exactly as for MiT-infected cells with no change in the placement of R3 or any other region. The values shown are the percent of CD4$^+$ cells that were alive after gene transduction and culture, averaged from triplicate cultures ± standard error of the mean (SEM). Relative survival was calculated using the values for % of cells alive and the formula 100 × (infected-uninfected)/uninfected. For this experiment, relative survival of MiT- or MiT-Bcl3-infected cells was 0.9 and 33, respectively.

by participating in higher-order protein complexes. Preliminary experiments also show that the subdomain responsible for the survival activity of Bcl-3 maps to the vicinity of the first and second ankyrin repeats.

A FLOW CYTOMETRIC METHOD OF ASSESSING T CELL SURVIVAL

In order to test for their effects on activated T cell survival, the cDNAs for Bcl-3 and mutant derivatives were cloned into the retroviral vector, MSCV-IRES-Thy1.1 (MiT).[1] This vector allows bicistronic expression of an introduced gene and of Thy1.1 (CD90.1) as an easily detected marker of retroviral transduction. Thy1.1, when compared to green fluorescent protein (GFP), proved to be superior for analyses of activated T cell death because GFP is rapidly lost from dead cells, while Thy1.1 is retained for at least 48 h after death on the cell surface where it can readily be detected with a high affinity monoclonal antibody.[27]

Superantigens (Sags) were used to activate nearly all T cells in T cell receptor (TCR) transgenic mice. Sags bind simultaneously to the variable portion of the β chain (Vβ) of TCR and to class II major histocompatibility complex (MHCII) on antigen-presenting cells (APC).[28] Both B and T cells are stimulated to proliferate by this interaction.[29] By using Sags in transgenic mice whose T cells expressed the same Vβ as part of their TCR (VβDO or DOTgR mice[1]), we were able to uniformly

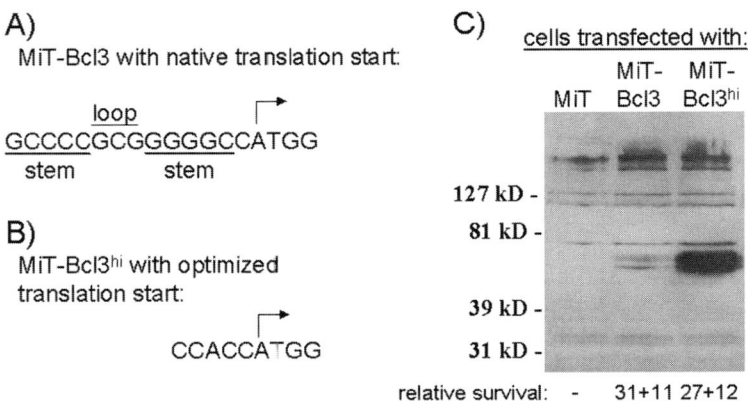

FIGURE 3. High levels of expression of Bcl-3 are not correlated with greater survival activity. Bcl-3 was cloned into the MiT retroviral vector with its native translation start (MiT-Bcl3, A) or an optimized translation start (MiT-Bcl3^{hi}, B). 293 cells were transfected with plasmids containing MiT, MiT-Bcl3, or MiT-Bcl3^{hi} and C) tested for levels of Bcl-3 expression by Western blot with a rabbit polyclonal antiserum specific for Bcl-3 (Santa Cruz Biotechnology Inc, catalogue no. sc-185) using standard methods. A potential stem-loop structure in the native translation start is indicated with *arrows* and *overline*. Relative survival after infection with MiT-Bcl3 or MiT-Bcl3^{hi} was averaged from seven experiments in which activated T cells were harvested and tested as described in FIGURE 2; values ± SEM are shown at the base of the Western blot. In general, SEM of the relative survival scored from triplicate infections in individual experiments was 25% or less of the average values observed.

activate T cells in order to infect them with MiT-derived retroviral vectors and test their ability to survive overnight culture in the absence of growth factors.

FIGURE 2 shows the gating method used for these assays. With sequential gating of flow cytometric data points we were able to track the fate of T cells—life or death —after they had expressed a given gene. To do so, T cells were activated in mice by injecting Sag and removed after they had just passed their peak of proliferation. In many of our assays, Bcl-3 was most active when introduced via retroviral vectors relatively late during activation, up to 66 h after Sag treatment (data not shown). Whole spleen or lymph node populations were exposed to virus for two hours, and then cultured for 20–24h in normal culture medium (RPMI supplemented with 10% fetal bovine serum and L-glutamine) containing no added T cell growth factors. After culture, bulk populations of both live and dead T cells were stained and analyzed for expression of Thy1.1 before being scored for survival. Because results from flow cytometric stains of dead or dying cells can be difficult to interpret, we adopted a protocol in which analytical gates were first set using comparisons of mock and parental vector-infected T cells, and then were left unchanged for analysis of cells exposed to Bcl-3 vector viruses (FIG. 2). We found that high frequencies of infection obscured results by increasing background staining, perhaps due to adherence of Thy1-bearing viral particles to cells, and so the percentages of cells infected was intentionally kept low, usually to less than 10%. As shown in FIGURE 2, and reported previously,[1] expression of Bcl-3 was associated with moderate but consistent increases in T cell survival.

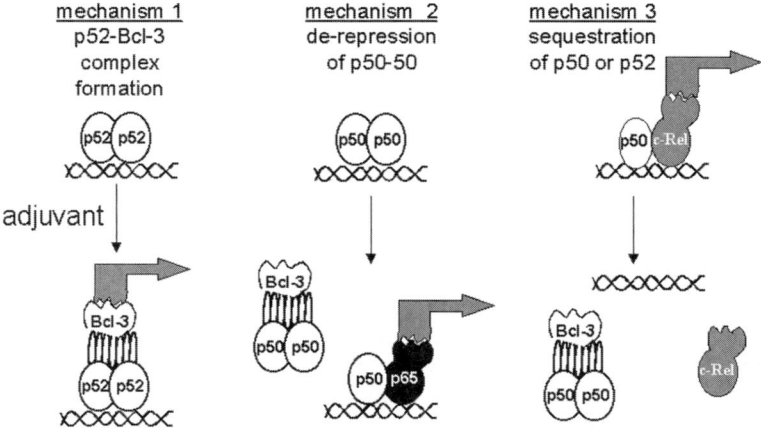

FIGURE 4. Three models for the mechanism of Bcl-3 induced survival of T cells. Bcl-3 may promote T cell survival via interaction with other members of the NFκB family of transcription factors. Bcl-3 has been shown elsewhere to increase transcription by either forming a higher order complex with p52 homodimers bound to DNA (Model 1), or by removing p50 homodimers from DNA, thereby relieving transcriptional repression (Model 2). Bcl-3 expression has been reported to shuttle p50 to the cytoplasm in some cell types.[20] This sequestration could decrease p50-dependent transcription, such as that of c-Rel-p50 heterodimers, in the nucleus (Model 3).

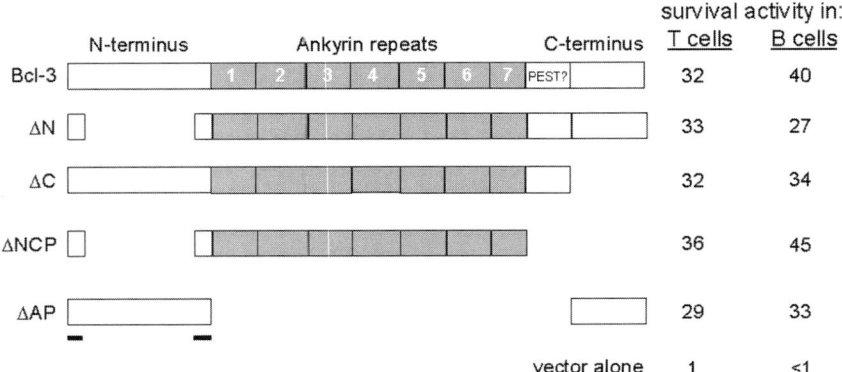

FIGURE 5. Survival activity of deletion mutants of Bcl-3 in T or B lymphocytes. Portions of Bcl-3 were deleted from MiT-Bcl3 using standard methods of PCR-assisted recombinant DNA cloning. All constructs were sequenced to verify that the mutations were as desired. Expressed regions are represented with boxes corresponding to the N-terminus, the seven ankyrin repeats, a putative PEST domain, or the C-terminus. All constructs contain amino acids 1–13 and 109–122 of mouse Bcl-3 (genbank accession AF067774). These residues are indicated by *black bars*, at bottom left. T and B cells were activated in VβDO or DOTgR mice with SEB superantigen, harvested after 40–48 h, infected with the indicated construct, and cultured for 20 h (T cells) or 40 h (B cells). Shown at right are values for the relative survival of activated T and B cells after culture, as calculated by comparison to mock-infected cells. The values are averaged from 2–9 experiments, depending on the construct. Relative survival induced by Bcl-2 expression was 40 and 59 in T and B cells, respectively.

OVEREXPRESSION OF BCL-3 IS NOT REQUIRED FOR T CELL SURVIVAL

Our initial experiments used retroviral promoter/enhancer elements for transcription of murine *Bcl3* and the native translation start site for protein synthesis. Because overexpression of genes can generate artifactual results, we sought to verify that appropriate levels of Bcl-3 were being expressed. In Western blots of transfected cells we found that expression levels were low unless the translation start site was optimized by being changed to that of the standard Kozak consensus sequence (see FIGURE 3). Interestingly, the native start site contains a GC-rich sequence that might form a stem-loop structure which could limit translation from the adjacent ATG initiation codon. Removal of these sequences led to much higher levels of expression, but the survival activity in infected T cells was not correspondingly increased. Although we cannot prove that the levels of Bcl-3 expressed in infected T cells are physiological using the reagents that are currently available, this result is consistent with the idea that Bcl-3 is effective in our model system without needing to be grossly overexpressed.

MOST OF BCL-3 CAN BE DELETED WITHOUT CHANGING ITS SURVIVAL ACTIVITY

FIGURES 5, 6, and 7 depict various mutant derivatives of Bcl-3 in cartoon form, along with measurements of their abilities to promote the survival of T cells from Sag-treated mice. Because Bcl-3 was originally discovered as a candidate oncogene in B lineage cells, survival activity in B220$^+$ B cells present in the same splenocyte population was also assessed.

Deletion mutants of Bcl-3 were generated by mutagenesis using selected oligonucleotides, PCR amplification, and standard restriction digest and ligation techniques. First, either the N- or C-terminus, or both termini, were removed (FIG. 5). These mutants, ΔN, ΔC, and ΔNCP, all promoted cell survival as effectively as wild-type when expressed in T or B cells. This result appears to preclude a role for mechanism 1 (FIG. 4), in which Bcl-3 drives transcription by interacting with both DNA-bound p52 and with elements of the RNA polymerase complex. Bcl-3-driven transcription via p52 has been reported to require both its N- and C-termini,[10] meaning that Bcl-3 is unlikely to promote lymphocyte survival via the formation of higher order complexes with p52.

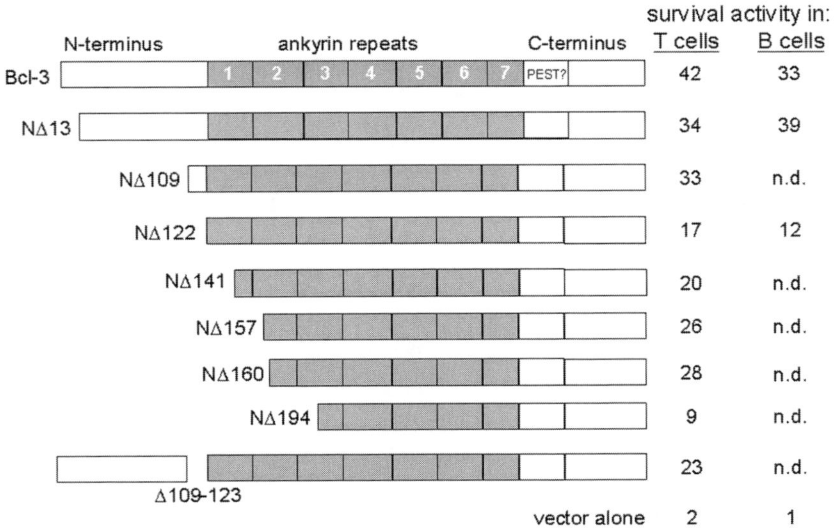

construct		survival activity in: T cells	B cells
Bcl-3	N-terminus / ankyrin repeats 1-7 / PEST? / C-terminus	42	33
NΔ13		34	39
NΔ109		33	n.d.
NΔ122		17	12
NΔ141		20	n.d.
NΔ157		26	n.d.
NΔ160		28	n.d.
NΔ194		9	n.d.
Δ109-123		23	n.d.
vector alone		2	1

FIGURE 6. Survival activity of amino-terminal deletion mutants of Bcl-3 in T or B lymphocytes. Increasing portions of the N-terminus of Bcl-3 were deleted from MiT-Bcl3 using standard methods of PCR-assisted recombinant DNA cloning, such that the first 13, 109, 122, 141, 157, 160, or 194 amino acids were not expressed. T and B cells were activated in VβDO or DOTgR mice with SEB superantigen, harvested after 40–48 h, infected with the indicated construct, and cultured for 20 h (T cells) or 40 h (B cells). Shown at right are values for the relative survival of activated T and B cells after culture, as calculated by comparison to mock-infected cells. The values are averaged from 1–3 experiments, depending on the construct. Relative survival induced by Bcl-2 in the same experiments was 54 and 44 for T and B cells, respectively. Not determined, n.d.

Next, the seven ankyrin repeat regions and the putative PEST domain were removed to generate mutant ΔAP, which, surprisingly, was also functional in the T and B cell survival assay. This result was unexpected for two reasons. First, the ankyrin repeat region of Bcl-3 provides the major interface for binding to p50 and p52,[30] and the activity of this construct apparently contradicted any role for such interactions in promoting lymphocyte survival. Second, removal of the the N- and C-termini, and then of the ankyrin repeat domain, ablated essentially all parts of the molecule making it unclear which regions would be required for activity. However, design of the constructs left in all of them a short stretch of 13 residues at the N-terminus, and residues internal residues 109–122, which are adjacent to the first ankyrin repeat.

In the next set of experiments, residues 1–13 and 109–122 of Bcl-3 were targeted for analysis (FIG. 6). Deletion of the first 13 amino acid residues produced a construct with full survival activity, showing they were not required. Deletion of residues 1–109 also had no effect, but deletion through to the residues adjacent to ankyrin repeat, 1–122, reduced activity by approximately half in both T and B cells. Deletion of internal residues 109–123, which left the rest of the N-terminus intact, produced a molecule with the same half-maximal activity. Because survival activity was not fully abolished by these deletions, further deletions were engineered in order

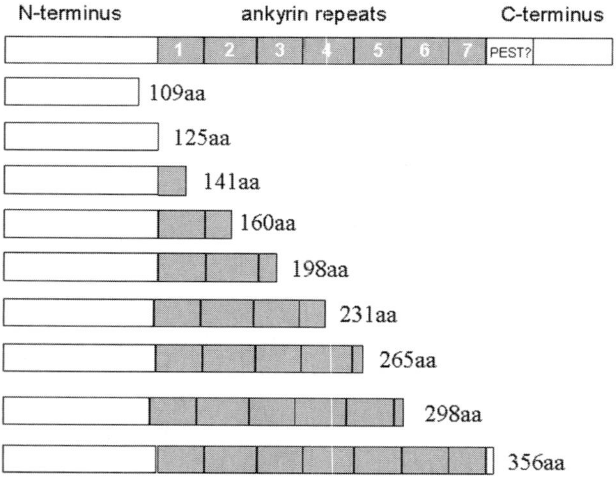

N-terminus	ankyrin repeats	C-terminus	survival activity in: T cells	B cells
	1 2 3 4 5 6 7 PEST?		85	30
	109aa		6	-2
	125aa		30	23
	141aa		21	14
	160aa		68	55
	198aa		69	18
	231aa		78	23
	265aa		88	36
	298aa		95	34
	356aa		68	n.d.

FIGURE 7. Survival activity of amino-terminal extension mutants of Bcl-3 in T or B lymphocytes. Increasing portions of the N-terminus of Bcl-3 were added to MiT using standard methods of PCR-assisted recombinant DNA cloning, such that the first 109, 125, 141, 160, 198, 231, 265, 298, or 356 amino acids were expressed. T and B cells were activated in VβDO mice with SEB superantigen, harvested after 64 h, infected with the indicated construct, and cultured for 20 h (T cells) or 40 h (B cells). Shown at right are values from one experiment performed with triplicate samples for the relative survival of activated T and B cells after culture, from separate experiments, as calculated by comparison to mock-infected cells. Relative survival induced by Bcl-2 in these experiments was 78 and 46 for T and B cells, respectively. Not determined, n.d.

TABLE 2. T cells but not B cells are killed by c-Rel and p50

Gene expressed	Relative survival[a] of:	
	T cells	B cells
Bcl-2	44 ± 3	14 ± 5
p50c	−9 ± 4	22 ± 3
p50-p50 forced dimer	−16 ± 4	17 ± 0.4
c-Rel-p50 forced dimer	−14 ± 4	20 ± 2
Empty vector	−0.6 ± 1.3	1.4 ± 0.5

[a]Relative survival± SD calculated as described in FIGURE 2 from triplicate samples in one experiment. Similar results were seen in two other experiments.

to find other active sites. Deletions through residues 141, 157, and 160 did not further decrease activity. However, deletion through residue 194 ablated most of the remaining survival activity of Bcl-3 in T cells.

Reciprocal experiments were performed in which increasing portions of the amino terminus and ankyrin repeat region were added back, in order to better determine which regions were sufficient for activity (FIG. 7). Here, expression of only the first 109 residues gave a molecule with no activity, as expected. Expression of residues 1–125 restored one-half to one-third of maximal activity, which was also expected. These results, together with those of FIGURES 5 and 6 suggested that Bcl-3 residues 109–122 are sufficient for significant survival activity in lymphocytes. Addition of the next 38 residues, to aa160, generated a molecule with high levels of T cell survival activity, which did not increase further with the addition of residues 161–198. Survival activity appeared to increase somewhat with further additions in the ankyrin repeat region, but the resolution of the assay was not sufficient to conclude whether or not these regions play a significant role. Similar patterns were seen in B cells, with no activity detected from aa1–109, intermediate activity with aa1–125, and high activity from the construct expressing residues 1–160. Some of these results did not agree exactly with the tests of N-terminal deletion mutants (FIG. 6) in which residues between aa160 and 194 seemed to be more important than residues between aa122 and 160. Overall, analyses of the deletion mutants showed that most of Bcl-3 could be deleted without abolishing its lymphocyte survival activity. All mutants generally behaved the same in both the T and the B cell populations, indicating that whatever interactions were occurring were likely to be the same in both cell types.

The proto-oncogene and NFκB factor c-Rel was shown previously to be lethal to T cells when expressed via retroviral transfer (Mitchell). This result was unexpected in light of reports that c-Rel has antiapoptotic activity in B cells.[31,32] In spite of these reports, the hypothesis that small fragments of Bcl-3 could somehow inhibit the activity of other transcription factors, such as Bcl-3's major binding partners p50 and p52, led us to test for the effects of expression of these molecules in both T and B lymphocytes. MiT retroviruses expressing p50 alone, or 'forced dimers' of p50 and c-Rel were constructed from gene cassettes encoding fusion proteins of cRel-p50, or p50-p50 (gift from William Sha and Deepta Battacharya, University of California,

Berkeley). These fusion proteins were expressed as a single polypeptide with each factor separated by a flexible linker of 10–20 amino acids, such that each half preferentially interacts with the other. Fusion of c-Rel and p50, for example forces dimerization of the two components, generating uniform populations of heterodimer molecules. When expressed, these proteins produced completely different results in T versus B lymphocytes (TABLE 2). In T cells, expression of p50 alone or as a homodimer was lethal, as was expression of the c-Rel-p50 heterodimer. In B cells however, each of these constructs prolonged survival, as expected. Hence, although Bcl-3 showed the same structural requirements for activity in T versus. B cells, the consequences of expression of at least some of the other members of the NFκB family was dramatically different, suggesting that these factors were not directly involved in mediating the survival effects of Bcl-3.

CONCLUSIONS

These experiments gave rise to the simple but useful conclusion that most of the Bcl-3 protein can be deleted without reducing its ability to prolong the survival of T and B lymphocytes. This observation seems to preclude mechanisms that involve multiple, simultaneous interactions of Bcl-3 with other proteins, such as the higher-order complex that is proposed to form when p52 homodimers are present.[10,14] For-

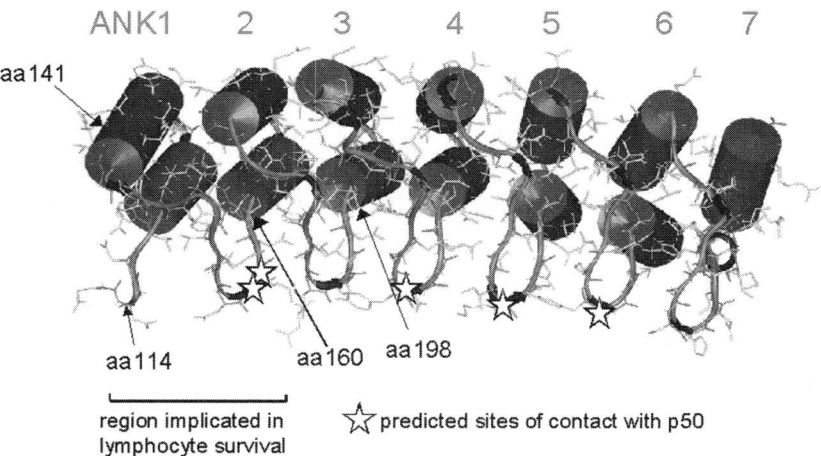

FIGURE 8. Structure of the ankyrin repeat domain of Bcl-3. A mouse Bcl-3 homology model was generated from the human Bcl-3 X-ray crystal structure 1K1A.pdb (Protein Database, www.pdb.org) using Modeller software.[42] Each ankyrin repeat contains two alpha-helical structures, which are depicted as solid cylinders, and a loop or 'finger' domain connecting each pair of helices. The structure begins with amino acid 114 of mouse Bcl-3; amino acids 160 and 198 are shown for comparison to the Bcl-3 mutants described in FIGURES 6 and 7. Predicted sites of contact with NFκB p50, indicated with stars, were identified by Michel et al.[30] by comparison of the sequence of Bcl-3 and the crystal structure of a complex of p50/p65 with the ankyrin repeat domain of IκBα.[39,40]

mation of this complex is important in other systems, such as human breast epithelium in which complexes of p52 and Bcl-3 were shown to induce cyclin D1 expression and alter cell cycle kinetics,[33] but such a complex does not seem to be required for lymphocyte survival. Our conclusion in no way precludes a role for p52 and Bcl-3 to operate together in generating immunity. In fact, mice engineered to lack Bcl-3 or p52 expression, or both, all show the same defects in antibody production and germinal center formation.[34,35]

Apart from finding that higher-order complexes of Bcl-3 with other proteins are unlikely to be involved, we cannot yet tell whether Bcl-3 acts on other genes by increasing or by decreasing their transcription. A small portion of Bcl-3 may be sufficient to increase gene expression through the removal of transcriptionally repressive p50-p50 homodimers from DNA, for example, or by increased shuttling of p50 or p52 between nuclear and cytoplasmic compartments. Accordingly, the models shown in FIGURE 4 need to be adjusted to reflect the possibility that small protein motifs are sufficient to alter the activities of other NFκB family members.

It is possible that Bcl-3's survival activity operates through nontranscriptional pathways. Indeed, Bcl-3 expression can be induced to high levels in platelets, which are anucleate.[36–38] It is interesting to note that Bcl-3 expression in human platelets was rapamycin-sensitive, a quality that is shared by relatively few transcripts and is associated with extensive secondary structure at 5' untranslated regions,[38] which may explain our observation that alterations in this region greatly increased translation (FIG. 4). Bcl-3 expression was correlated with increased platelet life spans in mice,[37] indicating that it is functionally relevant, but by a mechanism that cannot involve transcription of DNA.

An important future direction is to define exactly which subdomains of Bcl-3 are sufficient for prolonged lymphocyte survival, and then to determine which proteins or factors from activated T cells are bound to that subdomain. We have begun to achieve this goal by localizing the lymphocyte survival activity of Bcl-3 to the vicinity of the first and perhaps second ankyrin repeats. First, we can conclude that the region consisting of residues 109–122 are sufficient to induce significant survival, especially when that region is flanked by other residues as in mutant construct ΔAP (FIG. 5). Another region appears to have the same kind of activity, because several mutants had significant survival activity even when residues 109–122 were deleted, as with mutants Δ109–123, NΔ122, NΔ141, NΔ157, and NΔ160 (FIG. 6). The C-terminal boundary of the second region is in doubt, because one set of experiments implicated residues 161–194 (FIG. 6) and another, residues 142–160 (FIG. 7).

To make sense of these patterns, we used the the published crystal structure of the ankyrin repeat domain of human Bcl-3[30] to generate a homology model of the structure of mouse Bcl-3 (see FIGURE 8). As with the ankyrin repeat domain of IκBα,[39,40] the ankyrin repeat domain of Bcl-3 consists of a series of paired α-helices that are held in a stacked formation by hydrophobic patches. On the 'back' face of the structure shown in FIGURE 8 are short loops of sufficient length (2–3aa) to connect the two members of each α-helical pair, which are depicted as solid cylinders. On the 'front' face of this model are extended loops consisting of β-turn motifs (*ribbon arrows* in FIG. 8) within a total of 14–17 residues. It is on the loops of this face that most of the contacts between IκBα and the p50–p65 heterodimer were observed to occur.[39,40] Although the structure of a Bcl-3 molecule bound to p50 or p52 homodimers has not been solved, comparison of the sequence of IκBα to conserved residues in Bcl-3 indicated that many interactions are likely to be the same.[30] Conserved residues in Bcl-3 that are predicted to interact with p50 are indicated with stars in FIGURE 8. The survival activities of our deletion mutants did not correspond well with the presence or absence of these sites, leaving open the question of the importance of p50 and p52 in mediating lymphocyte survival.

Comparison of the structure of mouse Bcl-3 to the activities of its deletion mutants allowed us to visualize the structures likely to be involved in promoting lymphocyte survival. This comparison indicated that the lymphocyte survival activity of Bcl-3 maps to residues immediately upstream of the ANK1 α-helices (aa109–122) and to the first and perhaps second loops between ANK1-2 and ANK2-3 (FIG. 8). The 109–122 domain identified in our experiments corresponds to an acidic region in IκBα that binds to the basic nuclear localization sequence (NLS) of p65. The orientation of the acidic stretch in Bcl-3 is markedly different from that of IκBα.[30] Relative to IκBα, the acidic domain of Bcl-3 points in the opposite direction, such that it is oriented toward the loop between ANK1-2, rather than away from it. This different orientation is cited as one of the reasons for Bcl-3's decreased affinity for p65 because it makes contact with p65 less likely. The opposite course of the IκBα domain places two negatively charged aspartatic acid residues in juxtaposition to an argine and a lysine from the NLS of p65, which would not occur with Bcl-3. Moreover, the putative NLS binding site in Bcl-3 is much less acidic than that of IκBα,[30] making it unclear whether or not it would form a strong interaction with any NLS, including those of p50 or p52, which are Bcl-3's preferred binding partners. In fact, mutants of p50 lacking the NLS are still able to bind Bcl-3.[9]

Our results were ambiguous with respect to the relative roles played by the first and second loops between ANK1-2 and ANK 2-3, respectively. Successive deletions of the N-terminus of Bcl-3 did not abolish activity until residues 161–194, which contain the second loop and the α-helices of ANK2 (FIG. 8), had been removed. This pattern indicated that the first loop (corresponding to residues 141–160) was not required and that the second loop, or the second pair of α-helices, possessed the survival activity. In the reciprocal constructs, activity was increased greatly when residues 142–160 were restored to the rest of the N-terminus (FIG. 7), indicating that the first loop did contain activity. More constructs with focused deletions are required to resolve this ambiguity.

Although homodimers of p50 and p52 are the dominant binding partners for Bcl-3, several studies report that other factors bind Bcl-3. These include the src-family kinase c-fyn,[38] transcription factors c-jun and c-fos,[42] and transcription mediators Jab1, Pirin, Tip60, and Bard1.[14] It is possible that one of these factors, or others yet to be identified, underlie the survival activity of Bcl-3 rather than p50 or p52. Whatever the binding partner, it seems that small regions within Bcl-3 are effective at inducing prolonged lymphocyte survival. Small polypeptides can have inhibitory or stimulatory effects on other proteins, and in order to answer the fundamental question as to whether Bcl-3 needs to induce a gain or loss of function in order to prolong lymphocyte survival, it will be necessary to identify which secondary factor(s) are involved. Such experiments are underway, and we are optimistic that the important problem of understanding how immunological adjuvants promote T cell survival will be solved thereafter.

ACKNOWLEDGMENTS

This work was supported by USPHS AI5137, the Commonwealth of Kentucky Research Challenge Trust Fund and the Jewish Hospital Foundation. The authors are grateful to William Sha and Deepta Battacharya for their gift of p50-p50 and c-Rel-p50 forced dimer constructs.

REFERENCES

1. MITCHELL, T.C., D. HILDEMAN, R.M. KEDL, et al. 2001. Immunological adjuvants promote activated T cell survival via induction of Bcl-3. Nat. Immunol. **2:** 397–402.
2. OHNO, H., G. TAKIMOTO & T.W. MCKEITHAN. 1990. The candidate proto-oncogene bcl-3 is related to genes implicated in cell lineage determination and cell cycle control. Cell **60:** 991–997.
3. REBOLLO, A., L. DUMOUTIER, J.C. RENAULD, et al. 2000. Bcl-3 expression promotes cell survival following interleukin-4 deprivation and is controlled by AP1 and AP1-like transcription factors. Mol. Cell. Biol. **20:** 3407–3416.
4. BARKETT, M. & T.D. GILMORE. 1999. Control of apoptosis by Rel/NF-kappaB transcription factors. Oncogene **18:** 6910–6924.
5. GILMORE, T.D. 1999. The Rel/NF-kappaB signal transduction pathway: introduction. Oncogene **18:** 6842–6844.
6. SEDGWICK, S.G. & S.J. SMERDON. 1999. The ankyrin repeat: a diversity of interactions on a common structural framework. Trends Biochem. Sci. **24:** 311–316.
7. KERR, L.D., C.S. DUCKETT, P. WAMSLEY, et al. 1992. The proto-oncogene bcl-3 encodes an I kappa B protein. Genes Dev. **6:** 2352–2363.
8. HATADA, E.N., A. NIETERS, F.G. WULCZYN, et al. 1992. The ankyrin repeat domains of the NF-kappa B precursor p105 and the protooncogene bcl-3 act as specific inhibitors of NF-kappa B DNA binding. Proc. Natl. Acad. Sci. USA **89:** 2489–2493.
9. WULCZYN, F.G., M. NAUMANN & C. SCHEIDEREIT. 1992. Candidate proto-oncogene bcl-3 encodes a subunit-specific inhibitor of transcription factor NF-kappa B. Nature **358:** 597–599.
10. BOURS, V., G. FRANZOSO, V. AZARENKO, et al. 1993. The oncoprotein Bcl-3 directly transactivates through kappa B motifs via association with DNA-binding p50B homodimers. Cell **72:** 729–739.
11. NOLAN, G.P., T. FUJITA, K. BHATIA, et al. 1993. The bcl-3 proto-oncogene encodes a nuclear I kappa B-like molecule that preferentially interacts with NF-kappa B p50 and p52 in a phosphorylation-dependent manner. Mol. Cell. Biol. **13:** 3557–3566.
12. BLOM, N., S. GAMMELTOFT & S. BRUNAK. 1999. Sequence and structure-based prediction of eukaryotic protein phosphorylation sites. J. Mol. Biol. **294:** 1351–1362.
13. RECHSTEINER, M. & S.W. ROGERS. 1996. PEST sequences and regulation by proteolysis. Trends Biochem. Sci. **21:** 267–271.
14. DECHEND, R., F. HIRANO, K. LEHMANN, et al. 1999. The Bcl-3 oncoprotein acts as a bridging factor between NF-kappaB/Rel and nuclear co-regulators. Oncogene **18:** 3316–3323.
15. FRANZOSO, G., V. BOURS, V. AZARENKO, et al. 1993. The oncoprotein Bcl-3 can facilitate NF-kappa B-mediated transactivation by removing inhibiting p50 homodimers from select kappa B sites. EMBO J. **12:** 3893–3901.
16. FUJITA, T., G.P. NOLAN, H.C. LIOU, et al. 1993. The candidate proto-oncogene bcl-3 encodes a transcriptional coactivator that activates through NF-kappa B p50 homodimers. Genes Dev. **7:** 1354–1363.
17. INOUE, J., T. TAKAHARA, T. AKIZAWA & O.HINO. 1993. Bcl-3, a member of the I kappa B proteins, has distinct specificity towards the Rel family of proteins. Oncogene **8:** 2067–2073.
18. FRANZOSO, G., V. BOURS, S. PARK, et al. 1992. The candidate oncoprotein Bcl-3 is an antagonist of p50/NF-kappa B-mediated inhibition. Nature **359:** 339–342.

19. WATANABE, N., T. IWAMURA, T. SHINODA & T. FUJITA. 1997. Regulation of NFKB1 proteins by the candidate oncoprotein BCL-3: generation of NF-kappaB homodimers from the cytoplasmic pool of p50-p105 and nuclear translocation. EMBO J. **16:** 3609–3620.
20. BRASIER, A.R., M. LU, T. HAI, et al. 2001. NF-kappa B-inducible BCL-3 expression is an autoregulatory loop controlling nuclear p50/NF-kappa B1 residence. J. Biol. Chem. **276:** 32080–32093.
21. BEG, A.A., W.C. SHA, R.T. BRONSON, et al. 1995. Embryonic lethality and liver degeneration in mice lacking the RelA component of NF-kappa B. Nature **376:** 167–170.
22. BEG, A.A. & D. BALTIMORE. 1996. An essential role for NF-kappaB in preventing TNF-alpha-induced cell death. Science **274:** 782–784.
23. ABBADIE, C., N. KABRUN, F. BOUALI, et al. 1993. High levels of c-rel expression are associated with programmed cell death in the developing avian embryo and in bone marrow cells in vitro. Cell **75:** 899–912.
24. LIN, B., C. WILLIAMS-SKIPP, Y. TAO, et al. 1999. NF-kappaB functions as both a proapoptotic and antiapoptotic regulatory factor within a single cell type. Cell Death Differ. **6:** 570–582.
25. KIM, D., M. XU, L. NIE, et al. 2002. Helix-loop-helix proteins regulate pre-TCR and TCR signaling through modulation of Rel/NF-kappaB activities. Immunity **16:** 9–21.
26. SHEEHY, A.M. & M.S. SCHLISSEL. 1999. Overexpression of RelA causes G1 arrest and apoptosis in a pro-B cell line. J. Biol. Chem. **274:** 8708–8716.
27. HILDEMAN, D., B. WHITLOCK, S. GARDAI, et al. Intracellular expression of free radical scavengers protects activated T cells from death. Manuscript in preparation.
28. WHITE, J., A. HERMAN, A.M. PULLEN, et al. 1989. The V beta-specific superantigen staphylococcal enterotoxin B: stimulation of mature T cells and clonal deletion in neonatal mice. Cell **56:** 27–35.
29. MOURAD, W., P. SCHOLL, A. DIAZ, et al. 1989. The staphylococcal toxic shock syndrome toxin 1 triggers B cell proliferation and differentiation via major histocompatibility complex- unrestricted cognate T/B cell interaction. J. Exp. Med. **170:** 2011–2022.
30. MICHEL, F., M. SOLER-LOPEZ, C. PETOSA, et al. 2001. Crystal structure of the ankyrin repeat domain of Bcl-3: a unique member of the IkappaB protein family. EMBO J. **20:** 6180–6190.
31. GRUMONT, R.J., I.J. ROURKE & S.GERONDAKIS. 1999. Rel-dependent induction of A1 transcription is required to protect B cells from antigen receptor ligation-induced apoptosis. Genes Dev. **13:** 400–411.
32. TUMANG, J.R., A. OWYANG, S. ANDJELIC, et al. 1998. c-Rel is essential for B lymphocyte survival and cell cycle progression. Eur. J. Immunol. **28:** 4299–4312.
33. WESTERHEIDE, S.D., M.W. MAYO, V. ANEST, et al. 2001. The putative oncoprotein Bcl-3 induces cyclin D1 to stimulate G(1) transition. Mol. Cell. Biol. **21:** 8428–8436.
34. SCHWARZ, E.M., P. KRIMPENFORT, A. BERNS & I.M.VERMA. 1997. Immunological defects in mice with a targeted disruption in Bcl-3. Genes Dev. **11:** 187–197.
35. FRANZOSO, G., L. CARLSON, T. SCHARTON-KERSTEN, et al. 1997. Critical roles for the Bcl-3 oncoprotein in T cell-mediated immunity, splenic microarchitecture, and germinal center reactions. Immunity **6:** 479–490.
36. PABLA, R., A.S. WEYRICH, D.A. DIXON, et al. 1999. Integrin-dependent control of translation: engagement of integrin alphaIIbbeta3 regulates synthesis of proteins in activated human platelets. J. Cell Biol. **144:** 175–184.
37. PIGUET, P.F., C.VESIN & A.ROCHAT. 2001. Beta2 integrin modulates platelet caspase activation and life span in mice. Eur. J. Cell Biol. **80:** 171–177.
38. WEYRICH, A.S., D.A. DIXON, R. PABLA, et al. 1998. Signal-dependent translation of a regulatory protein, Bcl-3, in activated human platelets. Proc. Natl. Acad. Sci. USA **95:** 5556–5561.
39. JACOBS, M.D. & S.C.HARRISON. 1998. Structure of an IkappaBalpha/NF-kappaB complex. Cell **95:** 749–758.

40. HUXFORD, T., D.B. HUANG, S. MALEK & G.GHOSH. 1998. The crystal structure of the IkappaBalpha/NF-kappaB complex reveals mechanisms of NF-kappaB inactivation. Cell **95:** 759–770.
41. NA, S.Y., J.E. CHOI, H.J. KIM, *et al.* 1999. Bcl3, an IkappaB protein, stimulates activating protein-1 transactivation and cellular proliferation. J. Biol. Chem. **274:** 28491–28496.
42. SALI, A. & T.L. BLUNDELL. 1993. Comparative protein modelling by satisfaction of spatial restraints. J. Mol. Biol. **234:** 779–815.

Molecular Characterization of Antigen-Induced Lung Inflammation in a Murine Model of Asthma

MASSOUD DAHESHIA,[a] NIAN TIAN,[a] TIMOTHY CONNOLLY,[b] AMAR DRAWID,[a] QUIYAN WU,[c] JEAN-GUY BIENVENU,[d] JEAN CAVALLO,[c] RAY JUPP,[a] GEORGE T. DE SANCTIS,[a] AND ANNE MINNICH[a]

[a]*Department of Respiratory Disease and Rheumatoid Arthritis,* [b]*Cambridge Genomics Center, Aventis Pharmaceuticals Cambridge, Massachusetts, USA*

[c]*Functional Genomics,* [d]*Drug Safety Evaluation, Aventis Pharmaceuticals, Bridgewater New Jersey 08807, USA*

ABSTRACT: Asthma is one of the foremost contributors to morbidity and mortality in industrialized countries. Our objective was to characterize the acute response to allergen and to identify potentially novel molecular targets for pharmacological intervention in asthma. We therefore designed a study to identify genes whose regulation was altered following ovalbumin (OVA) challenge in the presence and absence of treatment with glucocorticoids in BALB/c mice. RNA was isolated from lungs for gene profiling from 8-week-old sensitized mice, 3 and 18 hours post OVA challenge on days 1, 4, and 7 of aerosol challenge. Taqman (real time RT-PCR) analysis of marker genes indicative of Th2 (IL-4, IL-13), eosinophil (RANTES, eotaxin), Th1/macrophage (IFNγ) and epithelial cell (MUC5AC) phenotypes were used to characterize responses to allergen challenge. Histological evaluation of lungs from additional challenged animals revealed inflammatory infiltrates on days 4 and 7, but not on day 1 post challenge. We postulate that expression of IL-4, IL-13 and other genes by OVA at day 1 probably reflects activation of resident cells, whereas the fivefold increase in the number of regulated genes at day 7 reflects the contribution of recruited cells. Of the regulated genes, only a subset was counterregulated by dexamethasone treatment. Although regulated genes included genes in many protein families, herein we report regulation of two proteases whose role in response to OVA challenge has not been characterized. This model will be used to generate disease hypotheses for which may play an important role in initiating disease pathology in this model.

KEYWORDS: asthma; cathepsin S; MMP-12; inflammation; microarray; lung

INTRODUCTION

Atopic asthma is a heterogenous disease characterized by an increase in airway inflammation and in airway reactivity to various nonspecific stimuli. Airway hyperreactivity (AHR), a hallmark of asthma, is commonly associated with several

Address for correspondence: Anne Minnich, Aventis Pharmaceuticals, Rt. 202/206, Bridgewater, NJ 08807. Voice: 908-231-5639; fax: 908-231-3052.
anne.minnich@aventis.com

pathological features in the lung including thickening of the basal membrane, epithelium hypertrophy/hyperplasia and exaggerated mucus secretions.[1] It is generally accepted that repeated exposure to aerosolized allergens in sensitized individuals generates an exaggerated immune response in the lung. It is widely accepted that both genetic and environmental factors influence the phenotypic expression of this disease. An area of intense debate concerns the cellular nature of the disease and contribution of the resident cell types to the pathobiology of the disease. While mast cells and eosinophils have been widely viewed as key contributors to the expression of the asthma phenotype, other cell types have been shown to participate in the disease processes. Specifically, it is becoming increasingly clear that T lymphocytes are the major orchestrators in this process[2] and that in the absence of T cells the disease phenotype is severely impaired.[3] In support of this, T cell depletion abrogates antigen-induced lung inflammation[4] and adoptive transfer of Ag-specific T cells restores the inflammation.[5] *In situ* hybridization studies have unequivocally shown that the majority of T cells in the lung at the onset of disease are of the Th2 phenotype.[6] Data generated from gene knockout and transgenic animal studies support a major role for the Th2 cytokines (reviewed in refs. 7 and 8) such as IL-4, IL-5 and IL-13 in the generation and expression of asthma. How Th2 cells are generated and how their secreted products are involved in lung pathogeneses are still under investigation. Moreover, it is clear that disease severity and duration are dependent on cells other than T cells and that many mediators and pathways contribute to the genesis of the asthma phenotype.

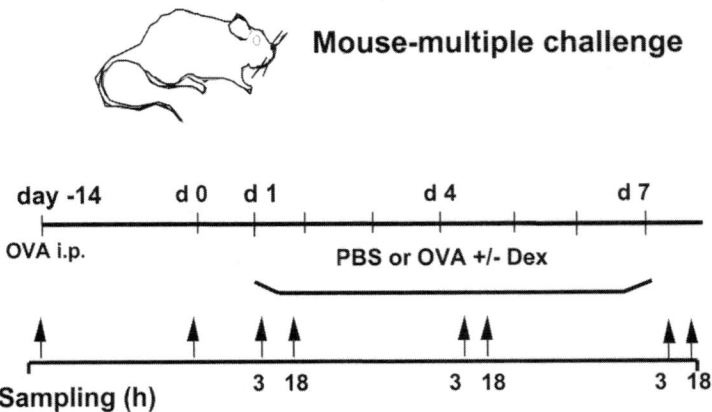

FIGURE 1. Design of OVA challenge study. Antigen sensitization and aerosol challenge: Six-week-old male BALB/c were intraperitonealy sensitized at day-14 and -7, with 10 µg of ovalbumin precipitated with 1 mg of aluminum hydroxide in 200 µL of PBS. This mode of immunization has been shown to generate peripheral Th2 cells and high serum IgE and IgG1. During days 1 to 7, mice were challenged with 6% aerosolized ovalbumin in 1/2×PBS for 25 min per day. Control mice were challenged with vehicle (PBS) alone. Dexamethasone was given intraperitoneally at 50 mg/kg. At days 1, 4, and 7, $n = 4$ animals were sacrificed 3 and 18 h post challenge and lungs taken for RNA extraction. All animal protocols conformed to institutional ethics committee criteria.

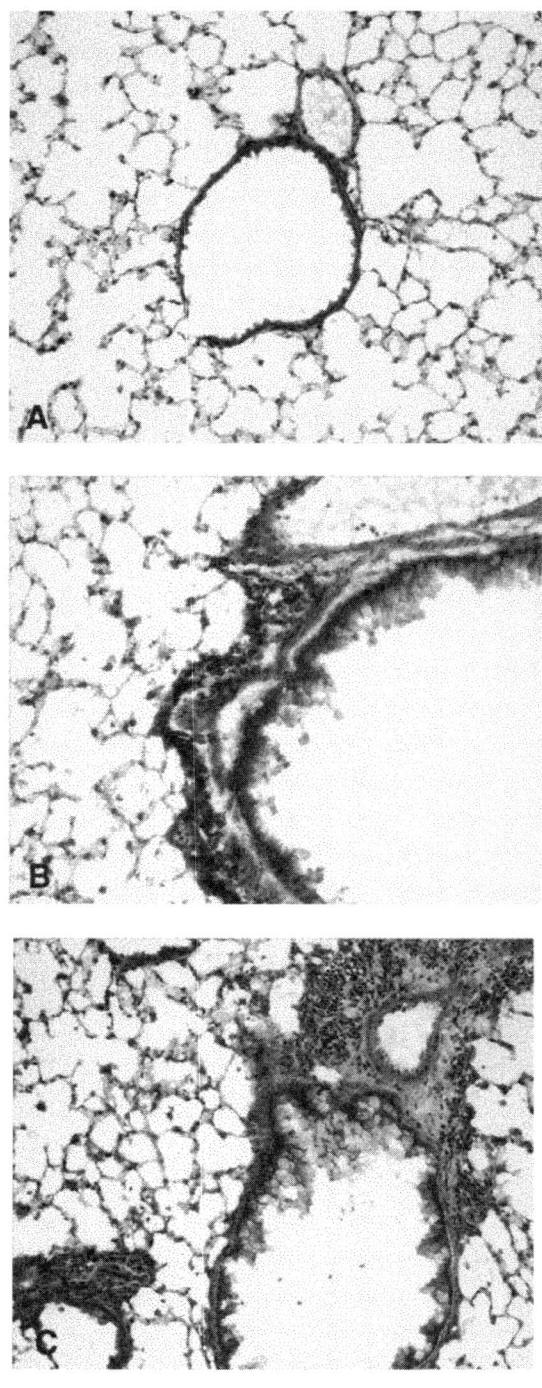

In this study, gene chip profiling of an established animal model of atopic asthma was used in order to characterize the molecular events underlying the acute and chronic inflammatory responses to allergen challenge. Protocols involving sensitization with and subsequent inhalation of ovalbumin (OVA) in BALB/c mice have been shown to recapitulate many of the features of human topic asthma.[9] The objectives of this study were:

1. to characterize the pathophysiological events involved in the early response to OVA challenge on a molecular level;

2. to characterize the ability of steroid treatment to diminish or abrogate the OVA-induced gene response to OVA challenge; and

3. to generate hypotheses regarding potentially novel molecular targets for pharmacological intervention using Affymetrix gene chip profiling methodologies and databases.

RESULTS AND DISCUSSION

Study Design

To mimic atopic asthma, a method of immunization was chosen which has previously been shown to generate serum IgE in BALB/c mice, which display an inclination to generate Th2 cytokines. To generate cell infiltration in the lung, immune mice were challenged by the airway mucosal route (with Ag or vehicle alone) for seven days, and lungs were sampled at different time points to reflect response to acute and chronic OVA challenge (see FIGURE 1). Naïve lungs served as the baseline control in the absence of any manipulation, and immunized but not challenged lungs as an internal control for the effect of systemic immunization on lung gene expression. For each day, two time points (3h and 18h), post challenge were chosen to cover gene expression with different kinetics (FIG. 1).

FIGURE 2. Histological analysis of murine lungs following acute and chronic OVA challenge. For tissue collection and histology, mice were anesthetized with CO_2 inhalation 5 min prior to tissue collection. For each mouse, the lungs were infused via the trachea with 4% formaldehyde/PBS, at a rate of 1.8 mL/min, until all pulmonary lobes were fully inflated. The lungs were tied off at the trachea, removed, and fixed in the same fixative for an additional 2 h at 4°C on a shaker. Subsequently, the lungs were rinsed twice in cold PBS, then trimmed. The lung samples were cryoprotected by immersion in 30% sucrose/PBS for 4 h at 4°C, on a shaker, followed by immersion in 1:1 OCT:30% sucrose/PBS overnight at 4°C, on a shaker. The cryoprotected lung samples were then placed in OCT, frozen on ground dry ice, and stored at −80°C. The frozen blocks were sectioned at −20°C to obtain seven-micron thick sections. Sections were stained with H&E, utilizing Harris's Hematoxylin (Poly-Scientific R&D Corporation) and Eosin (Poly-Scientific R&D Corporation). The H&E stained lung slides were then evaluated using light microscopy and representative digital images of histopathological changes were captured. Images shown are of mouse lung, frozen section, H&E, 200× magnification. **A:** Day 1, 3 h post OVA challenge. No inflammatory infiltrate or other histopathological changes are present. **B:** Day 4, 3 h post OVA challenge. Perivascular and peribronchiolar infiltrate of predominantly polymorphonuclear cells is present. Note hyperplasia of bronchiolar epithelial mucous cells. **C:** Day 7, 18 h post OVA challenge. Perivascular and peribronchiolar infiltrate of mixed inflammatory cells and bronchiolar epithelial mucous cell hyperplasia are present.

Gene profiling was performed on total lung RNA samples obtained from the respective treatment groups. Corrections for signal and noise of intensity values, and fold change calculations, were performed with a P-fold Bayesian model as previously described.[10] For each time point, the following fold changes in gene expression were calculated from the median of quadruplicate biological replicates: (1) OVA versus PBS challenge, and (2) OVA+DEX versus OVA treatment.

Phenotypic Characterization of OVA- versus PBS-Challenged Mice

Histological evaluation of sections from lungs of challenged and normal mice revealed no detectable inflammatory cell influx or phenotypic changes compared to PBS on day 1, three hours post OVA challenge and only a mild granulocytic influx after 18h on the same day (see FIGURE 2 and TABLE 1). In contrast, lung sections from mice challenged for four and seven days were characterized by perivascular and peribronchiolar infiltrate of mixed inflammatory cells and hyperplasia of bronchiolar epithelial mucous cells (FIG. 2).

Expression of Inflammatory Cytokine Expression in Lungs of OVA- versus PBS-Challenged Mice

As measured by real-time PCR with specific primer/probe sets, pulmonary expression of the Th2 cytokines IL-4 and IL-13, was significantly induced ($1,000\times$ and $15\times$, respectively, see FIGURE 3, *upper panel*) on day 1, three hours following acute OVA challenge. This response was maintained during the seven days of the study. The greater OVA-mediated upregulation of IL-4 and IL-13 mRNA following one-week challenge may reflect influx of inflammatory cells, whereas the early response reflects activation of resident cells. The cellular source of these Th2 cytokines, previously believed to be expressed exclusively in T cells, is unclear but may include mast cells, bronchial epithelium, or bronchus-associated lymphoid tissue (BALT). Expression of eotaxin-2, but not RANTES was also markedly induced, especially following chronic challenge. IFNγ and MUC5AC were induced only after chronic challenge (FIG. 3, *lower panel*). The marked mucin expression only after chronic challenge response may reflect airway phenotypic changes such as epithelial cell metaplasia (presence of goblet cells) and is likely driven by IL-13 (11;12). Late IFN-γ induction could be involved in resolution of inflammation as has been recently suggested.[13] Overall these results indicate that the transcriptional responses post OVA challenge in this mouse model may recapitulate phenotypic changes believed to be important in human allergic asthma. Of these genes however, only eotaxin-2 was identified as being regulated following analysis of the microarray data, highlighting the potential for false negative results with the latter technology.

Microarray analysis revealed that more genes were upregulated at early (3h) rather than later (18h) time points on each day of challenge; i.e., that induction of gene expression by aerosol antigen challenge is rapid, but that mRNA half-life of many of the induced genes is relatively short. The number of genes upregulated by OVA challenge tripled from 20 at day 1, 3h to 60 genes at day 4, 3h. Moreover, five times as many genes were upregulated by chronic (7 day) challenge compared to acute (1 day) challenge.

Because one of the aims of this study was to generate potential molecular targets for pharmacological intervention in asthma, the distribution of regulated genes among genes encoding so-called targetable classes of proteins was examined (see TABLE 2). Genes of all classes were regulated at least twofold, with numbers depending on the P-value criterion used.

The most highly regulated gene of any class was gob-5, thought to encode a calcium-activated chloride channel, consistent with a previous report which identified this gene by suppression subtractive hybridization (SSH) in a similar model.[14]

TABLE 1. Semiquantitative evaluation of inflammatory infiltrate following acute and chronic OVA challenge

Microscopic Observations—Lung	Day 1		Day 4		Day 7	
$n = 5$ animals per time point examined	3h	18h	3h	18h	3h	18h
Infiltrate, PMN, perivascular						
Minimal		4				
Mild		—				
Infiltrate, PMN, interstitial/alveolar						
Minimal	1	3				
Mild	—	—				
Infiltrate, mixed cells, perivascular		3	—	—	—	
Minimal		3	—	—	—	
Mild		2	5	5	4	
Moderate						1
Infiltrate, mixed cells, interstitial/alveolar						
Minimal			5	1	—	
Mild			—	4	5	
Hyperplasia, bronchiolar epithelium						
Minimal			4	4	3	4
Mild			—	1	2	1
Hyperplasia, goblet cells, bronchiolar						
Minimal			2	2	3	4
Mild			—	1	2	1
Multinucleated giant cells						
Minimal				3	4	3
Mild				—	1	2
Subpleural mixed cell infiltrate						
Minimal				—	1	1
Mild				1	1	2

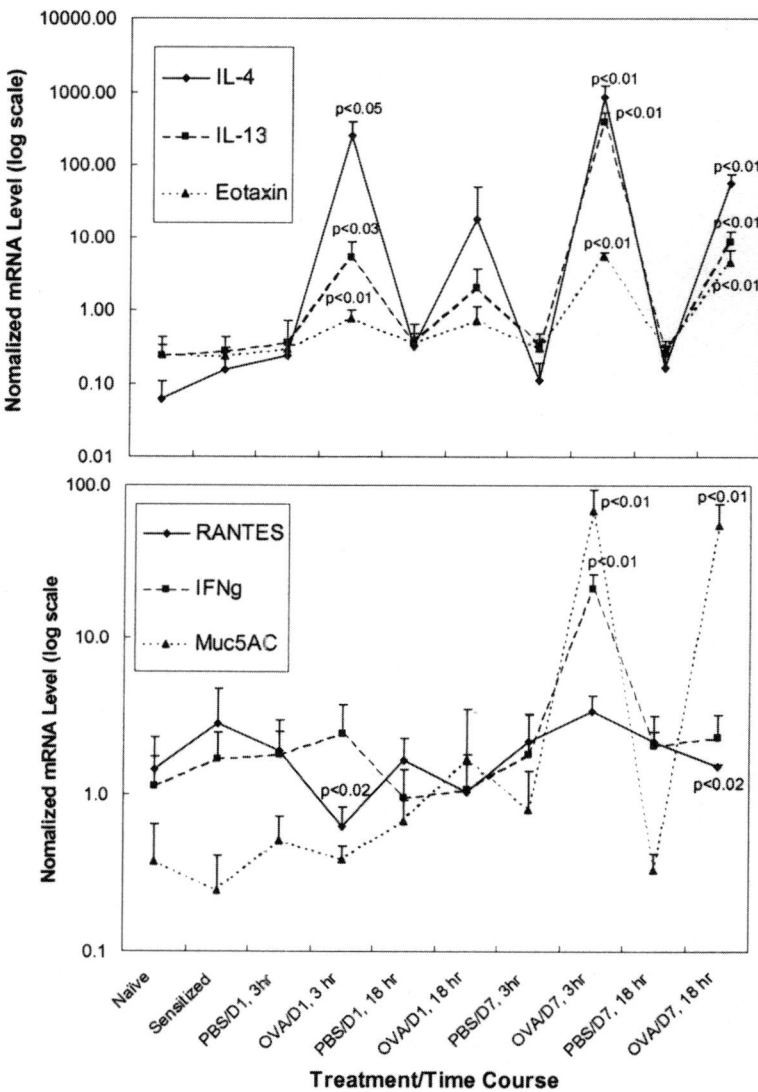

FIGURE 3. Real-time PCR quantitation of marker gene expression in murine lung following acute and chronic OVA challenge. Taqman®-PCR was used to characterize the effects of OVA challenge on pulmonary expression of indicated marker genes in the murine balb/c model. Lung total RNA was subjected to reverse transcription and Taqman PCR with primers and probes specific to targets indicated in figures. Gene expression was normalized to GAPDH. Error bars represent S.D. of $n = 4$ mice. P values represent comparison of OVA- to PBS-challenged mice.

TABLE 2. Distribution of protein family classes among regulated genes

Protein Family	OVA/PBS Any time point			
	up ($r \geq 2$) (no P value criterion)	down ($r \leq 0.5$) (no P value criterion)	up ($r \geq 2$, $P < 0.1$)	down ($r \leq 0.5$, $P < 0.1$)
Adhesion	26	8	14	2
Cytokine	28	16	16	5
GPCR	11	18	4	7
Protein kinase	16	11	5	4
Nuclear receptor	2	5	1	3
Phosphatase	4	4	0	2
Phospholipase/ Phosphodiesterase	4	1	3	0
Protease	16	10	9	3
Transporter-ion-channel	15	10	5	6
Unclassified	286	244	132	89
Total	409	330	190	122

Several proteases of different classes but with potential elastolytic activity were also regulated. The most highly upregulated protease was matrix metalloproteinase-12 (MMP-12; macrophage elastase), induced at day 4 by OVA, and stimulated as much as 13-fold following chronic challenge (see FIGURE 4, *upper panel*). Upregulation of this gene by OVA was corrected with dexamethasone (FIG. 4, *upper panel*). Although MMP-12 has been implicated in alveolar degradation in COPD[15,16] and acute lung injury,[17] its potential role in asthma has not been studied. In addition to MMPs, expression of cysteine proteases was stimulated by OVA. Though not as strongly induced as MMP-12, upregulation of cathepsin S (CatS) by OVA challenge (FIG. 4 *lower panel*) was confirmed by real-time PCR (data not shown). CatS overexpression was only partially counter-regulated by dexamethasone following chronic challenge (FIG. 4, *lower panel*).

In order to rapidly assess the potential tissue distribution of regulated genes of interest, a database was constructed following hybridization of RNAs from various murine tissues to the gene chip. Examination of the tissue distribution of cathepsin S (see FIGURE 5) revealed strong expression in lymphoid tissues and lung, with relatively little expression in heart, muscle, kidney, and central nervous system tissues. This distribution is consistent with the known role of cathepsin S in antigen presentation.[18]

In addition to proteolysis, TABLE 3 indicates that cellular processes and responses potentially implicated in the pathophysiology of asthma, such as inflammation, remodeling, increase in airway hyperreactivity, and epithelial hypertrophy and hyperplasia, are reflected in pulmonary gene regulation in response to OVA challenge.

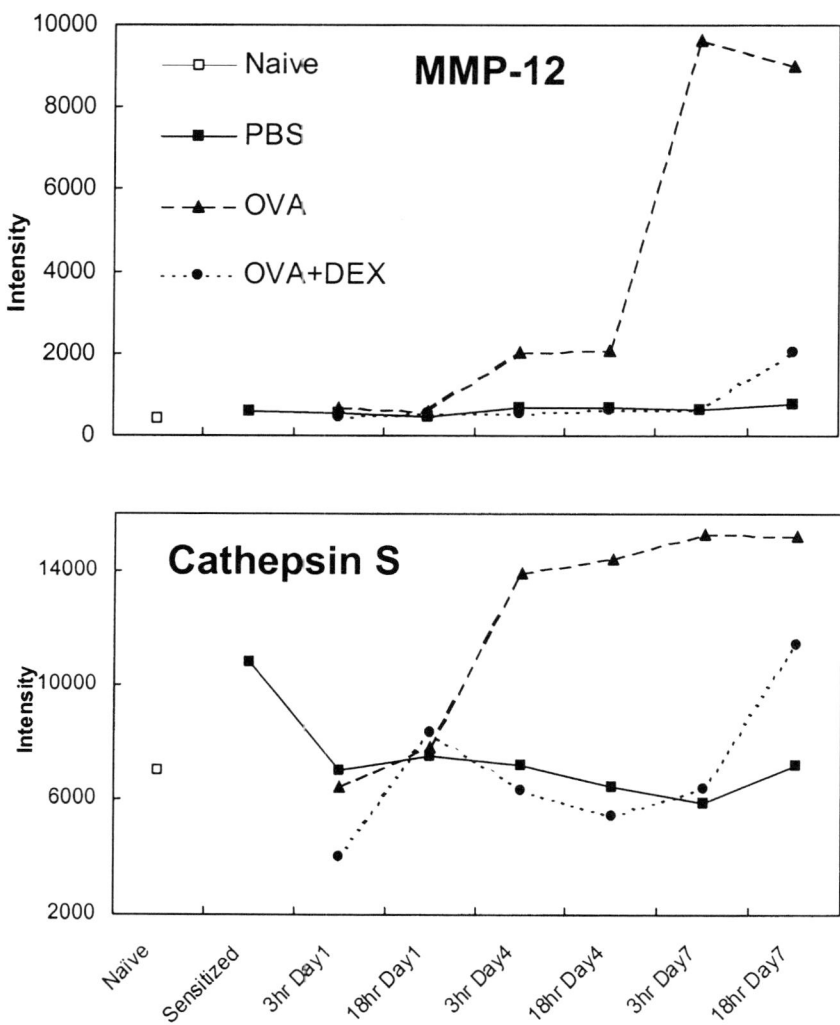

FIGURE 4. MMP-12 and cathepsin S upregulation by chronic and acute OVA challenge. Intensity (*y-axis*) values represent signals from microarray analysis of total lung RNA from $n = 4$ mice as described in FIGURE 1. Intensity values less than 700 were assigned absence calls by Affymetrix software.

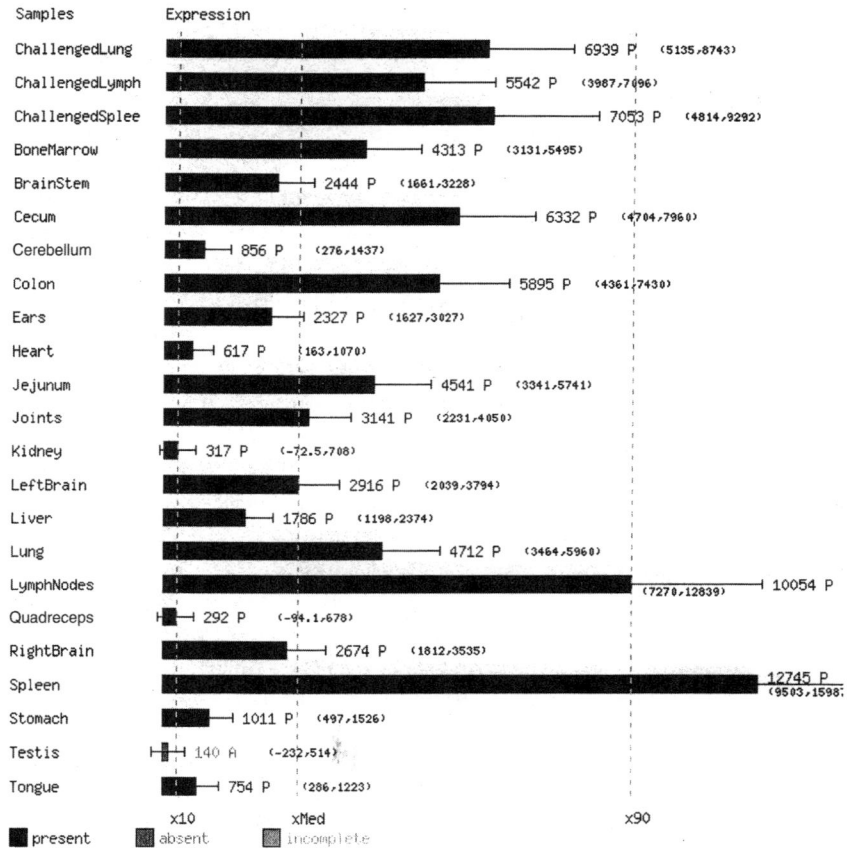

FIGURE 5. Cathepsin S expression in murine tissue expression database. *Error bars* represent range of values.

SUMMARY/CONCLUSIONS

1. The results of transcriptional gene profiling demonstrate that antigen challenge can induce changes in pulmonary gene expression prior to the initiation of inflammatory cell trafficking. Identification of cell types expressing genes regulated following acute challenge may elucidate the early pathophysiological events in this murine model of allergic asthma.

2. Induction/upregulation of several secreted proteases during OVA challenge (TABLE 2) suggests a role for elastolysis in the pathogenesis of airway hyperreactivity in this model.

3. In the context of allergic airway disease, transcriptional profiling has the potential to generate novel hypotheses regarding molecular targets amenable to pharmacological intervention.

TABLE 3. Genes upregulated following acute OVA challenge

Family	Upregulated at least twofold Day 1, 3 h	Fifty genes with highest fold regulation Day 7, 3 h
Adhesion	2	7
Antiinflammatory		1
Apoptosis/cell cycle	1	1
Cytokine	4	6
Chemokine receptor	0	1
Complement	0	2
Energy Metabolism	1	2
Extracellular Matrix	1	0
Ig	1	4
Ion transport	1	4
Metaplasia	2	3
Misc/unknown	2	12
Protease	1	3
Remodeling	1	
Signaling	1	1
Stress response	2	1
Transcription	3	2

Genes upregulated at least twofold are described. Only 23 genes were upregulated at Day1, 3 h with $P < 0.1$ (left data column). Right column contains 50 genes with highest fold upregulated at Day 7, 3 h.

REFERENCES

1. FAHY, J.V. 2001. Remodeling of the airway epithelium in asthma. Am. J. Respir. Crit Care Med. **164:** S46–S51.
2. ROMAGNANI, S. 2001. T-cell responses in allergy and asthma. Curr. Opin. Allergy Clin. Immunol. **1:** 73–78.
3. GARLISI, C.G., A. FALCONE, T.T. KUNG, et al. 1995. T cells are necessary for Th2 cytokine production and eosinophil accumulation in airways of antigen-challenged allergic mice. Clin. Immunol. Immunopathol. **75:** 75–83.
4. GAVETT, S.H., X. CHEN, F. FINKELMAN & M. WILLS-KARP. 1994. Depletion of murine CD4$^+$ T lymphocytes prevents antigen-induced airway hyperreactivity and pulmonary eosinophilia. Am. J. Respir. Cell Mol. Biol. **10:** 587–593.
5. WISE, J.T., T.J. BAGINSKI & J.L. MOBLEY. 1999. An adoptive transfer model of allergic lung inflammation in mice is mediated by CD4$^+$CD62LlowCD25$^+$ T cells. J. Immunol. **162:** 5592–5600.
6. ROBINSON, D.S., Q. HAMID, S. YING, et al. 1992. Predominant TH2-like bronchoalveolar T-lymphocyte population in atopic asthma. N. Engl. J. Med. **326:** 298–304.

7. ROMAGNANI, S. 2002. Cytokines and chemoattractants in allergic inflammation. Mol. Immunol. **38:** 881–885.
8. SCHWARTZ, R.S. 2002. A new element in the mechanism of asthma. N. Engl. J. Med. **346:** 857–858.
9. LLOYD, C.M., J.A. GONZALO, A.J. COYLE & J.C. GUTIERREZ-RAMOS. 2001. Mouse models of allergic airway disease. Adv. Immunol. **77:** 263–295.
10. THEILHABER, J., S. BUSHNELL, A. JACKSON & R. FUCHS. 2001. Bayesian estimation of fold-changes in the analysis of gene expression: the PFOLD algorithm. J. Comput. Biol. **8:** 585–614.
11. ZHU, Z., R.J. HOMER, Z. WANG, et al. 1999. Pulmonary expression of interleukin-13 causes inflammation, mucus hypersecretion, subepithelial fibrosis, physiologic abnormalities, and eotaxin production. J. Clin. Invest. **103:** 779–788.
12. SHIM, J.J., K. DABBAGH, I.F. UEKI, et al. 2001. IL-13 induces mucin production by stimulating epidermal growth factor receptors and by activating neutrophils. Am. J. Physiol. Lung Cell. Mol. Physiol. **280:** L134–L140.
13. SHI, Z.O., M.J. FISCHER, G.T. DE SANCTIS, et al. 2002. IFN-gamma, but not Fas, mediates reduction of allergen-induced mucous cell metaplasia by inducing apoptosis. J.Immunol. **168:** 4764–4771.
14. NAKANISHI, A., S. MORITA, H. IWASHITA, et al. 2001. Role of gob-5 in mucus overproduction and airway hyperresponsiveness in asthma. Proc. Natl. Acad. Sci. USA **98:** 5175–5180.
15. HAUTAMAKI, R.D., D.K. KOBAYASHI, R.M. SENIOR & S.D. SHAPIRO. 1997. Requirement for macrophage elastase for cigarette smoke-induced emphysema in mice. Science **277:** 2002–2004.
16. WANG, Z., T. ZHENG, Z. ZHU, et al. 2000. Interferon gamma induction of pulmonary emphysema in the adult murine lung. J. Exp. Med. **192:** 1587–1600.
17. WARNER, R.L., C.S. LEWIS, L. BELTRAN, et al. 2001. The role of metalloelastase in immune complex-induced acute lung injury. Am. J. Pathol. 158:2139–2144.
18. RIESE, R.J. & H.A. CHAPMAN. 2000. Cathepsins and compartmentalization in antigen presentation. Curr. Opin. Immunol. **12:** 107–113.

Unlocking the Mysteries of Virus–Host Interactions

Does Functional Genomics Hold the Key?

MARCUS J. KORTH AND MICHAEL G. KATZE

Department of Microbiology and Washington National Primate Research Center, University of Washington, Seattle, Washington 98195-8070, USA

ABSTRACT: The interactions between viruses and the cells they infect are complex and multifaceted. While viruses strive to usurp cellular functions to their advantage, the cell strives to thwart these efforts by mounting a variety of defensive responses. These responses may include the induction of interferon, stress response, or apoptotic pathways, all of which are accompanied by changes in gene expression. Some viruses consistently win this tug of war, whereas others succumb to cellular defense mechanisms. The viral and cellular factors that determine the outcome are for the most part still unknown. With the advent of functional genomics, potent new technologies are now available to probe the complexities of virus-host interactions in ever increasing depth and detail. We describe here our efforts to use microarrays, proteomics, and bioinformatics to focus in on the changes in gene expression and protein production that occur in a virus-infected cell and to use these technologies to unlock the mysteries of virus-host interactions.

KEYWORDS: simian immunodeficiency virus; hepatitis C virus; influenza virus; microarray; proteomics

Viruses are amazingly diverse. Some encode only a few genes, others encode hundreds. Some are little more than a nuisance, others are terrifying in their capacity to inflict disease and death. All too often, we have little or no ability to stop them once an infection has occurred. What is it about a given virus, or the cellular response to its presence, that determines the course of infection? Do all viruses elicit a common response, which varies in its effectiveness depending on the virus? Or, do certain viruses provoke a unique cellular response or perhaps even manipulate the response to their own advantage? Knowing the answers to these questions may yield many benefits, including new diagnostic techniques or the identification of novel targets for antiviral therapies. Now, the tools needed to answer these questions are also available. Microarrays, proteomics, and advances in information technologies all promise to deliver exciting new insights into the complex interaction between viruses and the cells they infect. In this article, we will provide an overview of our efforts to apply the technologies of functional genomics to the study of virus–host interactions. We will include a description of our experimental systems, a discussion of our

Address for correspondence: Michael G. Katze, Department of Microbiology, University of Washington, Box 358070, Seattle, WA 98195-8070. Voice: 206-732-6135; fax: 206-732-6056.
honey@u.washington.edu

data management and analysis scheme, and some thoughts on how to best exploit these powerful new technologies.

EXPERIMENTAL SYSTEMS FOR VIRUS–HOST INTERACTIONS

Influenza Virus

Influenza virus has been a mainstay of our research for over 18 years. This fascinating virus uses a number of clever strategies to overcome the innate immune response and to use the cellular protein synthesis machinery to its advantage. Naturally, we were eager to begin using microarrays to further our understanding of this virus. In our initial studies,[1] we infected HeLa cells with wild-type virus or with a heat-inactivated virus that was unable to replicate. We then examined cellular gene expression at four and eight hours postinfection. This strategy gave us the opportunity to profile the cellular transcriptional response to infection at multiple time points, and to determine whether viral replication was required for changes in gene expression. From these analyses, we observed that influenza virus infection alters the expression of numerous cellular genes, including genes involved in transcriptional regulation, growth-factor signaling, mRNA processing, protein synthesis, and protein degradation. The majority of these changes occur late in infection and represent a decrease in gene expression. Although to a lesser extent, we also observed changes in gene expression in cells infected with heat-inactivated virus, demonstrating that early events in the viral life cycle, such as attachment or entry, affect intracellular signaling pathways that result in changes in gene expression. In particular, we observed that infection with heat-inactivated virus results in the upregulation of several members of the metallothionein gene family, the increased expression of which may represent a protective response to virus-induced oxidative stress.

More recently, we have begun to capitalize on the ability to engineer recombinant forms of influenza virus, which has allowed us to focus on the effects of specific viral genes.[2] Using a reverse genetics technology, Dr. García-Sastre and colleagues have engineered viruses that lack the NS1 gene,[3] or which contain the NS1 gene from the 1918 pandemic strain,[4] a virus that killed over 500,000 Americans. The NS1 gene is of particular interest, because of the considerable evidence that NS1 functions as an interferon antagonist. When we infected a human lung epithelial cell line with influenza virus lacking the NS1 gene, we observed a significant increase in the expression of genes involved in interferon signaling. This increase was greater than that observed in cells infected with the wild-type virus, indicating that NS1 alters the cellular response to infection in a fashion that is consistent with a role in mediating resistance to the interferon response. Interestingly, there was no increase in interferon-pathway gene expression in cells infected with a virus containing the NS1 gene from the 1918 pandemic strain. This finding points to the possibility that the extreme virulence of the 1918 virus may have been due in part to the ability of its NS1 protein to act as a particularly efficient interferon antagonist. Given the interest in understanding the virulence of the 1918 pandemic strain, we are also examining the cellular response to recombinant influenza viruses containing the glycoproteins HA or NA from the 1918 virus. These studies, together with an examination of the virulence of these strains in animal models, should give us new insights into influenza virus pathogenesis.

Although the majority of our influenza virus studies have focused on the transcriptional response to infection, it is important to remember that this virus also has a significant impact on mRNA translation. An extra degree of caution must therefore be taken when interpreting the biological relevance of the transcriptional changes that occur in response to infection, since such changes may not be accompanied by similar changes in protein production. Clearly, the addition of proteomic analyses will eventually provide a much clearer picture of the events that occur in an influenza virus–infected cell. However, we also have found that microarrays can be used as a tool to examine changes in the translation state of cellular mRNAs. We are now combining polysome fractionation with cDNA microarray analyses in an attempt to identify cellular mRNAs that are selectively recruited to polyribosomes following infection. One goal of this approach is to determine whether such mRNAs contain specific sequence elements that contribute to their selective translation. In particular, we are interested in determining whether GRSF-1, a cellular mRNA-binding protein, plays a role in this process. We previously demonstrated that GRSF-1 specifically interacts with conserved sequences in the 5' UTR of influenza virus mRNAs and that it specifically stimulates translation of a viral 5' UTR-driven template in a cell-free translation system.[5] Our microarray studies may therefore help to determine whether GRSF-1 plays a similar role in the control of cellular mRNA translation.

Hepatitis C Virus

Our original interest in hepatitis C virus (HCV) stemmed from our research into the various strategies used by viruses to evade the interferon-mediated antiviral response. These efforts led to our demonstration that the HCV nonstructural 5A protein (NS5A) is a potent inhibitor of the interferon-induced protein kinase, PKR,[6] and that NS5A alters specific signal transduction pathways by binding to growth factor receptor-bound protein 2 (Grb2),[7] a cellular adapter protein that mediates growth factor–induced signaling. We have now expanded our studies of HCV to include microarray analyses of a broad range of HCV experimental systems, including NS5A-expressing cell lines, the HCV replicon system,[8] and cultured primary human fetal hepatocytes transfected with HCV RNA. Given the inability to culture this virus, these experimental systems provide several alternative approaches to study HCV replication and its impact on cellular processes.

Despite the many benefits of using *in vitro* systems—including abundant samples, defined variables, and ease of experimental manipulation—it is ultimately necessary to profile gene expression patterns in samples derived from HCV-infected individuals. Although such studies are fraught with challenges, they provide an essential look at gene expression changes in the setting of an actual human infection. In our first attempt at working with human samples, we have undertaken an extensive analysis of gene expression changes in tumors derived from patients with HCV-associated hepatocellular carcinoma. In these studies, we are comparing matched tumor and nontumor samples and evaluating observed changes in gene expression against similar comparisons of normal and cirrhotic liver. We also have the advantage of being able to correlate gene expression changes with patient clinical characteristics. This has allowed us to perform a variety of data analyses in which we are attempting to identify gene expression changes that could serve as novel markers of hepatocellular carcinoma and which could facilitate early detection of this malignancy.

In our latest endeavor, we have joined forces with Dr. Robert Carithers, Jr. and the liver transplantation group at the University of Washington to examine gene expression profiles in liver biopsies obtained from patients who have undergone liver transplantation due to HCV-associated liver disease. Chronic HCV infection is the most common indication for liver transplantation in the United States and Europe. The vast majority of patients with active HCV infection at the time of liver transplantation develop high-titer HCV viremia after the procedure. A few patients develop rapidly progressive disease, but most have mild degrees of liver injury, and at least a third show no biochemical or histological evidence of liver injury in the first 10 years after transplantation.[9] Thus, the outcome of HCV infection in liver transplant recipients resembles the clinical course of HCV infection in the nontransplant setting. By examining gene expression profiles in serial biopsies taken from transplant patients, we hope to increase our understanding of the basic relationships between HCV replication and liver disease.

NONHUMAN PRIMATES AND SIMIAN IMMUNODEFICIENCY VIRUS

Although nonhuman primates are used extensively in biomedical research, surprisingly little effort has been made to apply the technologies of functional genomics to research using these animals. One reason for this is the nearly complete absence of genomic information for nonhuman primate species. To begin to overcome this limitation, we have initiated a large-scale effort to increase the number of nonhuman primate nucleotide sequences available in public databases. We are focusing our efforts on the rhesus macaque (*Macaca mulatta*), because of its widespread use as a model for human physiology and disease and because of its importance as an animal model for AIDS.

As an initial step, we have constructed cDNA libraries from several rhesus macaque tissues. These libraries serve as a source of cDNA clones for expressed sequence tag (EST) sequencing, which is being performed through collaboration with Amersham Biosciences (Sunnyvale, CA). Our goal is to generate over 50,000 ESTs, which will be deposited into GenBank and used for the construction of macaque DNA microarrays. We anticipate that these genomic resources will be useful for a wide range of research endeavors, including studies aimed at providing insight into the evolutionary relationship between the human and macaque genomes. From our own vantage point, we see these resources as a significant opportunity to further our interest in virus-host interactions, specifically with regard to immunodeficiency virus pathogenesis.

As the most widely used animal in AIDS research, the rhesus macaque has greatly facilitated studies of immunodeficiency virus pathogenesis, antiretroviral therapy, and vaccine development. Still, despite the widespread use of this animal model, our understanding of the molecular events that occur during the course of infection, therapy, or vaccination and subsequent challenge remains limited. Through the technologies of functional genomics, we now have the capabilities to characterize and explore this model system in ways never before possible. We are currently working to develop experimental systems to profile cellular gene expression changes in response to simian immunodeficiency virus (SIV) infection. We have begun with analyses of SIV-infected human T-cell lines, and intend to progress to SIV-infected macaque peripheral blood mononuclear cells and eventually to samples derived from SIV-infected animals. By cataloging the changes in cellular gene expression that occur during SIV infection, we hope to greatly expand our understanding of the use of the rhesus macaque as a model in AIDS research and to gain new insights into immunodeficiency virus infection and pathogenesis in the human population.

DATA MANAGEMENT AND ANALYSIS

As our use of microarrays has extended to an increasing number of experimental systems, we have found ourselves buried in an avalanche of data. We view this as an enviable problem, since the more experimental data that can be compared the greater the likelihood that meaningful information will be obtained. But more and more data also comes with a price. It is difficult to manage and mine this amount of data, which leads us into the realm of data management and analysis.

Image Analysis

The first step in data analysis is to analyze the scanned microarray images for differentially expressed genes. This step is critical, since appropriate statistical analyses must be applied to accurately detect changes in gene expression. Although many commercial software packages for microarray image analysis are available, only a few provide methods for estimating error in the data. This makes it difficult to sort meaningful data from the reams of numbers produced in a typical microarray experiment. Our spot finding and image analysis is done using the Spot-On software package developed by Dr. Roger Bumgarner at the University of Washington. The image analysis component, Spot-On Image, processes images to extract intensities in each color, measures local background for each color, and estimates error in both local background and the ratio. The image analysis process produces nonnormalized expression ratios that are uncorrected for labeling, fluorescence detection efficiencies, or relative mRNA concentrations. The second component, Spot-On Unite, normalizes the data using a unique algorithm that corrects for the nonlinearity of two-color data and analyzes replicate data to produce mean ratios and error estimates across multiple measurements. The third component, Spot-On Select, selects genes that are differentially expressed to a statistically significant degree. This software has significantly enhanced our ability to obtain statistically meaningful data from our microarray experiments.

Expression Array Manager

Because microarray analyses typically generate tens of thousands of measurements for each experiment, effective data storage and management are essential. To manage the huge amounts of data generated from multiple array experiments, our bioinformatics group has developed a sophisticated gene expression database, which we call Expression Array Manager. Expression Array Manager consists of an Oracle database, a web server and servlet engine, a collection of software tools for uploading data to the database, and additional software for uploading data from Expression Array

Manager to a commercial data analysis system (described below). These tools can also be used to load data into public gene expression databases once such repositories become available. An important feature of Expression Array Manager is that it allows us to archive all information required by the proposed Minimum Information About a Microarray Experiment (MIAME) standards,[10] including experimental and array design, the samples used and the method of extract preparation, hybridization procedures and parameters, the raw image files, image analysis data, and normalization controls. This type of information is essential for ensuring that the data can be properly interpreted, independently verified, and available for comparison with other entries in the database. Once a project has been completed and the results published, all data outlined in the MIAME standards can be made available to the public through the Expression Array Manager Web site (http://www.expression.washington.edu/public).

Similarly, researchers in our laboratory access Expression Array Manager through their Web browser, from which they are able to register and organize RNA preparations, experiments, projects, and so on, and to load image analysis data obtained using Spot-On. The ability to integrate our image analysis and laboratory information management system is a key feature of this database, as is the ability to extend the database to accommodate other types of data. In this regard, we are working to extend Expression Array Manager to include proteomics data and to develop tools to generate integrated sets of protein and gene expression measurements. For higher order data analysis functions, experimental data are selected for subsequent automated loading from Expression Array Manager into a separate commercial database, described below.

Higher Order Analyses

A wide variety of individual software tools and algorithms are available in the public domain for the analysis of gene expression data. However, it is difficult to integrate these tools with one another, and working with data from a large number of experiments quickly becomes cumbersome. To get around these limitations, we have acquired access to the Rosetta Resolver System (Rosetta Biosoftware, Kirkland, WA), an enterprise system that combines advanced analysis software, a high-capacity database, and high-performance server hardware to facilitate the storage, retrieval, and analysis of large amounts of gene expression data.

A key feature of Resolver is that it has rigorous error modeling and calculates accurate P-values and error bars for every gene expression measurement. This error modeling is carried throughout the system's analysis tools, adding greater predictive power to the analyses. The system contains a variety of clustering algorithms, including agglomerative, divisive, K-means, K-medians, and self-organizing maps, as well as an assortment of clustering analysis visualization tools. Particularly useful is the Rosetta Array Search Tool, which can be used to search the database for expression patterns similar to an expression pattern of interest. For example, if a particular gene expression profile is observed in cells infected with influenza virus, it is a relatively straightforward process to query the database and determine if similar profiles are found in cells infected with other types of viruses. The more comprehensive the database, the more valuable this type of tool becomes.

We should note that Resolver and Expression Array Manager each require a significant infrastructure of highly specialized personnel and high-end computer resources. Our research group now includes a full-time System Administrator, a Database Administrator, and a number of software developers and bioinformatics specialists. Our computer resources are also substantial, including two Sun Enterprise 6500 systems and three Sun Enterprise 4500 systems, which are connected to a 4.5-terabyte RAID (Redundant Array of Independent Disks) system for data storage and are which are designed to provide fail-over file service. All data are backed up daily to a DLT tape robot. Although microarrays themselves are becoming ever more affordable, and their use is spreading to a growing number of laboratories, the difficulties and complexities of data management and analysis will remain an obstacle for many research groups.

A COMPREHENSIVE DATABASE OF VIRUS-HOST INTERACTIONS

In our first foray into global gene expression analysis, we compared cellular gene expression patterns in mock-infected and HIV-1–infected cells at two and three days postinfection.[11] Not surprisingly, we identified a number of differentially expressed genes, and this limited time course provided some insight into the temporal changes in gene expression. We quickly realized, however, that a single study with limited variables provides little opportunity for in-depth analysis. The best you can hope for is to pull from your list of differentially expressed genes some clue as to which cellular pathways are altered in response to infection. However, even this can be difficult, as all first-time users of microarrays quickly discover. How then, can we best use the tools of functional genomics to our advantage?

Most major advances in science result from the accumulation of knowledge obtained over time by many investigators using a variety of experimental approaches. Similarly, despite the tremendous data-generating power of microarrays and proteomics, a single experiment (or even series of experiments) is unlikely to yield truly significant advances in our understanding of the dynamics of virus-host interactions. Rather, we believe the only way to exploit the full power of functional genomics is to develop a comprehensive database of gene expression and proteomics data derived from a wide range of experimental systems. This should include data obtained from experiments using many different viruses, both *in vitro* and *in vivo*, and from humans and animal models. Only with such a database will it be possible to look at the "big picture" and determine whether a common cellular response to virus infection exists, or whether specific types of viruses elicit unique responses.

Although this article has focused on microarray analyses, we believe it is essential to also incorporate proteomics into our studies of virus-host interactions. Since mRNA translation rates or protein half-lives cannot be measured by microarrays, proteomics, with its focus on the systematic identification and quantification of proteins, is an essential component of a functional genomics approach. Protein analysis may be particularly important for studying virus-host interactions, since many viruses have well documented effects on cellular mRNA translation. Our work in this area is a collaborative effort with Dr. Ruedi Aebersold at the Institute for Systems Biology (Seattle, WA). Dr. Aebersold's group has developed a novel method for protein profiling, based on a new class of reagent termed the isotope-coded affinity tag (ICAT).[12] This method has the potential to identify and quantify most, if not all of the proteins present in a cell or tissue. The ability to obtain both gene expression and proteomic data from a given sample is an exciting prospect and should yield an important added dimension to our data analysis capabilities.

Where will all this lead? On a basic science level, to a clearer understanding of how cells respond to virus infection and how different viruses affect the response and its outcome. The wide diversity of viruses and their effects on the host promises that these studies will lead to many exciting discoveries. On a practical level, an understanding of the host response to specific viruses may lead to novel diagnostic techniques based on the "molecular signature" of a virus. This diagnostic potential has broad applications. For example, our studies of gene expression changes linked to HCV-associated hepatocellular carcinoma have pointed to several "marker genes," the expression of which may be diagnostic for the disease. An additional application that has garnered considerable interest of late is the potential of using microarrays as rapid-diagnostic tools to detect exposure to viral agents of bioterrorism. In this regard, we are working with Illumigen Biosciences, a Seattle-based biotechnology company, to examine the feasibility of diagnosing exposure to specific respiratory viruses based on gene expression profiling. Finally, a comprehensive database of virus-host interactions may lead to the identification of new viral or cellular gene targets for antiviral therapies. The identification of such targets is likely to be an important first step in developing drugs capable of acting against multiple members of a viral genus or family. The availability of broad-spectrum antivirals would clearly be of immense value. Although considerable work lies ahead, the tools of functional genomics promise to bring major advances to the field of virus-host interactions and to the diagnosis and treatment of viral diseases.

ACKNOWLEDGMENTS

We thank our many colleagues who have devoted considerable effort to building the research program described in this article. In particular, we note the contributions of Dr. Roger Bumgarner and Dr. Gary Geiss, who have been at the forefront of these efforts, and Jeff Furlong, the primary developer of Expression Array Manager. Funding in our laboratory is provided by National Institutes of Health awards AI22646, AI47304, AI48214, RR00166, and RR16354 and by Illumigen Biosciences, Seattle, Washington.

REFERENCES

1. GEISS, G.K., M.C. AN, R.E. BUMGARNER, et al. 2001. Global impact of influenza virus on cellular pathways is mediated by both replication-dependent and -independent events. J. Virol. **75:** 4321–4331.
2. GEISS, G.K., M. SALVATORE, T.M. TUMPEY, et al. 2002. Cellular transcriptional profiling in influenza A virus infected lung epithelial cells: the role of the nonstructural NS1 protein in the evasion of the host innate defense and its potential contribution to pandemic influenza. Proc. Natl. Acad. Sci. USA. **99:** 10736–10741.
3. GARCÍA-SASTRE, A., A. EGOROV, D. MATASSOV, et al. 1999. Influenza A virus lacking the NS1 gene replicates in interferon-deficient systems. Virology **252:** 324–330.

4. BASLER, C.F., A.H. REID, J.K. DYBING, et al. 2001. Sequence of the 1918 pandemic influenza virus nonstructural gene (NS) segment and characterization of recombinant viruses bearing the 1918 NS genes. Proc. Natl. Acad. Sci. USA **98:** 2746–2751.
5. PARK, Y.-W., J. WILUSZ & M.G. KATZE. 1999. Regulation of eukaryotic protein synthesis: selective influenza viral mRNA translation is mediated by the cellular RNA-binding protein GRSF-1. Proc. Natl. Acad. Sci. USA **96:** 6694–6699.
6. GALE, M., JR., M.J. KORTH, N.M. TANG, et al. 1997. Evidence that hepatitis C virus resistance to interferon is mediated through repression of the PKR protein kinase by the nonstructural 5A protein. Virology **230:** 217–227.
7. TAN, S.-L., H. NAKAO, Y. HE, et al. 1999. NS5A, a nonstructural protein of hepatitis C virus, binds growth factor receptor-bound protein 2 adaptor protein in a Src homology 3 domain/ligand-dependent manner and perturbs mitogenic signaling. Proc. Natl. Acad. Sci. USA **96:** 5533–5538.
8. LOHMANN, V., F. KÖRNER, J.-O. KOCH, et al. 1999. Replication of subgenomic hepatitis C virus RNAs in a hepatoma cell line. Science **285:** 110–113.
9. SHUHART, M.C., M.P. BRONNER, D.R. GRETCH, et al. 1997. Histological and clinical outcome after liver transplantation for hepatitis C. Hepatology **26:** 1646–1652.
10. BRAZMA, A., P. HINGAMP, J. QUACKENBUSH, et al. 2001. Minimum information about a microarray experiment (MIAME) toward standards for microarray data. Nature Genet. **29:** 365–371.
11. GEISS, G.K., R.E. BUMGARNER, M. AN, et al. 2000. Large-scale monitoring of host cell gene expression during HIV-1 infection using cDNA microarrays. Virology **266:** 8–16.
12. GYGI, S.P., B. RIST, S.A. GERBER, et al. 1999. Quantitative analysis of complex protein mixtures using isotope-coded affinity tags. Nature Biotechnol. **17:** 994–999.

Genetic Determinants of Coxsackievirus B3 Pathogenesis

BRUCE M. McMANUS,[a] BOBBY YANAGAWA,[a] NANA REZAI,[a] HONGLIN LUO,[a] LYDIA TAYLOR,[a] MARY ZHANG,[a] JANE YUAN,[a] JONATHAN BUCKLEY,[b] TIMOTHY TRICHE,[b] GEORGE SCHREINER,[c] AND DECHENG YANG[a]

[a]*UBC McDonald Research Laboratories/The iCAPTUR⁴E Center, Department of Pathology and Laboratory Medicine, St. Paul's Hospital/Providence Health Care-University of British Columbia, Canada*

[b]*Children's Hospital Los Angeles, Los Angeles, California, USA*

[c]*Scios Inc., Sunnyvale, California, USA*

ABSTRACT: The development of high throughput genomic and bioinformatic analysis tools, coupled with established molecular techniques, has allowed new insights into the pathogenesis of infectious diseases. In humans, coxsackievirus B3 (CVB3) is the primary etiological agent of viral myocarditis, an inflammatory disease process involving the heart muscle. Early host cellular survival and apoptotic mechanisms during viral infections, as well as immune events, affect myocarditis progression and outcome. Therefore, our laboratory has been keenly interested in infectomics, defined here as the transcriptional events of both virus and host. We first elucidated up- or downregulated transcriptional activities in CVB3-infected hearts by mRNA differential display. Further characterization of these regulated genes including Nip21, IP10, and IGTPase, and study of their role in CVB3-infection are underway. In further dissection of the stages of myocarditis—peak viremia, inflammatory infiltration and tissue repair—we used cDNA microarrays to probe differential gene expression in the myocardium following virus infection. Following virus infection, there are global decreases in metabolic and mitochondrial genes, increases in signaling genes and distinctive patterns in other functional groups. To establish early gene expression profiles in infected cells by themselves, we also used oligonucleotide arrays in an *in vitro* model of CVB3 infection. Notably, we have found increased expression of transcription factors *c-fos* and *c-jun* downstream of extracellular signal-related kinase, a pathway which is crucial for virus replication and pathogenesis. Our investigations based on gene profiling following CVB3 infection have thus far been fruitful in providing new experimental leads. High throughput genetic analysis has allowed us to simultaneously try on greater than 12,000 potential genetic "glass slippers." Our *in vitro* experimental plan has enabled us to chart prominent patterns of gene expression, analyzed by novel bioinformatic approaches, and to separate varied and potentially significant gene expression events.

KEYWORDS: genomic analysis; coxsackievirus B3; genetics; infectomics

Address for correspondence: Dr. Bruce M. McManus, UBC McDonald Research Laboratories/The iCAPTR⁴E Center, Department of Pathology and Laboratory Medicine, Rm. 292, 1081 Burrold St., St. Paul's Hospital/Providence Health Care-University of British Columbia, Canada, V6Z 146. Voice: 604-806-8586; fax: 604-806-8351.
  bmcmanus@mrl.ubc.ca

The combination of advances in both genomic analysis and bioinformatic screening tools has afforded potential for a greater understanding of complex multifactoral human diseases, such as cancer, atheromatous diseases and infections, including viral myocarditis. By screening the expression of thousands of genes simultaneously, followed with functional genomic validation, our groups and others are closing in on significant signaling events in disease settings. Expression levels of RNA and proteins are related to gene sequence variation. The concept of genetic uniqueness and its importance is of course not new. Even genomic manipulation was considered years ago. In 1928, preceding the discovery of the DNA double helix by 25 years, J.B.S. Haldane suggested that genetic modification may play a key role in the understanding of biology:

> Now, we know how the genes, or units which determine heredity, are arranged in the nucleus of the cell, and also about how big they are. If we magnified a hen's egg to the size of the world (which would make atoms rather larger than eggs and electrons barely visible) we could still get a gene into a room and probably on to a small table. But such magnification being impossible, the question [as to] how to alter a single gene without interfering with the others becomes serious, and some men have already spent their lives vainly on it; many more will.... (J.B.S. Haldane, *Possible Worlds*, 1928, pp.152–153.)

Indeed, Professor Haldane pioneered the studies of genetic susceptibility to infection relating high frequencies of thalassemia and human heterozygote selection against malaria.[1] Such observations laid a framework for the field of genomics when it finally arrived. The field of infectomics, defined as the genomics of microbial agents and target cells and their interactions, is now burgeoning.[2]

Contemporary infectomic analyses have catalogued transcriptional and proteomic events upon infection of host cells by a wide range of agents including human immunodeficiency virus,,[3] cytomegalovirus,[4] herpes simplex virus-1,[5] and hepatitis C virus.[6] Such studies are primarily focused on one fundamental issue in infectious diseases: how to comprehensively and integratively grasp the interactions between microbial pathogens and their hosts.

In our own pursuit of this question, we have focused on the infectomics of coxsackievirus B3 (CVB3) pathogenesis in the setting of viral infection of the heart and subsequent myocardial injury, inflammation, and repair. Utilizing a combination of strategies including differential display mRNA, cDNA arrays, and GeneChips® (Affymetrix, Inc., Santa Clara, CA), both in cell culture and *in vivo*, we are continuing to dissect out important host transcriptional events relevant to various stages of CVB3 pathogenesis, and in so doing we have greatly accelerated the hypothesis-driven research that follows.

Coxsackievirus B3 is an enterovirus in the picornavirus family and a major causative agent for diseases such as myocarditis, pancreatitis, and hepatitis. The CVB3 genome is a positive polarity, single-stranded RNA molecule approximately 7.4 kb in length that encodes for both structural and nonstructural proteins. Traditionally, the approach in the field of myocarditis, as in many infectious diseases, has focused primarily on the study of virus genomics, virulence factors and their direct injurious effects on host tissue architecture, organ function, and immune response. Also, owing to their smaller sizes, many microbial genomes, including that of coxsackieviruses have previously been sequenced.[7] Consequently, CVB3 studies have been in the "post-genomic" phase of investigation for almost 20 years. As mentioned earlier, the CVB3 genome is limited in size and complexity and all proteins are synthesized as a single virus polyprotein. Since the CVB3 RNA-dependent RNA polymerase has no proofreading function and thus a relatively high error rate (10^{-4}), it not only regulates virus replication, but also conveys mutations that ensure genomic variability in virus RNA populations. Phenotypes that reflect CVB3 mutations are reflected in the ability of a particular strain of virus, experimentally propagated in various cell lines, to rapidly diverge and develop preference for either one or both CVB3 receptors.[8] It would therefore be very informative to determine differences in host gene profiles in response to viruses that have a tropism for either the coxsackievirus and adenovirus receptor or the decay-accelerating factor coreceptor. To gain insight into the virus genome, we have used site-directed mutagenesis to construct over 30 different CVB3 mutants within the 5′-untranslated region (UTR). Our investigations have revealed the importance of the internal ribosomal entry sequence located in the 5′ UTR to virus translation initiation, infectivity and tissue tropism.[9,10] How mutations elsewhere in the CVB3 genome affect interactions with receptors remains to be determined.

In comparison with the coxsackieviral genome, the human genome is considerably more complex. As such, it represents a much greater computational and analytical challenge. Initial release of the draft sequences of the human genome from Celera and Ensembl predicted the total gene numbers at 30–35,000 genes.[11,12] Recent subsequent analyses have revealed that although there is overlap in known genes between the Celera and Ensembl sequences, that there are significant differences in novel sequences which suggests that this may be an underestimation.[13,14]

In focusing on the heart, Dr. C.C. Liew and his colleagues, key contributors to cardiovascular genomics, have attempted to characterize the set of genes expressed in the cardiovascular system in normal, disease, and developmental settings. Their group has estimated that 29,000 genes (an estimate based on 36,000 as the total number of human genes) are expressed in the cardiovascular system. Based on their findings, they have concluded that relatively few genes are tissue specific in expression, and that instead the majority are ubiquitously expressed.[15] High throughput genomics studies have already led to advances in the understanding of heart muscle injury in the setting of idiopathic dilated cardiomyopathy[16] and myocardial infarction.[17]

In early attempts to identify important genes differentially regulated by CVB3, we utilized differential mRNA display (reviewed in ref. 18) to identify host gene responses to virus infection in CVB3-infected mouse hearts. From these studies, we identified and partially sequenced 28 genes that were positively and negatively expressed in CVB3 hearts as compared to noninfected sham controls during the preimmune phase of infection.[19] We further confirmed differential expression of seven of these genes by Northern blot. Five of these genes were of particular interest, Nip21 among them, as well as previously uncharacterized genes in viral myocarditis such as interferon-inducible protein-10 (IP-10) and interferon-inducible GTPase (IGTPase). To probe deeper into the functional role of these proteins in viral myocarditis, we established Tet-On-inducible HeLa cells over-expressing Nip21, IGTPase and IP10. Several interesting observations have ensued. We found that Nip21, a Bcl-2 family member diminished in expression during infection, reduced CVB3 replication by inducing mitochondria-mediated and caspase-dependent apoptosis in target cells.[20] We are currently characterizing IP10 in the context of hypertrophy and apoptosis induction in the setting of viral myocarditis. Furthermore,

IGTPase is an antiapoptotic factor operating through activation of the PKB/Akt pathway. The role of this protein in CVB3 infection is also an area of intense study in our laboratory.

Following these initial studies, our next transcriptional investigations relied on cDNA microarrays to investigate, on a larger scale, murine host gene response profiles in virus infected mouse hearts, especially to dissect disease pathogenesis over time. We utilized a pool of RNA from 15 mouse hearts to hybridize onto two identical custom cDNA microarrays. Intensity values were then averaged over the two chips and any genes that exhibited either less than 2.5-fold expression over background or was derived from less than 40% of the spot were excluded from subsequent analysis. We then mined all known genes that expressed more than 1.8-fold change in RNA expression in virus samples over control for clustering and validatory analysis. Such analysis was performed to determine gene alterations during the course of acute and chronic disease.

Viral myocarditis is a disease composed of several quite distinct stages including viremic injury, immune infiltration and reclamation. The first phase is characterized by virus infection and direct damage of target myocardial cells in the absence of a visible host immune response. The immune phase of infection includes mobilization of innate responses and adaptive defenses and is most readily characterized by mononuclear inflammatory cell infiltration of susceptible target organs. The final phase consists of healing with various degrees of fibrotic reparation and cardiac dilation. The latter may occur in the presence or absence of chronic, low-level infection. Our proof-of-principle for this experiment was in the identification of genes known to be upregulated during most infectious processes. We showed a marked increase in RNA of such genes as MHC which are involved in antigen presentation, and heat shock proteins and the interferon response, all of which are part of an immediate early stress response. We also clustered known genes based on functional groups and found that most genes in these groups had similar temporal patterns of expression. Most notably, we found broad increases in RNA of genes involved in protein expression, cell architecture and cell cycle, and consistent decreases in expression of mitochondrial and cell metabolism genes during the inflammatory phase.[21] Comparative genomics must be used to relate those expression changes to human disease progression.[22]

The observed global decreases in mitochondrial and metabolic gene expression are of importance, considering the central role of mitochondria in energy production for contractile myocardial cells and the growing recognition of mitochondrial mechanisms in cell death. Thus, we considered the possibility that alterations in normal mitochondrial homeostasis may be targeted by CVB3. Having previously found that CVB3 infection in cell culture induces caspase-3-mediated apoptosis in susceptible cells,[23] we further found mitochondrial cytochrome c release and activation of downstream caspases in these cells. In addition, we determined that overexpression of Bcl-2 or Bcl-x_L markedly reduced cytochrome c release, depressed subsequent activation of caspases and delayed the loss of host cell viability following CVB3 infection. Overexpression of Bcl-2 and Bcl-x_L also decreased the amount of progeny virus released into the supernatant. Thus, we have determined mitochondrial participation in CVB3-induced cell death including release of cytochrome c as an important mechanism in caspase activation and, as such, perhaps an important factor in the release of progeny virus and host cellular injury.

Early studies in viral myocarditis, performed mainly by virologists and immunologists, focused on the immune phase of virus infection. More recently, however, the nature and extent of early direct virus injury to target myocytes has been appreciated in our laboratory as well as by others, and continues to be a phenomenon of great interest.[23,24] In order to focus on this direct injury, we have utilized a well-characterized *in vitro* HeLa (human cervical carcinoma) cell model of CVB3 infection to dissect target cell protective responses. The transcriptional profiles resulting from viral injury assayed by GeneChip® over time were analyzed based on coordinate expression or "guilt by association." In other words, a transcript from a known gene is found to be differentially regulated and compared with patterns of other genes whose expression values are similar over time. This is based on the theory that genes which are coordinately regulated and expressed may be involved in similar functional roles or pathways. Brown *et al.*[25] have shown, using 78 different experiments in *Saccharomyces cerevisiae*, that clustering based on eight different gene expression events was similar within functional groups. We have shown similar results by investigation of differential gene expression events in CVB3-infected mouse hearts wherein genes clustered into functional groups had strikingly similar temporal expression profiles.[21]

In CVB3-infected HeLa cell samples, we found significant transient expression of the *c-jun* and *c-fos* genes at early timepoints, consistent with previous data in Echovirus-1 infection.[26] There are several potential upstream signaling pathways, such as MAPK-ERK and Jak/Stat, which activate *c-jun* and *c-fos*, respectively. We have found that infection of HeLa cells with CVB3 induces both an early activation of Stat3 and a biphasic activation of the MAPK-ERK pathways. We have further shown that inhibition of ERK signaling significantly inhibits CVB3 progeny release and decreases virus protein production.[27] Furthermore, inhibition of ERK1/2 activation circumvents CVB3-induced apoptosis. Our data have suggested that ERK1/2 activation is necessary for CVB3 replication and contributes to CVB3 pathogenesis in host cells. Recently, Opavsky *et al.*[28] have also shown ERK activation both *in vitro* and *in vivo* models of CBV3 infection which is associated with increased virus pathogenesis. We are currently analyzing the oligonucleotide array results for further temporal patterns of expression in order to characterize potentially significant signaling partners activated during the infectious process.

In order to strengthen the inferences from our previous results, we used replicate samples using the Affymetrix GeneChip® platform.[29] Hence, the HeLa cell time-course experiment was repeated using triplicate samples for targeted and representative timepoints. To ensure reproducibility, we carefully screened our total RNA and intermediate products during subsequent processing steps to detect any contamination by spectrophotometry and ensured that samples showed no degradation through examination by gel electrophoresis. Once hybridized onto the GeneChip®, 3':5' ratios of the internal GAPDH and beta-actin controls were measured as indices of RNA degradation during hybridization, and a cutoff value for each chip was set at less than 3. Our minimum intensity value for any signal was 115 intensity units, minimum probe positivity required more than 16 of 20 pairs (in match *versus* mismatch probes) to be present, and our statistical difference threshold (intensity of perfect match/mismatch probes) was set at 1.5 or greater for confidence in expression values. Once all samples were quality controlled, each chip was ready for data analysis and bioinformatic investigation.

As supported by the growing literature and by personal accounts, the use of different bioinformatic tools can yield very different end results.[30] There are several bioinformatic strategies, and it remains to be seen which is the most sensitive and informative. Certainly, much of the debate on how to rationalize expression data lies in the biological context and the nature of the experiment being performed. Analysis of our results began by putting the gene expression profiles, as assessed on the Affymetrix platform, through several steps of normalization and data reduction. In our analysis, we chose to exclude genes with negative average difference (Avg Diff) values across all samples by truncating at 10 Avg Diff units. The Affymetrix algorithm takes into account the differences in fluorescence between the "perfect match" probes and its "mismatch" counterparts (containing a mismatch nucleotide). Each gene is probed by 16 sets of perfect match and mismatch pairs and the difference between these pairs is averaged, equaling the Avg Diff value (Affymetrix, Inc., Santa Clara, CA). Next, the data is transformed by taking the log function of the Avg Diff units. This was followed by data normalization by calculating a multiplicative factor for each sample in order to scale the sample mean for a subset ($n = 59$) of ribosomal mRNAs to a fixed value ($n = 8$). Once transformed, data analysis was performed using Genetrix™ (EpiCenter Software, Los Angeles, CA) and GeneSpring™ (Silicon Genetics, Redwood City, CA) software. For uncharacterized sequences, we have Blast searched against known human sequences with high sequence homology ($P < 0.1$). Using search databases such as Locus Link, which access OMIM to search Mendelian literature, PUBMED for articles, GenBank, Protein databases, and Unigene for clusters of known gene sequences, we are currently trying to characterize novel genes whose expression is regulated. Through the use of such analytical tools, we have found several potential signaling, contractile, cytoskeletal, and metabolic genes which may be important in the infectious process. Nonarray techniques are being used to dissect out potential mechanisms for genes with sufficient biological reason to suspect a functional pathogenetic relation.

To further identify which downstream ERK target genes were being transcribed due to virus infection, we utilized a specific MEK1 inhibitor (upstream of ERK) in an *in vitro* pharmacogenomic analysis of CVB3 infection. By uncovering downstream genes which are expressed following infection, but are repressed with the MEK1 inhibitor, we are identifying target genes and increasing our understanding of the apparent provirus effect of ERK signaling in target cells and organs. One such gene is the inflammatory mediator and CXC chemokine IL-8, which exhibits a 5-fold increase in expression in CVB3-infected cells, but a return to control levels following addition of the MEK1 inhibitor. Recently, infection with Adenovirus serotype 7 (Ad7), has been shown to induce expression of cytoprotective IL-8 activation in an ERK-dependent manner.[31] Since CVB3 and Ad7 share usage of the common coxsackievirus and adenovirus receptor and considering the early temporal expression of IL-8, it is possible that receptor binding may be responsible for this induction.

In light of altered transcriptional expression of cell cycle regulatory genes identified by oligonucleotide and by cDNA microarray analysis during CVB3 infection, we probed further into the effects of this pathogen on cellular replication in a cell culture model. Notably, our *in vitro* experiments revealed an early increase in cyclin D gene expression following CVB3 infection, which we confirmed by Northern blot analysis. We then continued to examine cell cycle progression and regulation when infection was initiated during the late G1 phase of the cell cycle. Decreased levels of G1 cyclins (cyclin D1 and cyclin E) protein expression, reduced G1 cyclin-associated kinase activities and phosphorylation of retinoblastoma protein were observed (in review). Using a general caspase inhibitor, we showed that the reduction of cyclin D1 is caspase-independent. Taken together, these results demonstrated that CVB3 infection disrupts host cell homeostasis by blocking the cell cycle at the G1/S boundary through inhibition of G1 cyclin kinases. Whether cell cycle disruption is a virus strategy for chronic infection has yet to be determined.[32]

Recent microarray data from cell lines and *in vivo* tissues, in concordance with work from our laboratory, suggests that there exist trends in early cellular stress responses[33] to a range of stimuli, such as virus infection, UV and IR ionizing radiation,[34] proteasome inhibition, and growth factor deprivation. Although the universality of stress responses is not a new phenomenon, global gene expression profiling suggests that this reaction may be more widespread than previously believed. Indeed, a ubiquitous stress response element, ATF3 (activating transcription factor 3), was found to be expressed both in our CVB3-infected cells and in array analysis done by others.[35] In most all cell stress responses, this protein is transcriptionally upregulated[36] and as such, can be considered part of a stereotypic stress response. Depending on the cellular milieu, ATF3 can either be a transcriptional repressor or can bind to *c-jun* in order to facilitate transcription. ATF3 can also bind to its own promoter to self-repress its transcription. This negative feedback mechanism may partially explain its early and transient expression post-stress induction.[37] The exact role of ATF3 has not been precisely determined. Rather, it possesses a wide range of known functions and the result of ATF3 activation likely depends on the cellular milieu. Our *in vivo* gene profiling in adolescent CVB3-infected mouse hearts has also revealed members of the ATF family of genes, including ATF4, which increases during the inflammatory phase of infection.[21]

Genomics is based on the premise that there is a relationship between the genes expressed by a cell and the proteins that are actually translated. However, a caveat for using genomics to study diseases is that there are several regulatory events downstream of transcription which contributes to the phenotype of cells and the portraits of disease. For instance, the coxsackievirus genome codes for viral proteases, necessary for cleavage of the virus polyprotein, and which selectively cleave host structural proteins and enzymes. Notably, viral proteases disrupt the host cell translational apparatus by inactivating eukaryotic initiation 4-γ (eIF4G)[38] and poly-(A)-binding protein immediately following virus entry.[39,40] Thus it is perhaps not surprising that in cells and tissues infected with CVB3 it is difficult to relate gene transcription to protein expression, to say nothing of protein function. Therefore, although host RNA expression can reveal which potentially relevant signaling pathways have been activated more in one system than in another, further validation is necessary to understand which proteins are translated and functional. Since there are many levels of cellular regulation, the presence of a differentially expressed gene may only imply involvement, while the absence of gene alterations simply suggests inactivity.[41] Interestingly, there are an increasing number of human genes that are known to undergo cap-independent translation, such as VEGF,[42] c-myc,[43] apoptotic protease activating factor-1,[44] death-associated protein 5,[45] X-linked inhibitor of apoptosis[46] and eIF4G.[47] Many such genes encode for proteins involved in apoptotic and survival mechanisms, suggesting that they may be part of a host stress response which can be activated regardless of disruption of the normal protein translational apparatus. To obtain a true appreciation for the benefit to virus or host of transcriptional or translational events, one must probe much deeper with specific molecular, cellular and organismal techniques in order to understand the functional genomics.

Like most other diseases, both infectious and noninfectious, an isolated genetic investigation is incomplete, since there are important non-genetic or environmental factors which affect disease pathogenesis. Presented as the population-attributable risk, genetic and environmental interactions can ultimately push an attributable risk well over 100%.[48] During coxsackieviral infection, host nutritional status has been shown to not only alter susceptibility to infection, possibly through reduced monocyte chemo-attractant protein-1, but also affect virus genomic regulation.[49,50] It has been shown that mice deficient in selenium and infected with a nonvirulent strain of CVB3 support a specific 6-nucleotide mutation to a virulence phenotype. In rural areas of southwestern China, there are selenium deficiencies in the population and incidence of an endemic cardiomyopathy, termed Keshan disease, from which various serotypes of coxsackievirus have been isolated.[51]

Novel high throughput techniques and bioinformatic tools are allowing investigators to play with differential gene patterns in an increasingly elegant sandbox. Our investigations into the pathogenesis of CVB3 have involved a synergistic effort between virologists, cell biologists, pathologists, and computer scientists. Ultimately, the goal of our genomics program is to improve the understanding, treatment and prevention of coxsackieviral myocarditis. A complete understanding of infectomics of CVB3-induced viral myocarditis may include a list of all virus and host genes, their spatial and temporal expression during the various stages of infection, and their interactions in all target organs. To this point, it would be useful to have a true infectomics chip which incorporates both host and virus genes to see the relative expression of both sets of genes together.[30] The use of such a chip would enhance our understanding of how various viral strains induce differences in pathogenesis and help explain which genes are responsible for resistance to disease as shown in select populations.[52]

ACKNOWLEDGMENXTS

This research is generously supported by the Canadian Institutes of Health Research, the Heart and Stroke Foundation of British Columbia and Yukon, the Heart and Stroke Foundation of Canada and the Michael Smith Foundation for Health Research.

REFERENCES

1. HALDANE, J.B.S. 1949. High frequencies of a-thalassemia are the result of natural selection by malaria. Nature **321:** 744–750.
2. HUANG, S.H., T. TRICHE & A.Y. JONG. 2002. Infectomics: Genomics and proteomics of microbial infections. Funct. Integr. Genomics **1:** 331–344.

3. GEISS, G.K., R.E. BUMGARNER, M.C. AN, et al. 2000. Large-scale monitoring of host cell gene expression during HIV-1 infection using cDNA microarrays. Virology **266**: 8–16.
4. ZHU, H., J.P. CONG, G. MAMTORA, et al. 1998. Cellular gene expression altered by human cytomegalovirus: global monitoring with oligonucleotide arrays. Proc. Natl. Acad. Sci. USA **95**: 14470–14475.
5. STINGLEY, S.W., J.J. RAMIREZ, S.A. AGUILAR, et al. 2000. Global analysis of herpes simplex virus type 1 transcription using an oligonucleotide-based DNA microarray. J. Virol. **74**: 9916–9927.
6. BIGGER, C.B., K.M. BRASKY & R.E. LANFORD. 2001. DNA microarray analysis of chimpanzee liver during acute resolving hepatitis C virus infection. J. Virol. **75**: 7059–7066.
7. KANDOLF, R. & P.H. HOFSCHNEIDER. 1985. Molecular cloning of the genome of a cardiotropic Coxsackie B3 virus: full-length reverse-transcribed recombinant cDNA generates infectious virus in mammalian cells. Proc. Natl. Acad. Sci. USA **82**: 4818–4822.
8. BERGELSON, J.M., J.F. MODLIN, W. WIELAND-ALTER, et al. 1997. Clinical coxsackievirus B isolates differ from laboratory strains in their interaction with two cell surface receptors. J. Infect. Dis. **175**: 697–700.
9. LIU, Z., C.M. CARTHY, P. CHEUNG, et al. 1999. Structural and functional analysis of the 5′ untranslated region of coxsackievirus B3 RNA: in vivo translational and infectivity studies of full-length mutants. Virology **265**: 206–217.
10. YANG, D., J.E. WILSON, D.R. ANDERSON, et al. 1997. In vitro mutational and inhibitory analysis of the cis-acting translational elements within the 5′ untranslated region of coxsackievirus B3: potential targets for antiviral action of antisense oligomers. Virology **228**: 63–73.
11. LANDER, E.S., L.M. LINTON, B. BIRREN, et al. 2001. Initial sequencing and analysis of the human genome. Nature **409**: 860–921.
12. VENTER, J.C., M.D. ADAMS, E.W. MYERS, et al. 2001. The sequence of the human genome. Science **291**: 1304–1351.
13. HOGENESCH, J.B., K.A. CHING, S. BATALOV, et al. 2001. A comparison of the Celera and Ensembl predicted gene sets reveals little overlap in novel genes. Cell **106**: 413–415.
14. WRIGHT, F.A., W.J. LEMON, W.D. ZHAO, et al. 2001. A draft annotation and overview of the human genome. Genome Biol. **2**: RESEARCH0025.
15. DEMPSEY, A.A., V.J. DZAU & C.C. LIEW. 2001. Cardiovascular genomics: estimating the total number of genes expressed in the human cardiovascular system. J. Mol. Cell. Cardiol. **33**: 1879–1886.
16. HAASE, D., M.H. LEHMANN, M.M. KORNER, et al. 2002. Identification and validation of selective upregulation of ventricular myosin light chain type 2 mRNA in idiopathic dilated cardiomyopathy. Eur. J. Heart Fail. **4**: 23–31.
17. TAKAHASHI, M., J. NISHIHIRA, M. SHIMPO, et al. 2001. Macrophage migration inhibitory factor as a redox-sensitive cytokine in cardiac myocytes. Cardiovasc. Res. **52**: 438–445.
18. ZHANG, J.S., E.L. DUNCAN, A.C. CHANG & R.R. REDDEL. 1998. Differential display of mRNA. Mol. Biotechnol. **10**: 155–165.
19. YANG, D., J. YU, Z. LUO, et al. 1999. Viral myocarditis: identification of five differentially expressed genes in coxsackievirus B3-infected mouse heart. Circ. Res. **84**: 704–712.
20. ZHANG, H.M., B. YANAGAWA, P. CHEUNG, et al. 2002. Nip21 gene expression reduces coxsackievirus B3 replication by promoting apoptotic cell death via a mitochondria-dependent pathway. Circ. Res. **90**: 1251–1258.
21. TAYLOR, L.A., C.M. CARTHY, D. YANG, et al. 2000. Host gene regulation during coxsackievirus B3 infection in mice: assessment by microarrays. Circ. Res. **87**: 328–334.
22. QURESHI, S.T., E. SKAMENE & D. MALO. 1999. Comparative genomics and host resistance against infectious diseases. Emerg. Infect. Dis. **5**: 36–47.
23. CARTHY, C.M., D.J. GRANVILLE, K.A. WATSON, et al. 1998. Caspase activation and specific cleavage of substrates after coxsackievirus B3-induced cytopathic effect in HeLa cells. J. Virol. **72**: 7669–7675.

24. KANDA, T., H. KOIKE, M. ARAI, et al. 1999. Increased severity of viral myocarditis in mice lacking lymphocyte maturation. Int. J. Cardiol. **68:** 13–22.
25. BROWN, A.J., R.J. PLANTA, F. RESTUHADI, et al. 2001. Transcript analysis of 1003 novel yeast genes using high-throughput northern hybridizations. EMBO J. **20:** 3177–3186.
26. HUTTUNEN, P., T. HYYPIA, P. VIHINEN, et al. 1998. Echovirus 1 infection induces both stress- and growth-activated mitogen-activated protein kinase pathways and regulates the transcription of cellular immediate-early genes. Virology **250:** 85–93.
27. LUO, H., B. YANAGAWA, J. ZHANG, et al. 2002. Coxsackievirus B3 replication is reduced by inhibition of the extracellular signal-regulated kinase (ERK) signaling pathway. J. Virol. **76:** 3365–3373.
28. OPAVSKY, M.A., T. MARTINO, M. RABINOVITCH, et al. 2002. Enhanced ERK-1/2 activation in mice susceptible to coxsackievirus-induced myocarditis. J. Clin. Invest. **109:** 1561–1569.
29. LEE, M.L., F.C. KUO, G.A. WHITMORE & J. SKLAR. 2000. Importance of replication in microarray gene expression studies: statistical methods and evidence from repetitive cDNA hybridizations. Proc. Natl. Acad. Sci. USA 97: 9834–9839.
30. KELLAM, P. 2000. Host-pathogen studies in the post-genomic era. Genome Biol. **1:** REVIEWS1009.
31. ALCORN, M.J., J.L. BOOTH, K.M. COGGESHALL & J. P. METCALF. 2001. Adenovirus type 7 induces interleukin-8 production via activation of extracellular regulated kinase 1/2. J. Virol. **75:** 6450–6459.
32. FEUER, R., I. MENA, R. PAGARIGAN, et al. 2002. Cell cycle status affects coxsackievirus replication, persistence, and reactivation in vitro. J. Virol. **76:** 4430–4440.
33. MANGER, I.D. & D.A. RELMAN. 2000. How the host 'sees' pathogens: global gene expression responses to infection. Curr. Opin. Immunol. **12:** 215–218.
34. AMUNDSON, S.A., M. BITTNER, Y. CHEN, et al. 1999. Fluorescent cDNA microarray hybridization reveals complexity and heterogeneity of cellular genotoxic stress responses. Oncogene **18:** 3666–3672.
35. LIANG, G., C.D. WOLFGANG, B.P. CHEN, et al. 1996. ATF3 gene. Genomic organization, promoter, and regulation. J. Biol. Chem. **271:** 1695–1701.
36. HAI, T., C.D. WOLFGANG, D.K. MARSEE, et al. 1999. ATF3 and stress responses. Gene Expr. **7:** 321–335.
37. WOLFGANG, C.D., G. LIANG, Y. OKAMOTO, et al. 2000. Transcriptional autorepression of the stress-inducible gene ATF3. J. Biol. Chem. **275:** 16865–16870.
38. LAMPHEAR, B.J., R. KIRCHWEGER, T. SKERN & R.E. RHOADS. 1995. Mapping of functional domains in eukaryotic protein synthesis initiation factor 4G (eIF4G) with picornaviral proteases. Implications for cap-dependent and cap-independent translational initiation. J. Biol. Chem. **270:** 21975–21983.
39. KEREKATTE, V., B.D. KEIPER. C. BADORFF, et al. 1999. Cleavage of Poly(A)-binding protein by coxsackievirus 2A protease in vitro and in vivo: another mechanism for host protein synthesis shutoff? J. Virol. **73:** 709–17.
40. KUYUMCU-MARTINEZ, N.M., M. JOACHIMS & R.E. LLOYD. 2002. Efficient cleavage of ribosome-associated poly(A)-binding protein by enterovirus 3C protease. J. Virol. **76:** 2062–2074.
41. BLACKWELL, J.M. 2001. Genetics and genomics in infectious disease susceptibility. Trends Mol. Med. **7:** 521–526.
42. AKIRI, G., D. NAHARI, Y. FINKELSTEIN, et al. 1998. Regulation of vascular endothelial growth factor (VEGF) expression is mediated by internal initiation of translation and alternative initiation of transcription. Oncogene **17:** 227–236.
43. NANBRU, C., I. LAFON, S. AUDIGIER, et al. 1997. Alternative translation of the proto-oncogene c-myc by an internal ribosome entry site. J. Biol. Chem. **272:** 32061–32066.
44. COLDWELL, M.J., S.A. MITCHELL, M. STONELEY, et al. 2000. Initiation of Apaf-1 translation by internal ribosome entry. Oncogene **19:** 899–905.
45. HENIS-KORENBLIT, S., N.L. STRUMPF, D. GOLDSTAUB & A. KIMCHI. 2000. A novel form of DAP5 protein accumulates in apoptotic cells as a result of caspase cleavage and internal ribosome entry site-mediated translation. Mol. Cell. Biol. **20:** 496–506.

46. HOLCIK, M. & R.G. KORNELUK. 2000. Functional characterization of the X-linked inhibitor of apoptosis (XIAP) internal ribosome entry site element: role of La autoantigen in XIAP translation. Mol. Cell. Biol. **20:** 4648–657.
47. GAN, W., M. LaCELLE & R.E. RHOADS. 1998. Functional characterization of the internal ribosome entry site of eIF4G mRNA. J. Biol. Chem. **273:** 5006–5012.
48. WILLETT, W.C. 2002. Balancing life-style and genomics research for disease prevention. Science **296:** 695–698.
49. BECK, M.A. & C.C. MATTHEWS. 2000. Micronutrients and host resistance to viral infection. Proc. Nutr. Soc. **59:** 581–585.
50. BECK, M.A., Q. SHI, V.C. MORRIS & O.A. LEVANDER. 1995. Rapid genomic evolution of a non-virulent coxsackievirus B3 in selenium-deficient mice results in selection of identical virulent isolates. Nat. Med. **1:** 433–436.
51. PENG, T., Y. LI, Y. YANG, *et al.* 2000. Characterization of enterovirus isolates from patients with heart muscle disease in a selenium-deficient area of China. J. Clin. Microbiol. **38:** 3538–3543.
52. HILL, A.V. 1999. Genetics and genomics of infectious disease susceptibility. Br. Med. Bull. **55:** 401–413.

A Functional Genomics Approach to Kaposi's Sarcoma

ASHLEE V. MOSES,[a] MICHAEL A. JARVIS,[a] CAMILO RAGGO,[a]
YOLANDA C. BELL,[b] REBECCA RUHL,[a] B.G. MATTIAS LUUKKONEN,[b]
DIANA J. GRIFFITH,[c] CECILY L. WAIT,[c] BRIAN J. DRUKER,[c]
MICHAEL C. HEINRICH,[c] JAY A. NELSON,[a] AND KLAUS FRÜH[a]

[a]*Vaccine and Gene Therapy Institute and Department of Molecular Microbiology and Immunology, Oregon Health & Science University, Portland, Oregon 97239, USA*

[b]*R.W. Johnson Pharmaceutical Research Institute, 3210 Merryfield Row, San Diego California 92121, USA*

[c]*Division of Hematology and Medical Oncology, Oregon Health & Science University and Portland Veterans Affairs Medical Center, Portland, Oregon 97239, USA*[d]

ABSTRACT: Kaposi's sarcoma (KS) is the most frequent malignancy afflicting acquired immune-deficiency syndrome (AIDS) patients. Tumor lesions are characterized by spindle cells of vascular origin and vascularization. Kaposi's sarcoma–associated herpes virus (KSHV) is consistently found in all forms of KS. Infection of dermal microvascular endothelial cells (DMVEC) with KSHV recapitulates spindle cell formation *in vitro*. We studied this transformation process by DNA microarray analysis comparing the RNA expression profiles of KSHV-infected and mock-infected DMVEC. Genes involved in tumorigenesis, angiogenesis, host defense, cell growth and differentiation, transcription, and metabolism were observed to change significantly upon infection with KSHV. One of the most consistently KSHV-induced genes was the receptor tyrosine kinase and proto-oncogene c-Kit. Inhibition of c-Kit activity with the pharmacological inhibitor of c-Kit signaling STI571 reversed the KSHV-induced morphological transformation of DMVEC. Moreover, overexpression studies showed that c-Kit was sufficient to induce spindle cell formation (Moses *et al.* J. Virol. 76(16): 8383–8399). These data demonstrate that microarrays are useful for the identification of pharmacological targets essential for KS tumorigenesis.

KEYWORDS: Kaposi's sarcoma–associated herpesvirus; microarray; c-kit; antisense

INTRODUCTION

Kaposi's sarcoma (KS) is a vascular neoplasm characterized by angioproliferative lesions on the skin and visceral organs.[1] KS lesions are distinguished by the presence of proliferating spindle-shaped tumor cells of endothelial origin and exhibit abnormal vascularization with extensive extravasation of inflammatory cells and

Address for correspondence: Klaus Früh or Ashlee V. Moses, 505 NW 185th Ave., Beaverton, OR 97006, USA. Voice: 503-418-2735; fax: 503-418-2701.
fruehk@ohsu.edu; mosesa@ohsu.edu

erythrocytes.[2,3] Although KS is a rare condition in immunocompetent individuals, the disease is the most common malignancy associated with the Acquired Immunodeficiency Syndrome (AIDS).[4,5] Kaposi's sarcoma–associated herpesvirus (KSHV), or human herpesvirus 8 (HHV8), is the infectious agent consistently associated with KS development[6] and is considered the etiologic agent of disease.

KSHV is a type 2 γ-herpesvirus found in all forms of KS, in primary effusion lymphoma (PEL/BCBL), a rare form of AIDS-associated B cell lymphoma,[7] and in variants of multicentric Castleman's disease (MCD).[8] In the KS lesion, KSHV infects the majority of spindle cells as well as lesional endothelial cells and infiltrating leukocytes.[9–12] KSHV genes with the potential to deregulate cellular growth have been described, many of which are homologous to cellular genes.[13] Despite the recognition that KSHV encodes a variety of proteins that could conceivably induce and/or maintain KS lesions, the mechanisms of virus-induced oncogenesis remain unclear. Relevant *in vitro* models are thus urgently required to elucidate mechanisms of tumorigenesis.

In vitro studies with KSHV were initially performed with established PEL cell lines.[7,14,15] When considering studies of KS pathogenesis, however, endothelial cells are clearly a more relevant cell type in which to study the disease, since they are the likely precursors of KS spindle cells.[16–19] Furthermore, the gene expression program of KSHV in endothelial/spindle cells may differ from that mapped in KSHV-infected PEL cells. Interestingly, spindle cells cultured from KS tumors do not stably maintain the KSHV genome *in vitro*,[20,21] and the early consequences of cellular transformation are inaccessible via the study of fully transformed tumor cells. Thus, *in vitro* endothelial cell models of KSHV infection constitute appropriate systems in which to dissect the role of KSHV in KS spindle cell development and growth. Development of endothelial-based models of KSHV infection has proved to be challenging, and to date only a handful of such systems have been described. A pioneer system described by Flore *et al.* highlights the role played by paracrine signaling, since only a percentage of cells harbor the viral genome.[22] Other systems describe endothelial cell cultures in which the majority of cells become infected, latent infection predominates, and cells develop a spindle phenotype reminiscent of KS spindle cells. Our laboratory was the first to describe such a system based on infection of dermal microvascular endothelial cells (DMVEC).[25] Two additional fully permissive models have since been described.[23,24] Both our system and the one described by Lagunoff and colleagues[24] utilize MVEC lines immortalized by HPV gene products or telomerase respectively. Immortalization has the advantage of allowing long-term maintenance of age- and passage-matched cultures, since primary endothelial cells have a limited *in vitro* lifespan. Here we describe the results of global transcriptional profiling of the changes occurring in host cell mRNA levels during spindle cell formation. We also describe methods of target validation in this system and the identification of one particular target for therapeutic intervention.

RESULTS

The KSHV Culture System

The KSHV-permissive *in vitro* culture system used by our group[25] utilizes dermal microvascular endothelial cells that are immortalized with the E6 and E7 proteins of

HPV16 introduced via the recombinant retrovirus LXSN16 E6/E7. The immortalized cells, referred to hereafter as DMVEC, are infected with KSHV derived from the BCBL-1 PEL cell line or with a recombinant strain of KSHV that expresses green fluorescent protein (GFP) under the control of the cellular EF-1 promotor.[26] Infection can be readily demonstrated by expression of KSHV latent nuclear antigen-1 (LANA-1/ORF73), identified by immunofluorescent assay (IFA), or, in the case of GFP-KSHV, evaluation of green fluorescent cells. Following KSHV infection, DMVEC develop phenotypic features that have been associated with KS spindle cells *in vivo*. These include the loss of some endothelial phenotypic markers (e.g., von Willebrand factor), but retention of others (e.g., CD31 and VE-cadherin).[25] In addition, KSHV-infected DMVEC lose the typical cobblestone morphology that is characteristic of DMVEC, and develop a spindle phenotype. When spindle cell cultures are grown to confluence, the confluent monolayers display loss of contact inhibition, with cells growing on top of one another to form multilayered, disorganized foci. When placed into soft agar, spindle cells are able to form colonies. Mock-infected DMVEC, while immortalized with E6/E7, do not exhibit any of the standard features of transformation. Specifically, they grow with a flat profile in monolayer culture, maintain a normal cobblestone shape and do not exhibit anchorage-independent growth. The characteristic phenotypes of mock- and KSHV-infected DMVEC are illustrated in FIGURE 1 A–C. Infection of cells with GFP-KSHV at a low multiplicity of infection (MOI) and visualization of GFP confirms that spindling is

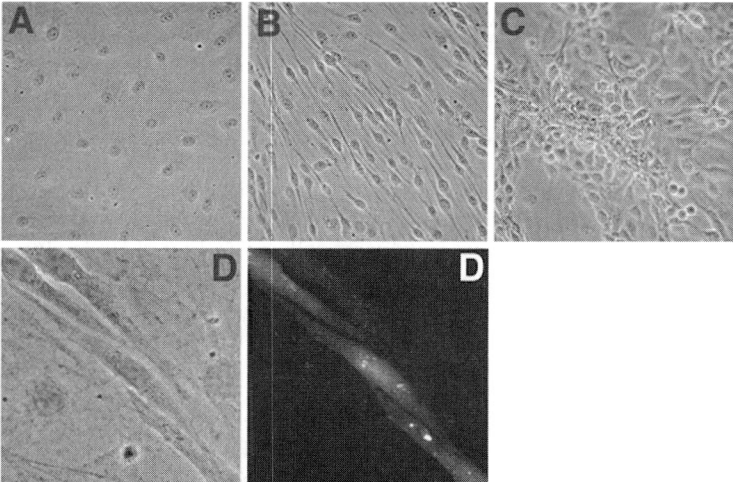

FIGURE 1. KSHV-infection induces cell spindling and focus formation in DMVEC. (**A**) Mock-infected DMVEC exhibit a cobblestone shape and flat profile. (**B**) KSHV-infected DMVEC develop spindle morphology. (**C**) KSHV-infected DMVEC cultured postconfluence exhibit lack of contact inhibition and grow in disorganized multilayered foci. In the image shown, only cells in the top layers are in focus. (**D**) Infection of DMVEC with GFP-KSHV at low MOI confirms that spindling is restricted to infected (GFP$^+$) cells. Phase and fluorescent fields are shown.

restricted to the KSHV-infected cells (FIG. 1D). In summary, KSHV-induced cellular phenotypes are reminiscent of KSHV spindle cells *in vivo*. Thus, this culture system provides a valid means to elucidate viral mechanisms of tumorigenesis.

The Study of KSHV Pathogenesis via Gene Expression Profiling

Gene expression profiling by DNA microarray analysis enables evaluation of transcriptional alterations in thousands of host genes in response to the stimulus or pathological state under investigation. To identify cellular genes that may contribute to KSHV-induced transformation, we used cDNA arrays as well as Affymetrix GeneChips for gene expression profiling of age- and passage-matched KSHV-infected and uninfected DMVEC. The results from cDNA arrays were recently published.[27] In addition, we performed several Affymetrix GeneChip experiments. We used the recently launched U133 A and B Affymetrix GeneChips which together contain approximately 45,000 individual probe sets with 39,000 individual transcripts. However, many of theses sets of probes are for different parts of the same genes so that the total number of defined genes is estimated to be about 33,000 genes. We used two KSHV-infected and their respective mock-infected cell lines for comparison. The results are shown in TABLE 1. Common to both experiments were a total of 583 genes which were up or downregulated more than twofold and scored as induced or decreased by the Affymetrix software. However, after removal of duplicates, this number was reduced to 472 genes. Of these, 215 (45%) were genes of unknown function. Genes with known function that were significantly altered by KSHV infection could be classified into several functional groups. A breakdown of these groups by gene numbers and up- or downregulation is shown in FIGURE 2. Strikingly, more than 50 genes involved in angiogenesis or cell adhesion were regulated during KSHV-infection. This is consistent with the extreme vascularization observed in KS tissue. The transforming properties of KSHV were also reflected in the large number of genes that were significantly regulated and that have known functions in signal transduction/transcription and tumorigenesis. More than 80 genes belonged to one of these groups. Thus, KSHV seems to induce a massive change in the cellular environment consistent with the drastic changes in the morphological and growth properties of KSHV-infected DMVEC. These data now form the basis of ongoing studies to elucidate the individual pathways regulated by KSHV in these endothelial cells.

TABLE 1. Transcriptional changes in KSHV-infected versus mock-infected DMVEC monitored by Affymetrix U133 array

Number of genes	Increased	Decreased
A Array		
Experiment 1	233	317
Experiment 2	297	417
B Array		
Experiment 1	156	187
Experiment 2	197	231

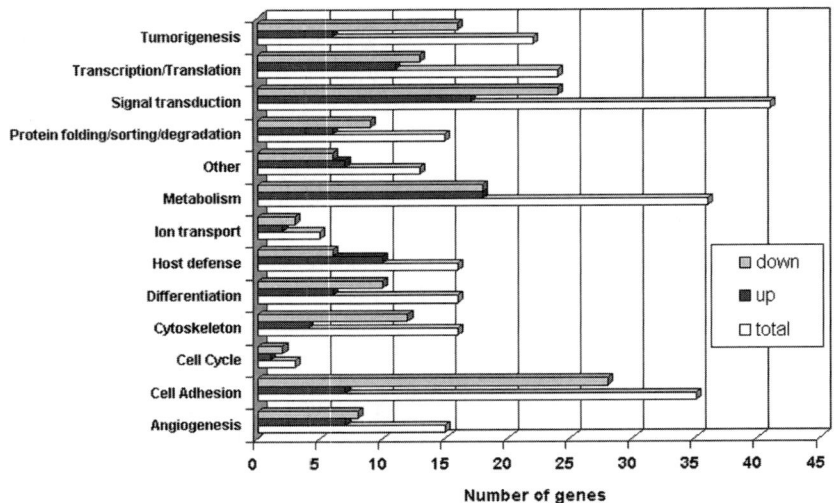

FIGURE 2. Functional groups in KSHV-infected cells. Approximately 33,000 genes were tested with two independent KSHV-infected or two independent mock-infected DMVEC cell lines. Genes with known function that changed more than twofold and were scored as increased or decreased by the Affymetrix software MAS 5.0 in both experiments were grouped according to their function.

Identification of c-Kit as a Gene of Interest

For several of the strongly upregulated genes, we have quantified their changes in mRNA levels by real-time PCR.[27] Since one of the characteristic features of KS is the presence of tumors of endothelial origin, we were particularly interested in further validating KSHV-induced genes with a known function in tumorigenesis in other systems. One of the genes of particular interest was that for the tyrosine kinase receptor (TKR) c-Kit, since Kit expression has been documented in a variety of human cancers including angiosarcomas and KS.[28] Abnormal c-Kit signaling due to receptor overexpression and/or constitutive activation has been causally implicated in the pathophysiology of many of these cancers,[29,30] and several TKR inhibitors that inhibit Kit activity are currently in clinical trials as antitumor agents.[28] We therefore evaluated the role of c-Kit in the transformation of DMVEC. The results were recently published[27] and will be summarized briefly.

Upregregulation of c-Kit mRNA and protein in KSHV-infected DMVEC was confirmed by RT-PCR and immunofluorescent analysis (IFA), respectively. To confirm that c-Kit induction was not unique to E6/E7-immortalized DMVEC, protein expression was also examined in primary KSHV-infected DMVEC. For these experiments we utilized the GFP-KSHV strain at a low MOI, since this enabled us to evaluate adjacent infected and uninfected cells in the monolayer, and verify the KSHV-infected cells by GFP visualization. As shown in FIGURE 3, enhanced expression of c-Kit was observed on GFP-positive, KSHV-infected cells in the virus-exposed culture, but not on adjacent GFP-negative uninfected cells.

To determine whether DMVEC expressed the ligand of c-Kit, stem cell factor (SCF) in addition to c-Kit, we performed qPCR analysis for SCF mRNA. Although SCF mRNA was readily detected in both KSHV-infected and uninfected DMVEC, indicating coexpression of receptor and ligand in these cells, no virus-induced change in SCF expression levels was noted.[27] Thus, KSHV infection did not alter the type or total amount of SCF produced, suggesting that, if KSHV infection alters c-Kit/SCF regulated signaling pathways, the contribution of virus infection is at the level of c-Kit expression.

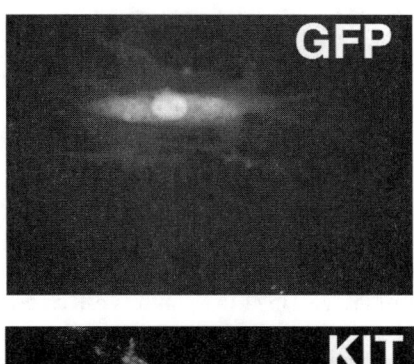

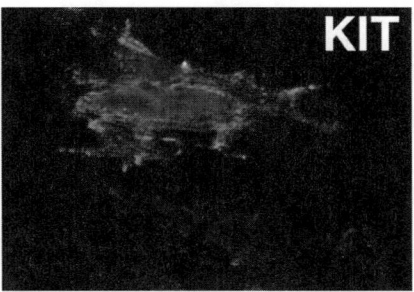

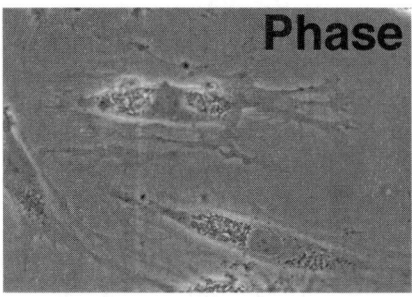

FIGURE 3. c-Kit upregulation is restricted to KSHV-infected cells. Primary DMVEC were infected with GFP-KSHV and c-Kit expression evaluated when less than 50% of the culture was infected (GFP+). Only GFP+ cells expressed increased surface Kit (Red). Low constitutive c-Kit levels were observed on the surface of uninfected (GFP−) cells in the same culture.

c-Kit Overexpression Induces DMVEC Spindle Cell Formation

In murine fibroblasts, ectopic expression of c-Kit induces cellular transformation and tumorigenicity in nude mice. Addition of exogenous SCF was required for the transformation, since the c-Kit receptor alone was transduced into the murine cells. To determine whether c-Kit upregulation was sufficient to induce morphologic changes reminiscent of those caused by KSHV infection of DMVEC, we overexpressed c-Kit in normal DMVEC in the absence of any KSHV genes. Overexpression was achieved by infecting DMVEC with a recombinant adenovirus expressing wild type c-Kit protein (Ad/c-KitWT). Interestingly, c-Kit overexpression in DMVEC had a dose-dependent effect on spindle morphology that was comparable to that observed following KSHV infection.[27] Antibody staining confirmed that only those cells that overexpressed c-Kit developed spindle morphology. Ad/c-KitWT-infected cells became elongated and disorganized, with overgrowth of the monolayer and a loss of discrete cell borders. This suggested that c-Kit is not only necessary but also sufficient for spindle cell formation in our model.

To test whether KSHV-induction of c-Kit plays an essential role in virus-induced transformation, the consequence of inhibiting c-Kit activity in KSHV-transformed DMVEC was evaluated. To inhibit c-Kit signaling, cells were treated with the tyrosine kinase inhibitor (TKI) STI571 that inhibits c-Kit activity.[31] Control KSHV-infected DMVEC exhibited disorganized growth, loss of contact inhibition and focus formation in monolayer culture, but in the presence of STI571, focus formation was inhibited and cells displayed an organized growth pattern with maintenance of distinct cellular margins.[27] This effect was dose-dependent and completely achieved at a drug concentration of $1\mu M$. The loss of transformed growth characteristics was not due to drug-induced cytotoxicity since doses of up to $10\mu M$ did not induce cell death, and removal of STI571 allowed gradual regeneration of the transformed phenotype.[27] Uninfected DMVEC exhibited normal growth with an organized cobblestone phenotype when maintained at confluence, and exposure of uninfected DMVEC to STI571 had no effect on cell morphology or viability.

STI571, (also known as imatinib mesylate; Gleevec™, Norvartis Pharmaceuticals, East Hanover, NJ), has proved to be remarkably effective for the treatment of chronic myelogenous leukemia (CML) through its inhibition of the TK activity of the BCR-ABL gene product. Gleevec was also recently FDA approved for the treatment of gastrointestinal stromal tumor (GIST), where c-Kit is the rational target. Clinical trials with c-Kit inhibitors have not revealed any adverse side-effects for normal hematopoiesis, pigmentation or mast cell activity (reviewed in ref. 28). It has been postulated that sufficient TKR activity for normal cellular processes may be retained in cells exposed to therapeutic concentrations of c-Kit inhibitors. This implies that c-Kit inhibitors would have the greatest therapeutic potential for diseases in which the tumor cells exhibit a preferential response to c-Kit activation, as was seen in the KSHV-infected DMVEC response to exogenous SCF. Indeed in our system, STI571 only returned cell growth to the levels seen in uninfected cells and no cytotoxic effect was observed. Thus, KS may be a cancer that would respond to doses of a c-Kit inhibitor that would not adversely affect normal Kit activity and function.

Inhibition of DMVEC Transformation with Antisense against c-Kit

Since STI571 is also active against a handful of other TKR receptors (e.g., c-Abl, BCR-Abl, PDGF-R), we wanted to confirm the specificity of action against c-Kit by an independent method. We planned a strategy based on specific inhibition of c-Kit mRNA translation through the use of antisense RNA molecules. The antisense strategy we selected is based on the use of phosphorodiamidate morpholino antisense oligomers (PMO-AS).[32] PMO-AS are 15–18 base pair oligonucleotides complementary to a specific mRNA start codon that prevent message translation through steric hindrance.[33] Intracellular delivery of the molecules is accomplished using a proprietary delivery system based on an EPEI delivery reagent developed by GeneTools, LLC (details at www.gene-tools.com). A PMO-AS complementary to the c-Kit start codon was obtained from GeneTools (Corvallis, OR) and KSHV-infected DMVEC were treated with an anti-KIT oligomer-EPEI delivery reagent complex. Control DMVEC cultures were loaded with EPEI reagent and sterile water or sterile water alone. Upon removal of the oligomer-EPEI solution, cell monolayers were cultured postconfluence to allow for focus formation, and examined by phase microscopy for evidence of phenotypic change. As expected, loss of contact inhibition and the capacity to grow in disorganized multilayered foci was evident in control KSHV-infected

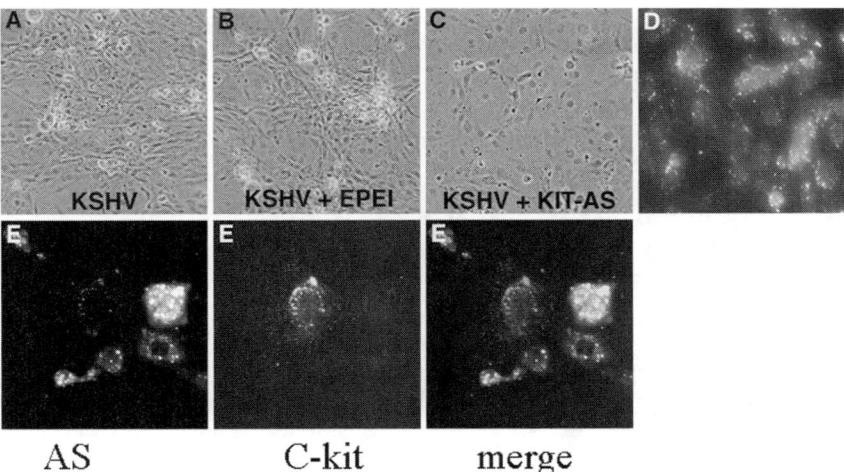

FIGURE 4. Inhibition of c-Kit expression with an antisense (AS) oligomer prevents KSHV-induced DMVEC transformation. (**A**) KSHV-infected DMVEC were cultured at confluence for 5 days to allow formation of multilayered foci. (**B**) KSHV-infected DMVEC treated with AS delivery reagent alone (EPEI) retained the ability to form foci. (**C**) Focus formation was inhibited by treating KSHV-infected DMVEC with an anti-Kit-AS. (**D**) Visualization of the FITC tag on the oligomer revealed efficient and stable cellular uptake. (**E**) In cell cultures loaded with less anti-Kit-AS, the reduction of c-Kit protein is evident only on AS-loaded/FITC$^+$ cells. *Left panel:* FITC-labeled AS; *middle panel:* Rhodamin-stained c-Kit; *right panel:* Merge of c-Kit and AS. Note that only the cell on the upper left does not contain AS and expresses c-Kit whereas all other cells in this field contain AS and do not express c-Kit.

DMVECs cultured for a five-day period (see FIGURE 4A). KSHV-infected DMVEC treated with the delivery agent (EPEI) alone showed similar focus formation at five days postloading (FIG. 4B). In contrast, cells loaded with 1.25 nM of the anti-c-Kit oligomer did not develop foci, but maintained a quiescent contact-inhibited monolayer (FIG. 4C). A FITC tag on the oligomer revealed uptake by more than 90% of DMVEC and stable persistence of the oligomer for the seven-day culture period examined (FIG. 4D). In dishes loaded with only 0.75nM of oligomer (where FITC expression was observed in ± 60% of cells), partial inhibition of focus formation was observed. These cultures were used to verify that the c-Kit oligomer was able to functionally downregulate c-Kit protein, since adjacent FITC/oligomer-positive and FITC/oligomer-negative cells could be observed in the same field. FIGURE 4E clearly demonstrates that c-Kit downregulation occurred in, but was specifically restricted to, FITC/oligomer-positive cells. These studies demonstrate that the PMO-AS are efficiently taken up and retained in DMVEC and are effective in reducing expression of the target protein. Thus, the antisense strategy will prove an effective means of specifically inhibiting expression of genes of interest and evaluating the consequence of inhibition in functional assays.

DISCUSSION

In summary, by employing gene expression profiling to an *in vitro* KS model, we have identified a group of genes induced by KSHV infection. The potential role of one of these induced gene products, the proto-oncogene c-Kit, was subsequently investigated in more detail. Experiments with recombinant adenovirus vectors demonstrated that overexpression of c-Kit induced spindle formation in normal DMVEC. KSHV-infected DMVEC displayed a growth advantage in response to the c-Kit ligand, SCF, that was inhibited by a pharmacological inhibitor of c-Kit TK activity, STI571. Moreover, inhibition of c-Kit signaling with STI571 abrogated focus formation by KSHV-infected cells, suggesting a role for c-Kit in DMVEC transformation. Validation of c-Kit as an important gene in KS tumorigenesis was greatly facilitated by the availability of STI571. To elucidate the mechanisms through which other genes induced by KSHV orchestrate the phenotypic change in DMVEC cells, we will now systematically investigate a functional role for these genes by inhibiting their expression using the antisense approach first developed with c-Kit.

To our knowledge, only one study has specifically examined KS tissue for c-Kit expression.[34] This study evaluated archived frozen KS tissue samples by immunohistochemistry and identified c-Kit expression in 2 of 13 samples examined. However, since fresh tissue was not available for examination via more sensitive quantitative methods, c-Kit expression in additional samples may have been beyond the sensitivity limits of the assay used. In addition, no information was presented regarding the presence of the KSHV genome or the clinical staging of the tumors. In ovarian cancers for example, Kit reactivity is high in Stage I cancers but decreased in Stage III cancers, implying a more important role for c-Kit in the earlier stages of tumor progression.[35] Despite the limits of the report, detection of c-Kit in at least some of the archival specimens supports a role for c-Kit in KS. While c-Kit expression and function has not to date been stringently examined in KS cells, c-Kit is known to be functionally expressed on endothelial cells, the cell type considered the precursor of the KS spindle cell. Interestingly, EC also express the c-Kit ligand SCF[36–38] and can thus sustain autocrine growth loops. In several small cell lung cancer (SCLC) and breast cancer studies, the observed coexpression of c-Kit and SCF is thought to generate an autocrine growth loop that contributes to malignant growth.[39–43] Cells that express c-Kit and SCF are often minimally responsive to exogenous SCF, suggesting maximal or preferential stimulation by endogenous cell-associated ligand.[40,43,44] In an intriguing study, examination of SCF-positive breast cancer subclones engineered to express different levels of c-Kit demonstrated a direct correlation between the level of c-Kit expressed and the growth response to exogenous SCF.[42] Our gene profiling and RT-PCR studies[27] have confirmed that KSHV-infected DMVEC express SCF as well as c-Kit, but that SCF levels are unaffected by infection. Therefore, the virus-associated defect is at the level of c-Kit expression. Elevated c-Kit levels could thus confer on KSHV-infected cells a preferential ability to respond to soluble SCF produced by neighboring cells. *In vivo*, the paracrine influence could be supplied by macrophages and/or mast cells, both cell types that are potent producers of SCF and extensively infiltrate KS lesions. These data make a compelling role for the c-Kit/SCF axis in promoting KS lesion growth.

Our study is a good example of the power of functional genomics approaches to answer important biological questions. The microarray analysis allowed for the detection of many genes that changed in the presence of KSHV. The known role of c-Kit in tumor formation, and the fact that GIST tumors also form spindle cells, implied an important role for c-Kit in the spindle cell formation induced by KSHV infection. Thus, the array results allowed for the formulation of new hypotheses that could subsequently be tested. Importantly, since multiple cellular genes were regulated by KSHV infection, it can be assumed that c-Kit is just the tip of the iceberg, and that additional oncogenic pathways remain to be discovered.

REFERENCES

1. TEMPLETON, A.C. 1981. Kaposi's sarcoma. Pathol. Annu. **16**(Pt.): 315–336.
2. ROTH, W.K., H. BRANDSTETTER & M. STURZL. 1992. Cellular and molecular features of HIV-associated Kaposi's sarcoma [editorial] [published erratum appears in AIDS 1992 Nov; **6**(11):following 1410]. Aids **6**(9): 895–913.
3. TAPPERO, J.W., M.A. CONANT, S.F. WOLFE, *et al*. 1993. Kaposi's sarcoma. Epidemiology, pathogenesis, histology, clinical spectrum, staging criteria and therapy. J. Am. Acad. Dermatol. **28**(3): 371–395.
4. GILL, P.S., B.M. ESPINA, T. MOUDGIL, *et al*. 1994. All-*trans* retinoic acid for the treatment of AIDS-related Kaposi's sarcoma: results of a pilot phase II study. Leukemia **8**(Suppl. 3): S26–S32.
5. GOEDERT, J.J., T.R. COTE, P. VIRGO, *et al*. 1998. Spectrum of AIDS-associated malignant disorders. Lancet **351**(9119): 1833–1839.
6. CHANG, Y., E. CESARMAN, M.S. PESSIN, *et al*. 1994. Identification of herpesvirus-like DNA sequences in AIDS-associated Kaposi's sarcoma [see comments]. Science **266**(5192): 1865–1869.
7. CESARMAN, E., Y. CHANG, P.S. MOORE, *et al*. 1995. Kaposi's sarcoma-associated herpesvirus-like DNA sequences in AIDS-related body-cavity-based lymphomas [see comments]. N. Engl. J. Med. **332**(18): 1186–1191.

8. SOULIER, J., L. GROLLET, E. OKSENHENDLER, et al. 1995. Kaposi's sarcoma-associated herpesvirus-like DNA sequences in multicentric Castleman's disease. Blood 86(4): 1276–1280.
9. BOSHOFF, C., T.F. SCHULZ, M.M. KENNEDY, et al. 1995. Kaposi's sarcoma-associated herpesvirus infects endothelial and spindle cells. Nat. Med. 1(12): 1274–1278.
10. LI, J.J., Y.Q. HUANG, C.J. COCKERELL, et al. 1996. Localization of human herpes-like virus type 8 in vascular endothelial cells and perivascular spindle-shaped cells of Kaposi's sarcoma lesions by in situ hybridization. Am. J. Pathol. 148(6): 1741–1748.
11. STASKUS, K.A., W. ZHONG, K. GEBHARD, et al. 1997. Kaposi's sarcoma-associated herpesvirus gene expression in endothelial (spindle) tumor cells. J. Virol. 71(1): 715–719.
12. STURZL, M., C. BLASIG, A. SCHREIER, et al. 1997. Expression of HHV-8 latency-associated T0.7 RNA in spindle cells and endothelial cells of AIDS-associated, classical and African Kaposi's sarcoma. Int. J. Cancer 72(1): 68–71.
13. DAMANIA, B. & J.U. JUNG. 2001. Comparative analysis of the transforming mechanisms of Epstein-Barr virus, Kaposi's sarcoma-associated herpesvirus, and *Herpesvirus saimiri*. Adv. Cancer Res. 80: 51–82.
14. ARVANITAKIS, L., E.A. MESRI, R.G. NADOR, et al. 1996. Establishment and characterization of a primary effusion (body cavity-based) lymphoma cell line (BC-3) harboring kaposi's sarcoma-associated herpesvirus (KSHV/HHV-8) in the absence of Epstein-Barr virus. Blood 88(7): 2648–2654.
15. BOSHOFF, C., S.-J. GAO, L.E. HEALY, et al. 1998. Establishing a $KSHV^+$ cell line (BCP-1) from peripheral blood and characterizing its growth in nod/SCID mice. Blood 91(5): 1671–1679.
16. BECKSTEAD, J.H., G.S. WOOD & V. FLETCHER. 1985. Evidence for the origin of Kaposi's sarcoma from lymphatic endothelium. Am. J. Pathol. 119(2): 294–300.
17. RUTGERS, J.L., R. WIECZOREK, F. BONETTI, et al. 1986. The expression of endothelial cell surface antigens by AIDS-associated Kaposi's sarcoma. Evidence for a vascular endothelial cell origin. Am. J. Pathol. 122(3): 493–499.
18. SCULLY, P.A., H.K. STEINMAN, C. KENNEDY, et al. 1988. AIDS-related Kaposi's sarcoma displays differential expression of endothelial surface antigens. Am. J. Pathol. 130(2): 244–251.
19. ROTH, W.K., S. WERNER, W. RISAU, et al. 1988. Cultured, AIDS-related Kaposi's sarcoma cells express endothelial cell markers and are weakly malignant in vitro. Int. J. Cancer 42(5): 767–773.
20. ALUIGI, M.G., A. ALBINI, S. CARLONE, et al. 1996. KSHV sequences in biopsies and cultured spindle cells of epidemic, iatrogenic and Mediterranean forms of Kaposi's sarcoma. Res. Virol. 147(5): 267–275.
21. AMBROZIAK, J.A., D.J. BLACKBOURN, B.G. HERNDIER, et al. 1995. Herpes-like sequences in HIV-infected and uninfected Kaposi's sarcoma patients. Science 268(5210): 582–583.
22. FLORE, O., S. RAFII, S. ELY, et al. 1998. Transformation of primary human endothelial cells by Kaposi's sarcoma- associated herpesvirus. Nature 394(6693): 588–592.
23. CIUFO, D.M., J.S. CANNON, L.J. POOLE, et al. 2001. Spindle cell conversion by Kaposi's sarcoma-associated herpesvirus: formation of colonies and plaques with mixed lytic and latent gene expression in infected primary dermal microvascular endothelial cell cultures. J. Virol. 75(12): 5614–5626.
24. LAGUNOFF, M., J. BECHTEL, E. VENETSANAKOS, et al. 2002. De novo infection and serial transmission of Kaposi's sarcoma-associated herpesvirus in cultured endothelial cells. J. Virol. 76(5): 2440–2448.
25. MOSES, A.V., K.N. FISH, R. RUHL, et al. 1999. Long-term infection and transformation of dermal microvascular endothelial cells by human herpesvirus 8. J. Virol. 73(8): 6892–6902.
26. VIEIRA, J., P. O'HEARN, L. KIMBALL, et al. 2001. Activation of Kaposi's sarcoma-associated herpesvirus (human herpesvirus 8) lytic replication by human cytomegalovirus. J. Virol. 75(3): 1378–1386.

27. MOSES, A.V., M.A. JARVIS, C. RAGGO, et al. 2002. KSHV-induced upregulation of the c-kit proto-oncogene, as identified by gene expression profiling, is essential for the transformation of endothelial cells. J. Virol. **76**(16): 8383–8399.
28. HEINRICH, M.C., C.D. BLANKE, B.J. DRUKER, et al. 2002. Inhibition of KIT tyrosine kinase activity: a novel molecular approach to the treatment of KIT-positive malignancies. J. Clin. Oncol. **20**(6): 1692–1703.
29. LINNEKIN, D. 1999. Early signaling pathways activated by c-Kit in hematopoietic cells. Int. J. Biochem. Cell Biol. **31**(10): 1053–1074.
30. BOISSAN, M., F. FEGER, J.J. GUILLOSSON, et al. 2000. c-Kit and c-kit mutations in mastocytosis and other hematological diseases. J. Leukocyte Biol. **67**(2): 135–148.
31. HEINRICH, M.C., D.J. GRIFFITH, B.J. DRUKER, et al. 2000. Inhibition of c-kit receptor tyrosine kinase activity by STI 571, a selective tyrosine kinase inhibitor. Blood **96**(3): 925–932.
32. SUMMERTON, J. & D. WELLER. 1997. Morpholino antisense oligomers: design, preparation, and properties. Antisense Nucleic Acid Drug Dev. **7**(3): 187–195.
33. GHOSH, C., D. STEIN, D. WELLER, et al. 2000. Evaluation of antisense mechanisms of action. Methods Enzymol. **313**: 135–143.
34. MIETTINEN, M., M. SARLOMO-RIKALA, J. LASOTA. 2000. KIT expression in angiosarcomas and fetal endothelial cells: lack of mutations of exon 11 and exon 17 of C-kit. Mod. Pathol. **13**(5): 536–541.
35. PARROTT, J.A., G. KIM, M.K. SKINNER. 2000. Expression and action of kit ligand/stem cell factor in normal human and bovine ovarian surface epithelium and ovarian cancer. Biol. Reprod. **62**(6): 1600–1609.
36. MIYAMOTO, T., Y. SASAGURI, T. SASAGURI, et al. 1997. Expression of stem cell factor in human aortic endothelial and smooth muscle cells. Atherosclerosis **129**(2): 207–213.
37. MIYAMOTO, T., Y. SASAGURI, K. SUGAMA, et al. 1994. Expression of the c-kit mRNA in human aortic endothelial cells. Biochem. Mol. Biol. Int. **34**(3): 513–520.
38. HEINRICH, M.C., D.C. DOOLEY, A.C. FREED, et al. 1993. Constitutive expression of steel factor gene by human stromal cells. Blood **82**(3): 771–783.
39. MATSUDA, R., T. TAKAHASHI, S. NAKAMURA, et al. 1993. Expression of the c-kit protein in human solid tumors and in corresponding fetal and adult normal tissues. Am. J. Pathol. **142**(1): 339–346.
40. TURNER, A.M., K.M. ZSEBO, F. MARTIN, et al. 1992. Nonhematopoietic tumor cell lines express stem cell factor and display c-kit receptors. Blood **80**(2): 374–381.
41. INOUE, M., S. KYO, M. FUJITA, et al. 1994. Coexpression of the c-kit receptor and the stem cell factor in gynecological tumors. Cancer Res. **54**(11): 3049–3053.
42. HINES, S.J., C. ORGAN, M.J. KORNSTEIN, et al. 1995. Coexpression of the c-kit and stem cell factor genes in breast carcinomas. Cell Growth Differ. **6**(6): 769–779.
43. KRYSTAL, G.W., S.J. HINES & C.P. ORGAN. 1996. Autocrine growth of small cell lung cancer mediated by coexpression of c-kit and stem cell factor. Cancer Res. **56**(2): 370–376.
44. BROUDY, V.C., N.L. KOVACH, L.G. BENNETT, et al. 1994. Human umbilical vein endothelial cells display high-affinity c-kit receptors and produce a soluble form of the c-kit receptor. Blood **83**(8): 2145–2152.

Chlamydiae Host Cell Interactions Revealed Using DNA Microarrays

JAMES B. MAHONY

Department of Pathology and Molecular Medicine, McMaster University, Regional Virology and Chlamydiology Laboratory, St. Joseph's Healthcare, Hamilton, Ontario, Canada L8N 4A6

ABSTRACT: Chlamydiae are obligate intracellular bacterial parasites that infect eukaryotic cells and live their entire life cycle within a cytoplasmic vacuole or inclusion. We have employed cDNA microarray and conventional biological approaches to study the pathogen-host cell interaction during *C. pneumoniae* infection of eukaryotic cells. Two host cell signaling pathways, MEK/ERK and PI 3-kinase/Akt, were activated within 5 and 20 minutes, respectively, following infection with chlamydiae. Pharmacological inhibition of these pathways blocked invasion of HEp2 cells indicating that activation of these pathways was required for infection. Rho family GTPase activity was essential for invasion, since the pan-Rho GTPase inhibitor, compactin, blocked infection of HEp2 cells. cDNA microarrays and reverse transcriptase PCR were used to study host cell and chlamydial gene expression during the replication cycle. Analysis of host cell gene expression following infection with *C. pneumoniae* indicated that genes coding for cytokines, growth factors, and signaling molecules were upregulated, as early as 2 hours postinfection. Analysis of chlamydial gene expression indicated a temporal regulation of transcription with distinct early-, mid-, and late-cycle classes of RNA transcripts. Newly discovered genes encoding three Ser/Thr protein kinases and one protein phosphatase were upregulated 6–12 hours postinfection. One protein kinase, designated CpnPK1, was first detected at 12 hours postinfection, accumulated in the inclusion throughout the replication cycle, and may be a type III effector molecule. An increased understanding of chlamydial host cell interactions, in particular the role of various chlamydial proteins in infection and identification of essential virulence factors should provide novel targets for the development of new antimicrobials.

KEYWORDS: chlamydiae; invasion; pathogen-host cell interactions; cDNA; microarrays

INTRODUCTION

Chlamydiae are members of the Chlamydiaceae family and are highly evolved pathogens capable of infecting a wide range of warm- and cold-blooded animals and a variety of cell types ranging from soil protists to brain microglial cells. In man, *C. trachomatis* is the world's leading cause of preventable blindness and the most

---

Address for correspondence: James B. Mahony, Director, Regional Virology and Chlamydiology Laboratory, St. Joseph's Healthcare, 50 Charlton Ave., East, Hamilton, Ontario, Canada L8N 4A6. Voice: 905-521-6021; fax: 905-521-6083.
mahonyj@mcmaster.ca

common sexually transmitted bacterial agent causing mucopurulent endocervicitis, endometritis, pelvic inflammatory disease, salpingitis, and involuntary infertility in women, urethritis in men, and conjunctivits, proctitis and pneumonitis in both genders. *C. pneumoniae* infections are common worldwide with seroepidemiological studies indicating that up to 70% of the general population is infected with this bacteria. Manifestations include pharyngitis, bronchitis, pneumonia, and exacerbations of asthma.[1] *C. pneumoniae* has been associated with atherosclerosis, coronary artery disease and stroke, and *C. pneumoniae* DNA has been detected in about 50% of atheromas in several published studies.[2] *C. pneumoniae* DNA has also been detected in CSF specimens of multiple sclerosis patients and in post mortem studies of brains of Alzheimer's disease patients in two small studies, but these findings have yet to be confirmed.

Chlamydiae are gram-negative, obligate, intracellular pathogens that possess a unique biphasic replication cycle which begins with infectious, nonmetabolically active elementary bodies (EB) binding to surface receptors which results in their uptake.[3] Chlamydiae direct their uptake into nonphagocytic cells by commandeering several host cell signaling pathways to induce a rearrangement of the actin cytoskeleton and formation of microvilli.[4] Once inside a vacuole, EB transform into metabolically active but noninfectious reticulate bodies (RB) that multiply by binary fission and undergo a transformation back into EB prior to release from the infected cell (see FIGURE 1). Chlamydial gene expression begins within two hours after infection, and RNA transcripts can be grouped into early- (genes coding for proteins involved in RNA, DNA and protein synthesis), mid- (genes coding for enzymes of intermediate metabolism) and late-cycle (genes involved in chromosome partitioning and cytokinesis).[5] Chlamydial transcription patterns appear to differ during an active replicating and nonreplicating persistent infection. Chlamydiae are auxotrophic for some amino acids and ribonucleoside triphosphates and have several ABC transporters for the uptake of these essential nutrients across the inclusion membrane. Under sub-optimal growth conditions (iron deprivation, heat shock, IFN-γ or antibiotics) chlamydiae transform into large persistent bodies which stop dividing (see FIGURE 2). A newly discovered family of Inc proteins that are incorporated into the inclusion membrane may act as porins or transporters for the uptake of

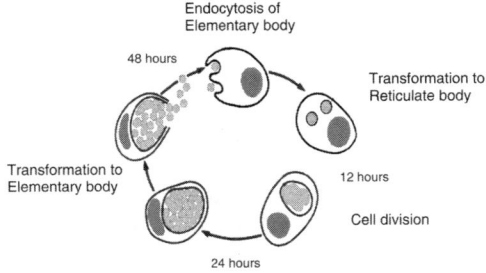

FIGURE 1. Chlamydiae replication cycle showing attachment and endocytosis of EB, transformation of EB to RB (2 h), cell division (12–24 h), transformation of RB to EB (24–48 h) and release of infectious EB (48–72 h).

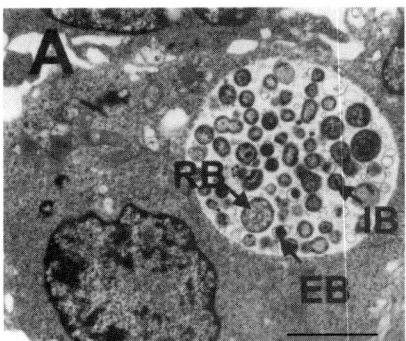
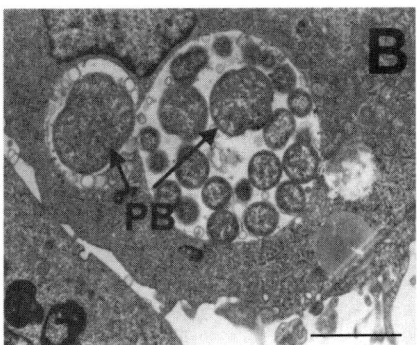

FIGURE 2. Chlamydial inclusions viewed by electron microscopy. Panel **A**, *C. pneumonie*-infected HEp2 cell showing reticulate body (RB), elementary body (EB), and intermediate body (IB); Panel **B**, *C. pneumoniae*-infected HEp2 cell pretreated with IFN-γ showing persistent body (PB). *Bar* = 1 μm.

nutrients.[6] Chlamydiae are susceptible to many broad spectrum antibiotics. The complete genome sequences of five chlamydiae including *C. trachomatis* and *C. pneumoniae* have been revealed.[7,8]

INVASION OF HOST CELLS

It is now clear that chlamydiae possess the required machinery to infect both professional phagocytes and nonprofessional phagocytic cells of several lineages including epithelial, endothelial, and smooth muscle cells. Efforts directed at understanding how chlamydiae attach to susceptible host cells have yet to reveal specific host cell receptors and to date, no adhesin has been shown to unequivocally mediate binding to and invasion of susceptible cells. Of the two predominant types of invasion sequences described for intracellular bacteria (trigger and zipper mechanisms), scanning electron microscopic studies reveal chlamydial invasion to resemble more closely the zipper-type process involving filopodia or microvilli, where the host cell membrane is in close juxtaposition around EB being internalized (see FIGURE 3). For some bacteria binding and internalization events have been shown to be multifaceted, requiring at least one other secondary receptor to facilitate invasion. A similar bipartite mechanism of invasion may also exist for chlamydiae, whereby initial attachment to the cell surface is followed by receptor activation, or interaction with a secondary receptor leading to uptake. Such a mechanism is supported by experimental evidence describing the ability to block chlamydial internalization without affecting binding to the cell surface. Experiments in our laboratory have recently shown that inhibition of specific host cell signal transduction cascades and actin polymerization can abrogate *C. pneumoniae* uptake without blocking attachment to the surface of HEp2 cells, suggestive of additional steps in the invasion process subsequent to initial attachment that are required for internalization.[4]

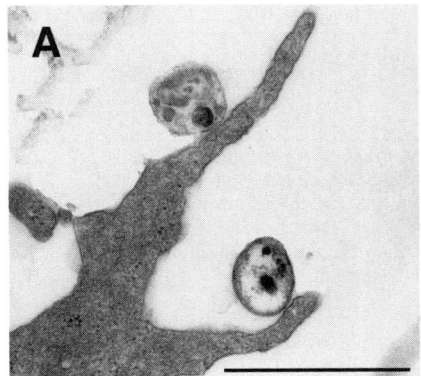
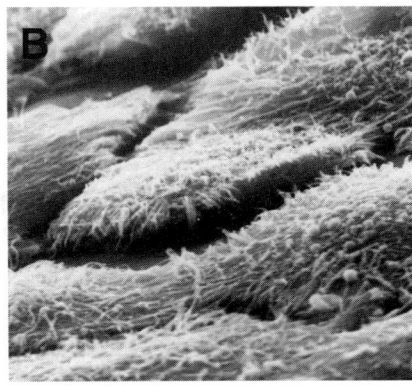

FIGURE 3. Induction of microvilli by *C. pneumoniae* into HEp2 cells. Panel **A**, transmission EM of microvilli 15 minutes after infection; Panel **B**, scanning EM of surface of HEp2 cells 15 minutes after infection. *Bar* = 1 µm.

Invasion by pathogenic bacteria relies heavily on manipulation of host cell signaling pathways in order to commandeer the cytoskeleton for uptake or for full virulence *in vivo*.[9] Often the molecular mediators to activate and deactivate specific cellular signaling cascades are delivered at the cell surface in the form of bacterial type III secretion effector proteins. Signal transduction pathways in mammalian cells are comprised of a collection of kinases, phosphatases, and adaptor molecules that collectively regulate diverse cellular processes including cytoskeletal rearrangements. Intracellular bacteria have evolved mechanisms to selectively activate and

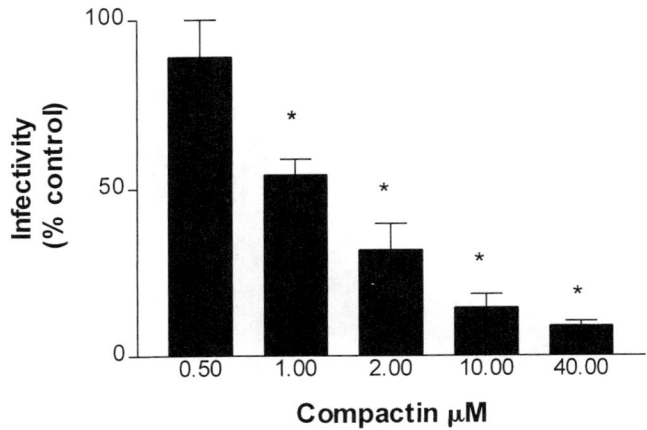

FIGURE 4. Effect of compactin on infectivity of *C. pneumoniae*. Data are expressed as the mean ± S.E. of duplicate determinations performed in three separate experiments. *$P < 0.01$, compared to no drug.

TABLE 1. Identification of *C. pneumoniae*–induced genes in HMEC-1[10] by cDNA array

Gene	cDNA probe accession number[a]	Major function(s)	Relative mRNA expression ratio[b]
Heparin-binding EGF-like growth factor	M60278	Blastocyst implantation, wound healing, tumor growth, smooth muscle cell hyperplasia, atherosclerosis; membrane-bound and soluble forms; soluble form is mitogenic and chemotactic for smooth muscle cells and fibroblasts	17.3
Insulin-like growth factor binding protein-4	M62403	Transport of IGFs in circulation; modulation of IGF binding to receptors and growth-promoting actions	15
Stromal-derived factor 1A	L36034	CXC chemokine; B-lymphophoiesis, cardiogenesis	13.0
Growth-associated protein-43	M25667	Neuronal growth; intracellular signaling molecule involved in cytoskeletal reorganization	10
Interferon α receptor	J03171	Jak tyrosine kinase-associated; STAT transcription factor activation	8.0
Insulin-like growth factor I receptor	X04434	Signal transduction component; a transmembrane tyrosine kinase linked to the ras/raf-MAPK cascade; antiapoptotic effects *in vivo* and *in vitro*	7.5
Interferon regulatory factor-1	X14454	Interferon-inducible transcription factor, regulates the transcriptional activation of IFN genes and genes involved in cell cycle progression and apoptosis	5.8
PDGF-α receptor	M21574	Member of the protein tyrosine kinase family of receptors	4.1
MCP-1	M24545	C-C chemokine; monocyte chemoattractant	3.5
Brain-derived neurotrophic factor	M61176	Involved in neuron integrity, stimulates the synaptic strength and survival of neurons	3.0
IL-8	Y00787	Chemotactic for neutrophils; neutrophil activation	2.7
IL-1β	K02770	T-cell activation, macrophage activation	2.5
Platelet-derived growth factor–associated protein	U41745	Binds PDGF with low affinity and enhances the mitogenic effect of PDGF-A, but not PDGF-B	2.5
PDGF-B chain	X02811	Mitogenic for connective tissue cells, chemokine for smooth muscle cells, fibroblasts, BB homodimer biologically active	2.5

TABLE 1/continued.

Gene	cDNA probe accession number[a]	Major function(s)	Relative mRNA expression ratio[b]
Erythroid differentiation protein	J03634	Also called Activin A; member of TGF-β superfamily, acts as paracrine and autocrine mediator of host defenses	2.4
FMLP-related receptor	M76673	Seven-transmembrane receptor, linked to G protein-coupled receptors, to activate chemotaxis and exocytosis	2.3
Basic fibroblast growth factor	M27968	Widespread mitogenic and neurotrophic activities, activates receptor tyrosine kinases	2.3
TNF-inducible hyaluronate-binding protein (TSG-6)	M31165	Cytokine-inducible secreted glycoprotein, antiinflammatory activity, plasmin inhibitor, possibly involved in SMC growth	2.1
Coagulation factor II receptor	M62424	Seven-transmembrane, G protein-coupled receptor for thrombin	2.0

cDNA microarrays were analyzed by scanning densitometry, and gene signals were normalized to the β-actin housekeeping gene.
[a]cDNA probe accession numbers correspond to gene sequences from GenBank.
[b]Relative mRNA expression is a ratio of the normalized optical density gene signal from *C. pneumoniae*-infected cells/normalized optical density gene signal from uninfected control cells. mRNA expression was assessed at 18 h postinfection.

deactivate cellular signaling cascades in order to manipulate the intracellular environment in a way that is compatible with invasion, growth, and intracellular residency. We have recently shown that *C. pneumoniae* infection of HEp2 cells induces phosphorylation and activation of specific host cell signaling pathways involving phosphoinositide (PI) 3-kinase, Akt, MEK1/2, extracellular signal–regulated kinase (ERK) 1/2, focal adhesion kinase (FAK) and the adaptor protein Shc.[4] The activity of PI 3-kinase and MEK, together with actin polymerization were necessary for bacterial entry into host cells, but not for attachment to the cell surface, suggesting that one outcome of *C. pneumoniae*-induced activation of PI 3-kinase and MEK1/2 signaling may be to facilitate cytoskeleton rearrangements and microvilli formation necessary for bacterial uptake. This is supported by the finding that treatment of cells with cytochalasin D reproduced both the inhibitory effect on *C. pneumoniae* entry without affecting binding to the cell surface, and the inhibition of microvilli formation during *C. pneumoniae* invasion in the presence of PI 3-kinase and MEK inhibitors. The critical involvement of the cytoskeleton is further indicated by the activity of the Rho-family GTPase inhibitor, compactin, which also blocks infection (see FIGURE 4). These data confirm the importance of cytoskeletal rearrangement for chlamydial invasion. We suspect that the diversity of chlamydial usage of host cell signaling to the benefit of the bacteria will become more complex as type III effector proteins in these bacteria are identified.

HOST CELL GENE EXPRESSION

Complete genome sequences of both microbial pathogens and host cells form the basis of microarray technology to study host-pathogen interactions. We have used a host gene cDNA array to characterize the mRNA expression profiles for 268 human genes following infection with *C. pneumoniae*.[10] *C. pneumoniae* infection upregulated mRNA expression for approximately 20 (8%) of the genes studied, some within two hours following infection (see TABLE 1). Genes coding for cytokines (interleukin-1), chemokines (monocyte chemotactic protein 1 and interleukin-8), and cellular growth factors (heparin-binding epidermal-like growth factor, basic fibroblast growth factor, and platelet-derived growth factor B chain) were the most prominently upregulated. While this study was modest in nature compared to the high density arrays containing thousands of host-cell genes, it provided the first exploration of host response to infection at the level of gene expression. Larger studies using high density arrays to analyze host gene profiling in response to chlamydial infection are anticipated in the very near future.

CHLAMYDIAL GENE EXPRESSION

Chlamydial microarrays to monitor chlamydial gene expression inside host cells are under development. These arrays will undoubtedly offer valuable information about microbial gene expression in a bacterial system that is notoriously difficult to work with. We have used RT-PCR analysis to study the temporal expression of selected genes during the replication cycle of *C. pneumoniae* (see FIGURE 5). Gene expression is regulated during the cycle with selected genes being upregulated during early- (16S rRNA, hsp60, omcB, adt1, ompA), mid- (polA, Cpn0095, Cpn0148, Cpn0703) or late-cycle (hctA, ftsK, parB).[11] A molecular description of the bacterial transcriptional program during infection could provide novel predictions about functions of unknown genes during the developmental cycle, characterize the adaptive response of chlamydiae following environmental perturbation, define a global gene signature of persistent bodies, and make hypothesis-driven predictions about putative virulence-associated genes during natural infections. However, genomic data generated from such studies will require careful molecular and biochemical experimentation in order to confirm the biological role of upregulated proteins.

The initial interaction between Gram-negative bacteria and host cells is at the level of membrane proteins and proteins that are secreted into the host cell. Evidence is mounting that chlamydiae contain a type III secretion apparatus. In addition to the observation of pili-like structures on the EB membrane initially observed in 1982 by Matsumoto, recent genomic analysis has revealed the presence of homologues of both structural and regulatory genetic components of a type III apparatus. Many gram-negative pathogenic bacteria direct their uptake into host cells with type III effectors. Several type III effectors are protein kinases and protein phosphatases that commandeer host signaling pathways to induce uptake and/or intracellular survival. We have shown recently that three Ser/Thr protein kinase genes in *C. pneumoniae* (Cpn0095, Cpn0148, Cpn0703) are upregulated 6–12 hours postinfection.[11] One of the kinases, CpnPK1 (Cpn0148), which first appears at 24 hours postinfection, accumulates into "preloaded" RB/EB throughout the cycle, suggesting a possible role for this protein as a type III effector during invasion (see FIGURE 6). Experiments are currently in progress to elucidate the role of these protein kinases in pathogenesis.

SUMMARY

Much has been learned about chlamydial biology since the sequencing of the entire genomes of *C. trachomatis* and *C. pneumoniae*. The availability of the complete genome sequence for chlamydia has provided a welcome opportunity for gene discovery and elucidation of roles that newly discovered proteins play in the pathogenesis of a bacteria for which tools of genetic manipulation are lacking. Availability of both human and chlamydial gene arrays will provide a greater understanding of

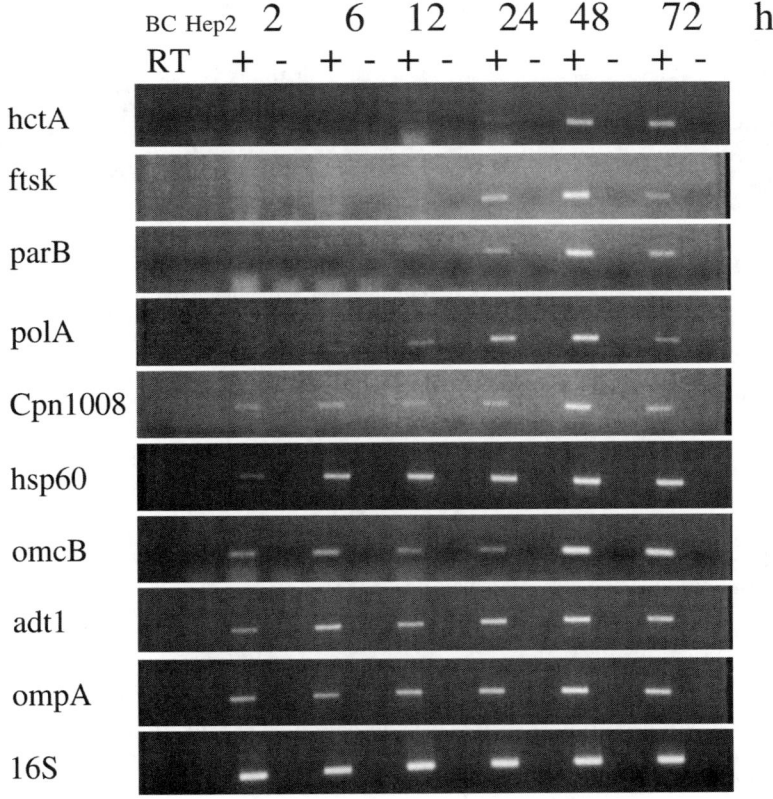

FIGURE 5. Temporally regulated expression of early- (16S rRNA, omp A, adt 1, omc B, hsp 60, Cpn1008) mid-(pol A), and late-cycle genes (ftsk, par B, hct A) during the replication cycle of *C. pneumoniae*. BC = no RNA control, RT$^-$ = no reverse transcriptase control.

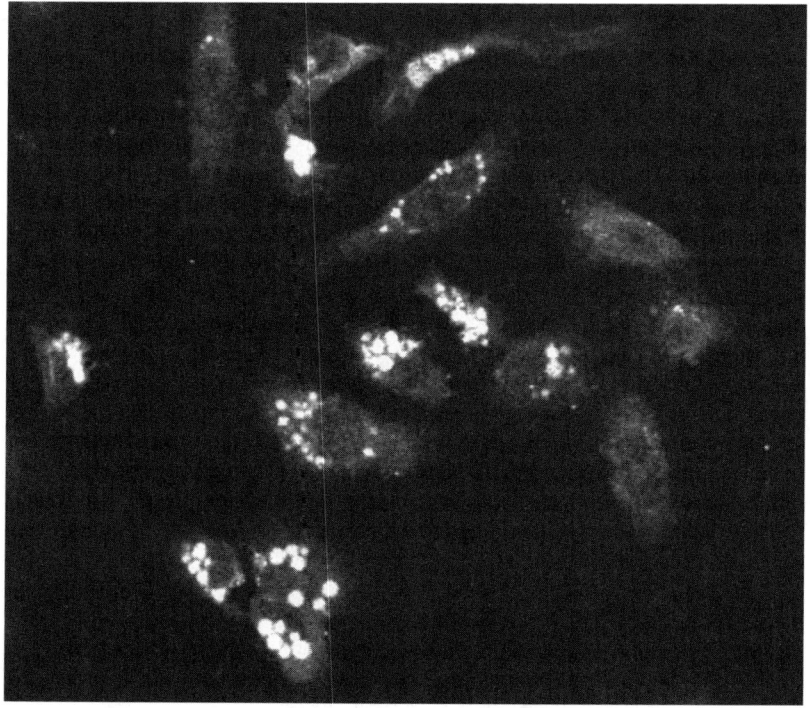

FIGURE 6. Expression of Cpn0148 Ser/Thr protein kinase in infected HEp2 cells. Cpn0148 was detected by indirect IF staining using mouse polyclonal antiserum to recombinant Cpn0148 and Alexa 488-conjugated anti-mouse IgG antibody at 48 h postinfection.

the intimate interaction between pathogen and host and may reveal increasing usage of host cell signaling by this highly evolved bacteria.

REFERENCES

1. KUO, C.C., L.A. JACKSON, L.A. CAMPBELL & J.T. GRAYSTON. 1995. *Chlamydia pneumoniae* (TWAR). Clin. Microbiol. Rev. **8:** 451–461.
2. GRAYSTON, J.T. 2000. Background and current knowledge of *Chlamydia pneumoniae* and atherosclerosis. J. Infect. Dis. **181**(Suppl. 3) S402–S410.
3. MOULDER, J.W. 1984. Order Chlamydiales and family Chlamydiaceae. *In* Bergey's Manual of Systematic Bacteriology, Vol. **1:** 729–739. N.R. Krieg & J.G. Holt, Eds. The Williams & Wilkins Co. Baltimore, MD.
4. COOMBES, B.K. & J. B. MAHONY. 2002. Identification of MEK- and phosphoinositide 3-kinase-dependent signalling as essential events during *Chlamydia pneumoniae* invasion of Hep2 cells. Cell. Microbiol. **4:** 447–460.
5. SHAW, E.I., C.A. DOOLEY, E.R. FISCHER, *et al.* 2000. Three temporal classes of gene expression during the *Chlamydia trachomatis* developmental cycle. Mol. Microbiol. **37:** 913–.
6. ROCKEY, D.D., M.A. SCIDMORE, J.P. BANNATINE & W.J. BROWN. 2002. Proteins in the chlamydial inclusion membrane. Microbes Infect. **4:** 333–340.

7. KALMAN, S., W.P. MITCHELL, R. MARATHE, et al. 1999. Comparative genomes of *Chlamydia pneumoniae* and *C. trachomatis*. Nat. Genet. **21:** 385–391.
8. STEPHENS, R.S., S. KALMAN, C. LAMMEL, et al. 1998. Genome sequence of an obligate intracellular pathogen of humans: *Chlamydia trachomatis*. Science **282:** 754–759.
9. FINLAY, B.B. & P. COSSART. 1997. Exploitation of mammalian host cell functions by bacterial pathogens. Science **276:** 718–725.
10. COOMBES, B.K. & J.B. MAHONY. 2001. cDNA array analysis of altered gene expression in human endothelial cells in response to *Chlamydia pneumoniae* infection. Infect. Immun. **69:** 1420–1427.
11. MAHONY, J.B., D. JOHNSON, B. COOMBES & X. SONG. 2002. Expression of a novel protein kinase gene (Cpn0148) during the replication cycle of *Chlamydia pneumoniae*. *In* Chlamydial Infections. J. Schachter, G. Christianson, I. Clarke, et al., Eds.: 559–562. Basim Yeri, Turkey.

Gene Expression Profile in *Neisseria meningitidis* and *Neisseria lactamica* upon Host-Cell Contact

From Basic Research to Vaccine Development

R. GRIFANTINI,[a] E. BARTOLINI,[a] A. MUZZI,[a] M. DRAGHI,[a] E. FRIGIMELICA,[a] J. BERGER,[b] F. RANDAZZO,[b] AND G. GRANDI[a]

[a]*Chiron SpA, Siena, Italy*

[b]*Chiron Corporation, 4560 Horton Street, Emeryville, California, USA*

ABBREVIATIONS: MenB–*Neisseria meningitidis* group B; STM–signature tagged mutagenesis; D-MEM–Dulbecco's Modified Eagle l Medium; GAPDH–glyceraldehyde 3-phosphate dehydrogenase; ORF–open reading frame; FCS–fetal calf serum

ABSTRACT: Differential gene regulation in the human pathogen *Neisseria meningitidis* group B (MenB) and in *Neisseria lactamica*, a human commensal species, was studied by whole genome microarray after bacterial interaction with epithelial cells. Host-cell contact induced changes in the expression of 347 and 285 genes in MenB and *N. lactamica*, respectively. Of these, only 167 were common to MenB and *N. lactamica*, suggesting that a different subset of genes is activated by pathogens and commensals. Change in gene expression was stable over time in *N. lactamica*, but short-lived in MenB. A large part (greater than 30%) of the regulated genes encoded proteins with unknown function. Among the known genes, those coding for pili, capsule, protein synthesis, nucleotide synthesis, cell wall metabolism, ATP synthesis, and protein folding were downregulated in MenB. Transporters for iron, chloride and sulfate, some known virulence factors, GAPDH and the entire pathway of selenocysteine biosynthesis were upregulated. Gene expression profiling indicates that approximately 40% of the regulated genes encode putative surface-associated proteins, suggesting that upon cell contact *Neisseria* undergoes substantial surface remodeling. This was confirmed by FACS analysis of adhering bacteria using mouse sera against a subset of recombinant proteins. Finally, a few surface-located, adhesion-activated antigens were capable of inducing bactericidal antibodies, indicating that microarray technology can be exploited for the identification of new vaccine candidates.

KEYWORDS: gene regulation; *Neisseria meningitidis*; *Neisseria lactamica*; vaccine development; microarray

Address for correspondence: Guido Grandi, Chiron SpA, Via Fiorentina 1, 53100 Siena, Italy. Voice: +39 (0577) 243506; fax: +39 (0577) 278514.
guido_grandi@chiron.it

INTRODUCTION

Neisseria meningitidis and *Neisseria lactamica* are related gram-negative bacteria, which colonize the human nasopharynx, but differ in the final outcome. *N. lactamica* is a commensal, which never causes disease. Conversely, *N. meningitidis* eventually spreads from the nasopharynx to the bloodstream and the meninges causing severe meningitis and sepsis in children and young people. The disease is fatal in 5 to 15% of cases and causes severe neurological sequelae in up to 25% of survivors.

Although enormous progress has been made over the last several years, our understanding of meningococcal invasion and infection is still incomplete (for recent reviews see refs. 1 and 2). New genomic technologies and the recent elucidation of *N. meningitidis* group B (MenB) genome sequence[3] are now expected to facilitate the study of *Neisseria* interaction with its human host.

In this study, DNA microarrays carrying the entire gene repertoire of the MC58 strain have been exploited to analyze changes in gene expression induced in *N. lactamica* and MenB upon interaction with human 16HBE14 epithelial cells. With this kind of analysis, three interesting pieces of information were obtained. First of all, the comparison of the gene activation profiles in MenB and *N. lactamica* led to the identification of genes regulated in both organisms and genes, which are specific for MenB. This latter set of genes is expected to play an important role in MenB virulence and pathogenicity. Secondly, several regulated genes (approximately 40%) encoded peripherally located proteins, indicating that host interaction induces a profound remodeling of the bacterial cell membrane. This observation was confirmed by FACS analysis of MenB cells using antibodies against selected recombinant surface proteins. Finally, when 12 upregulated proteins were tested for their capacity to induce bactericidal antibodies, five of them were positive in this assay indicating that DNA microarray technology can represent a valid approach to new vaccine discovery.

DNA microarrays have been used recently to study the gene expression profile in eukaryotic cells infected with different pathogens,[4–7] however studies focusing on the bacterial genes have not been published so far.[8] This work not only provides an overall picture of the transcriptional changes induced in bacteria upon host interaction, but also reveals novel aspects of meningococcal pathogenicity and paves the way to important applications of this technology.

MATERIALS AND METHODS

Bacterial Strains and Cell Cultures

MenB MC58 and *N. lactamica* NL19 were grown on GCB agar (BD Biosciences, Franklin Lakes, NJ) supplemented with 4g/L glucose, 0.1g/L glutamine, 2.2mg/L cocarboxylase at 37°C in 5% CO_2 for 16 hours. Adhesion assays were performed on 16HBE14, a polarized human bronchial epithelial cell line transformed with SV40 large T-antigen, kindly provided by R. Moxon (Oxford University, UK). Cells were cultured in Dulbecco's Modified Eagle Medium (D-MEM) supplemented with 10% fetal calf serum (FCS), 1.5mM glutamine and 100μg/mL kanamycin sulfate.

Adhesion Experiments

Bacteria colonies from 16-hour old plates were suspended in D-MEM medium at a final OD_{600} value of 1 and 0.4 mL of suspension (about 10^9 bacteria) were added to epithelial cells (2×10^6) and incubated at 37°C in 5% CO_2 at different times. Cell-adhering bacteria were colony counted after extensive washing (four times) of epithelial cells with 5 mL Hanks' Balanced Salt Solution (HBSS)-2% FCS (Life Technologies, Paisley, Scotland), followed by cell lysis with 1% saponin in HBSS for 10 min at 37°C. Nonspecific binding of bacteria to plastic was estimated following the same procedure described above in the absence of epithelial cells.

Microarray Preparation

DNA microarrays were prepared using DNA fragments of each annotated open reading frame (ORF) in the MenB MC58 genome, as published by Tettelin et al.[3] (http:www.tigr.org). PCR primers were selected from a MULTIFASTA file of the genomic ORFs using either Primer 3 (http://www.genome.wi.mit.edu/genome_software/other/primer3.html) or Primer Premier (Premier Biosoft, Ca, USA) software, and the support of locally developed "PERL" scripts for handling multiple nucleotide sequence sets. The majority of PCR primer pairs were 17–25 nucleotides long and were selected within the ORF sequences so as to have an average annealing temperature of around 55°C (range 50 to 60°C) and produce amplified products of 250–1,000 bp (when possible a length of 600–800 bp was selected). For ORFs shorter than 250 bp, primers annealing as close as possible to the start and stop codons were selected. In total, 2,121 out of 2,158 genes were amplified. Considering that the nonamplified genes correspond to duplicated sequences, 100% of the identified ORFs were represented on the chips. Amplification reactions were performed on MC58 genomic DNA with a Gene Amp PCR System 9700 (PE Applied Biosystems, Foster City, CA), and using Taq polymerase (ROCHE Diagnostic, Mannheim, Germany) as recommended by the manufacturer. PCR products were purified using Qia-Quick spin columns (Qiagen, Chatsworth, CA) and quantified spectrophotometrically at OD_{260}.

Array printing was performed using a Gen III spotter (Amersham Biosciences, Uppsala, Sweden) on type VII aluminum coated slides (Amersham Biosciences, Uppsala, Sweden) according to the manufacturer's protocol. Thirty-seven different eukaryotic and prokaryotic genes were included in the chips as positive and negative controls. To establish the stringency of hybridization conditions, six sequences in the 73–100% homology range to a spiked control RNA were also included as controls. Hybridization conditions were set to detect hybridization signals of sequences having at least 73% homology.

Microarray Hybridization and Analysis

Microarray analysis was carried out comparing the profile of total RNA extracted from bacteria growing in D-MEM–10% FCS culture medium and bacteria adhering to epithelial cells. Cell-adhering bacteria were prepared as described above. Total RNA was extracted from bacterial pellets using RNeasy spin columns (Qiagen, Chatsworth, CA). Bacterial RNA was quantified by one-step quantitative RT PCR of the 16S rRNA using LightCycler equipment (ROCHE Diagnostic, Mannheim,

Germany). For RNA labeling, 1.5 μg was reverse transcribed using Superscript II™ reverse transcriptase (Life Technologies, Paisley, Scotland), random 9-mer primers and the fluorochromes Cy-3 dCTP and Cy-5 dCTP (Amersham Biosciences, Uppsala, Sweden). Cy-3 and Cy-5 labeled cDNAs were copurified on Qia-Quick spin columns (Qiagen, Chatsworth, CA). The hybridization probe was constituted by a mixture of the differently labeled cDNAs derived by cell-adhering bacteria and bacteria growing in liquid medium. Probe hybridization and washing were performed as recommended by the slide supplier (Amersham Biosciences, Uppsala, Sweden). Slides were scanned with a GIII scanner (Amersham Biosciences, Uppsala, Sweden) at 10 μm per pixel resolution. In each experiment the two RNA samples were labeled in the direct (Cy3–Cy5) and reverse (Cy5–Cy3) labeling reaction to correct for dye-dependent variation of labeling efficiency. The resulting 16-bit images were processed using the Autogene program (version 2.5, BioDiscovery, Inc., Los Angeles, CA). For each image, the signal value of each spot was determined by subtracting the mean pixel intensity of the background value, and normalizing to the median of all spot signals. The spots, which gave a negative value after background subtraction, were arbitrarily assigned the standard deviation value of negative controls. The data resulting from direct and reverse labeling were averaged for each spot. Expression ratios were obtained at each timepoint dividing hybridization signals from adhering bacterial RNA by nonadhering bacterial RNA. The data from each timepoint represents the average of at least four independent experiments. Genes whose expression ratios changed by at least twofold (P-values < 0.01) were considered up- or down-regulated. Expression pattern analysis and data visualization were done using GeneSpring software (version 3.1.0, Silicon Genetics, Redwood City, CA).

Protein Expression and Immunization Procedures

Genes were PCR-amplified from MC58 chromosomal DNA by using 30-nucleotide-long specific primers annealing at the 5′ and 3′ ends of each gene. In all cases, the leader sequence for secretion was replaced with the ATG codon to drive the expression of the recombinant proteins in the cytoplasm of *E. coli*. Cloning and purification were performed as already described.[9] Briefly, proteins were expressed as His-tagged and GST fusions. His-tagged recombinant proteins were purified by metal ion affinity chromatography (IMAC), whereas glutathione-Sepharose 4B resin (Amersham Pharmacia Biotech, Inc., Piscataway, NJ) was used for GST-fusion purification. 20 μg of each purified protein was mixed with Freund's adjuvant and used to immunize CD1 mice at days 1, 21 and 35. Blood samples were taken on day 34 and 49.

For Western blot analysis, total bacterial extracts were separated on 12–15% polyacrylamide-SDS gels and proteins were detected with 1:100 mouse sera dilutions.

FACS Analysis

Adhering bacteria were collected after saponin treatment, washed with PBS-1% BSA and centrifuged. The bacterial capsule was permeabilized by dropwise addition of cold 70% EtOH directly on the pellet at −20°C for one hour. Bacteria were washed, resuspended with PBS-1% BSA at the desired density and incubated either with sera from mice immunized with meningococcal recombinant proteins or with pre-immune sera[9] for two hours on ice. After washing, bacteria were subsequently incubated with R-phycoerythrin-conjugated goat F(ab)$_2$ anti-mouse IgG (Cedar Lane Laboratories, Hornby, Canada) for 1 hour on ice to detect antibody binding. Bacteria were washed and finally fixed with 0.25% *para*-formaldehyde and analyzed for cell-bound fluorescence using a FACScalibur flow cytometer (Becton Dickinson, Franklin Lakes, NJ). Negative controls included noninfected human 16HBE14 epithelial cells subjected to the procedures described above.

Bactericidal Assay

Bactericidal activity of immune sera was tested against strains MC58, 2996 and mutants using pooled baby rabbit serum (Cedar Lane Laboratories, Hornby, Canada) as complement source, as described.[9] Essentially, bacteria were grown in Mueller-Hinton broth containing 0.25% Glucose, to OD620 of 0.23, and diluted to 105 CFU/mL in assay buffer (50 mM phosphate buffer, 10 mM MgCl2, 10 mM CaCl2, and 0.5% BSA, ph7.2). The serum bactericidal activity assay was performed using 25 mL of test serum dilutions, 12.5 µL of diluted bacteria and 12.5 µL of baby rabbit complement. Controls included bacteria incubated with preimmune serum and with heat-inactivated serum complement. For colony counting, 10 µL bacteria were plated on Mueller-Hinton agar plates at time 0 and after one-hour incubation at 37°C. Bactericidal titers were given as the reciprocal of the serum dilution yielding at least 50% bacterial killing.

RESULTS

Kinetics of Adhesion of Neisseria Strains to Epithelial Cells

Adhesion to the epithelial cells of the nasopharyngeal tract represents the first step of *Neisseria* infection. To study the kinetics of bacterial adhesion and find the optimal conditions for microarray experiments, *N. meningitis* and *N. lactamica* were incubated with the 16HBE14 human cell line. Samples were taken at time 0 and after 30, 60, 120, and 180 minutes of cocultivation. As shown in FIGURE 1, adhesion kinetics were similar for the two bacteria. After one hour of cocultivation, approximately 5–10 bacteria were found associated to each cell. This number increased with time, to reach 70–150 bacteria/cell after three hours, and paralleled the growth rate of MC58 in D-MEM culture medium. A large part of the time-dependent increase in cell-associated bacteria was due to new adhesion events taking place between cells and bacteria freely growing in the medium. In fact, when bacteria were incubated with the cells for one hour and the nonadhering bacteria were removed, the proliferation of cell-associated bacteria was negligible.

Panoramic View of Cell Contact–Induced Changes in Gene Expression

To study the changes in gene expression induced by host cell contact, RNA was purified from cell-adhering bacteria and bacteria grown in 16HBE14 culture medium. FIGURE 2 is a color-coded representation of the whole microarray analysis of MenB and *N. lactamica* during interaction with 16HBE14 epithelial cells. Overall,

347 and 285 genes altered their expression in MenB and in *N. lactamica*, respectively.

Only 167 of the regulated genes were common to both bacteria, indicating that while a common set of genes responds to cell-contact, the different behavior of the two bacteria most likely resides in the 180 and 118 genes specifically regulated in MenB and *N. lactamica*, respectively.

A relevant difference between MenB and *N. lactamica* is the time of persistence of RNA species in a cell-adhering population. As clearly evident from the comparison of FIGURE 2A and B, while the number of regulated RNA species markedly decreased with time in MenB, 30% of the adhesion-specific *N. lactamica* RNAs remained regulated throughout the analysis and most of the regulated genes remained either in the activation or in the downregulation state for a longer period of time.

The difference in mRNA levels between the two strains may be a consequence of different mechanisms of transcription regulation and/or RNA stability. It is interesting to note that six transcription regulators were found regulated during adhesion in MenB as opposed to the three regulators (NMB1561, NMB1511 and crgA

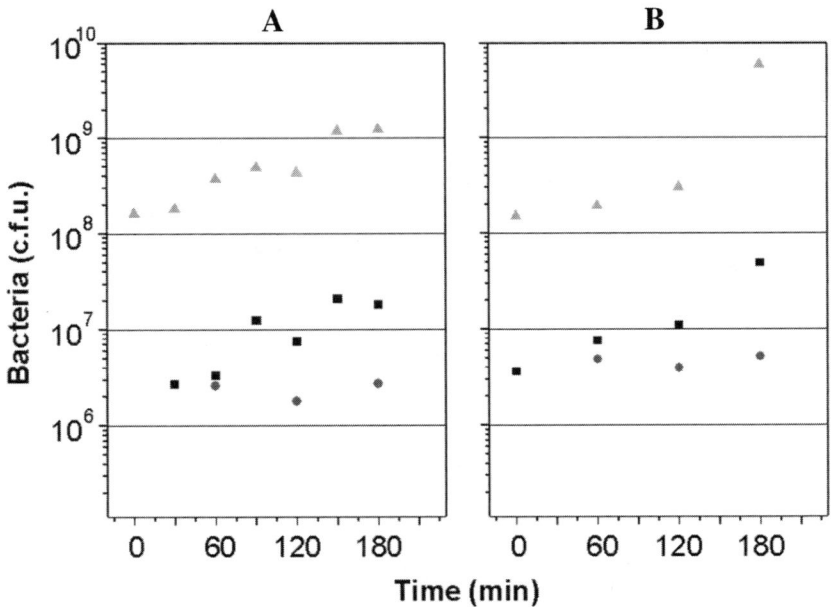

FIGURE 1. Adhesion and growth kinetics of MenB (**A**) and *N. lactamica* (**B**). Bacterial growth in D-MEM-10% FCS medium (▲) was determined by plating aliquots of the culture at different times. To evaluate the growth rate of cell-adhering bacteria, both strains were incubated with HBE14 epithelial cells for 1 hour and nonadhering bacteria were removed by extensive washing. Fresh sterile medium was added and adhering bacteria were counted at different times after lysis of epithelial cells (●). Finally, the kinetics of bacterial association was determined by adding bacteria to epithelial cells and cell-adhering bacteria were counted at different times after cell lysis (■).

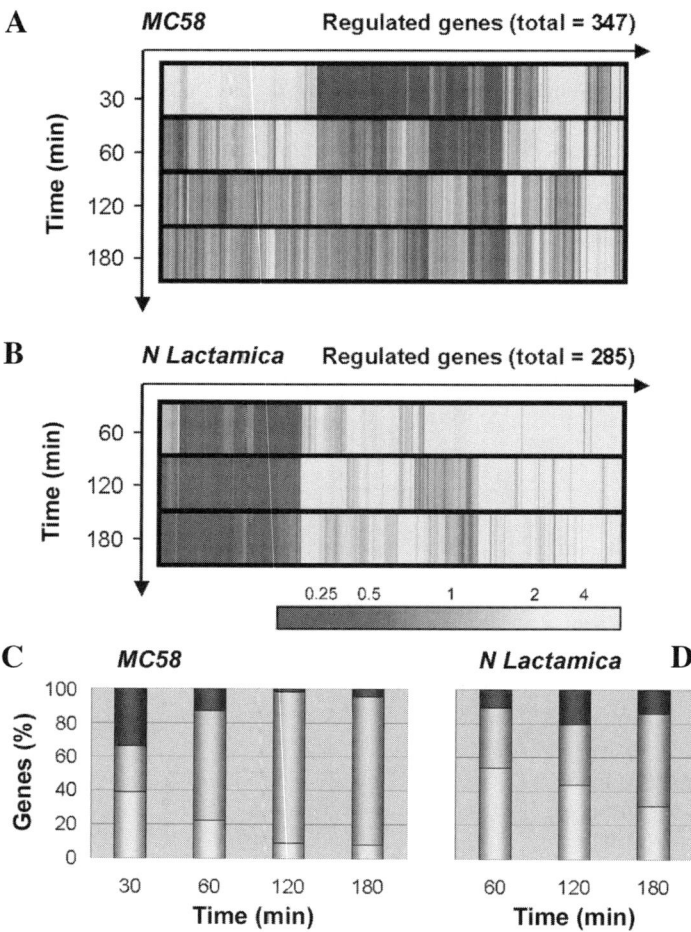

FIGURE 2. Kinetics of the gene expression pattern in MenB (**A**) and *N. lactamica* (**B**) adhering to epithelial cells. Bacteria (10^9) were added to 16HBE14 epithelial cells (2×10^6) and RNA was prepared at different times from adhering and freely growing bacteria. *Top panels* show clustered expression profiles of genes whose regulation differs from freely growing bacteria by at least twofold at any timepoint. *Bottom panels* group the same regulated genes as in the top panels according to their activation state (upregulated genes, *light gray*; downregulated genes, *dark gray*) to give a visual indication of the persistence of gene regulation.

(NMB1856)) regulated in *N. lactamica*. Furthermore, STM analysis by Sun et al.[10] has shown that inactivation of the RNAse genes NMB0686 and NMB0758 conferred an attenuated phenotype to MenB, suggesting the need for rapid RNA turnover.

While the biological significance of the difference in RNA persistence between MenB and *N. lactamica* remains to be thoroughly investigated, it is tempting to speculate that the phenomenon is linked to the different relationship the two bacteria have with the human host. *N. lactamica* has evolved to become commensal and nasopharyngeal epithelium represents its final destination. Therefore one would expect that once the bacterium comes into contact with epithelial cells the program of RNA and protein synthesis would remain more or less unaffected until substantial environmental variations occur. In contrast, MenB has the potential of moving from the epithelium to the endothelium and eventually of invading the blood stream and the meninges. This implies a transient interaction with epithelial cells and a propensity to reorganize its transcription and translation profiles to rapidly adapt itself to new environmental situations.

A Close View of Cell Contact–Induced Changes in Gene Expression

Cell Contact Induces Reduced Metabolism

An interesting observation derived from the microarray analysis of the transcriptional events occurring after cell contact is that, in agreement with the growth reduction curve shown in FIGURE 1, both *N. meningitidis* and *N. lactamica* reduce the activity of many growth-dependent genes. The list of downregulated genes in MenB includes 34 genes involved in protein synthesis, five genes implicated in nucleotide synthesis, and seven genes of cell wall septation and synthesis. Reduction of transcription activity also involved the gene cluster encoding the ATP synthase F1 and F0 subunits (atpC (NMB1933), atpD (NMB1934), atpG (NMB1935), atpA (NMB1936), atpH (NMB1937), atpF (NMB1938), and atpB (NMB1940)). This can be explained by an overall lower demand for ATP due to the reduced bacterial growth once associated to the cells. Alternatively, it is tempting to speculate that, once cell associated, bacteria are able to utilize part of the ATP synthesized by the host. Many of these metabolic genes (27 genes) were also downregulated in *N. lactamica*, indicating that in both species the interaction with epithelial cells is at least partially mediated by similar events and a reduced metabolic demand.

Upregulation of Transporters

A second common event occurring in the two species appears to be the activation of some transport systems involved in transmembrane trafficking of different compounds. Commonly upregulated transport machineries include the amino acid transporter gene NMB0177, the ABC transporters NMB0098 and NMB0041, the sulfate transporter gene cysT (NMB0881) and the ABC Fe^{3+} transporter gene NMB1990. Activation of genes involved in iron transport is intriguing since our experimental conditions were not iron limiting. Considering that, together with the ABC transporter gene, the transferrin binding protein gene (tbp1 (NMB0461)) and the oxygen-independent coprophorphyrinogen III oxydase gene (NMB0665) were also activated in both species, the data would suggest that of the three possible iron acquisition pathways,[11] adhering bacteria preferentially take up iron from transferrin.

Activation of transmembrane trafficking appears to be more pronounced in MenB. In fact, other transporter genes were specifically regulated in this organism and include the ABC cassette constituted by the three genes NMB0787, NMB0788, NMB0789, the amtB (NMB0615) transporter for ammonium, the ABC sulfate transporter (cysA (NMB0879), cysW (NMB0880), cysT (NMB0881), sbp (NMB1017)), the iron ABC transporter fbpA (NMB0634), the efflux pump gene NMB1719 and the chloride transporter gene NMB2006. It is interesting to note that NMB2006 is one of the 73 genes whose inactivation conferred an attenuated phenotype to MenB.[10] Furthermore, activation of the sulfate transport system, which is strictly linked to sulfur-containing amino acid metabolism, is probably the most evident difference between cell-adhering MenB and *N. lactamica* (see below).

Adhesion

In studying the biology of MenB invasion, a large number of experimental data have shown that after a first phase of localized adherence in which pili play an essential role, the genes of pili biosynthesis are downregulated to allow intimate attachment and diffuse adherence.[12] Our data show that the pilE gene (NMB0018), whose product contributes to the interaction with epithelial cells and the induction of cortical plaques, was slightly upregulated after 30 minutes. Furthermore, the pilC (NMB1847) transcript, encoding the major pilus adhesin involved in initial attachment to cells, was also marginally present in cell-associated bacteria after 30 minutes. However, at 30-minute incubation, crgA /NMB1856), the negative regulator of pilC1 expression,[13] was already clearly upregulated. In addition, pilT (NMB0052) RNA, whose product is responsible for pili retraction,[14] although not upregulated, was one of the most abundant RNA species among total bacterial RNAs (data not shown). As for the other pili genes, they appeared poorly transcribed and pilP (NMB1811) was downregulated.

Intimate attachment requires the involvement of membrane-associated proteins interacting with specific cellular receptors. Several bacterial proteins have been proposed, the best candidates being the Opa/Opc proteins, porins, and adhesins. Our microarray data on MenB show that the opa/opc genes and the porin genes were not regulated during adhesion but were very actively transcribed throughout the three-hour incubation (data not shown). Furthermore, MafA adhesins (mafA-1 (NMB0375), mafA-2 (NMB0652)) were upregulated at the beginning of our kinetics analysis and the macrophage infectivity potentiator (MIP)-related protein (NMB0995) was constantly upregulated. The expression of MIP genes is characteristic of intracellular pathogens and is known to increase their survival inside infected host cells.[15–17]

When expression of adhesion genes was analyzed in *N. lactamica*, a similar transcriptional pattern was observed, with the exception of mafA-1 that is MenB specific. Therefore, apart from mafA-1 and a few additional pilin genes specific for *N. lactamica* (data not shown), the overall expression profile would indicate that the two bacterial species utilize similar mechanisms of adhesion to epithelial cells.

Upregulation of Amino Acids and Selenocysteine Biosynthesis

IVET and STM technologies have shown that amino acid metabolism plays an important role in the infective process of many pathogens, including *Staphylococcus aureus, Pseudomonas aeruginosa, Streptococcus pneumoniae, Salmonella typhimurium*, and *Brucella suis*.[18] In agreement with these observations, our microarray analysis indicates that 16HBE14-associated MenB and *N. lactamica* upregulated some of the genes involved in the synthesis of several amino acids. In MenB, a more pronounced activation involves histidine, methionine, cysteine, and their selenoderivatives. Overall, 17 genes (including sulfate uptake genes) are implicated in the synthesis of adenosylmethionine, methionine and *N*-formylmethionyl-*t*RNA (see FIGURE 3). Considering that 13 of these genes were upregulated together with the siroheme synthase gene ([cysG-2] NMB1194, siroheme is the cofactor of sulfite reductase), our data unambiguously indicate that sulfur acquisition and metabolism play a key role in the adhesion process of MenB and represent one of the most striking metabolic differences between the two adhering bacteria.

Hypothetical Proteins

The most represented gene family responding to cell contact is the family of genes coding for hypothetical proteins (107 genes in MenB, 54 of which are also found in *N. lactamica*). This observation confirms that we still have no knowledge of many genes involved in virulence and cell contact. The list of genes that respond directly to host-cell contact in the two bacteria may provide a useful starting point for further studies. Particularly interesting are the 53 genes specifically induced in *N. meningitidis* since they are likely to play a role in virulence.

Glyceraldehyde 3-Phosphate Dehydrogenase

One of the genes upregulated in both MenB (4.8-fold) and *N. lactamica* (2.7-fold) is gapA-1 (NMB0207), the gene coding for the metabolic enzyme glyceraldehyde 3-phosphate dehydrogenase (GAPDH). The normal function of GAPDH in cellular metabolism is the conversion of glyceraldehyde 3-phosphate to 1, 3-diphosphoglycerate with the concomitant production of NADH. However, in some grampositive bacteria, the enzyme is exported to the bacterial surface. In *Streptococcus pyogenes*, GAPDH represents a major surface exposed protein and acts as an ADP-ribosylating enzyme.[19,20] In *Streptococcus pneumoniae*, the enzyme may be directly involved in the active efflux mechanism of erythromycin.[21] Furthermore, the enzyme plays an important role in cellular communication by activating host protein phosphorylation mechanisms.[22] Finally, in *Staphylococcus*, the cell-surface-associated GAPDH serves as a surface receptor for transferrin and binds different human serum proteins.[23] In MenB, the presence of two GAPDH genes in the chromosome, and the upregulation of one of the two genes following cell contact, suggest a special role for GAPDH. This role was confirmed by FACS analysis, which showed that following cell contact GAPDH is exported to and accumulated on the bacterial surface (data not shown). To our knowledge, this is the first time that GAPDH has been found on the surface of a gram-negative bacterium.

Other Genes

Other genes, belonging to different categories, respond to cell contact and are worth mentioning. For instance, the catalase gene (kat (NMB0216)) was found upregulated in both bacteria. This is consistent with the fact that producing oxygen

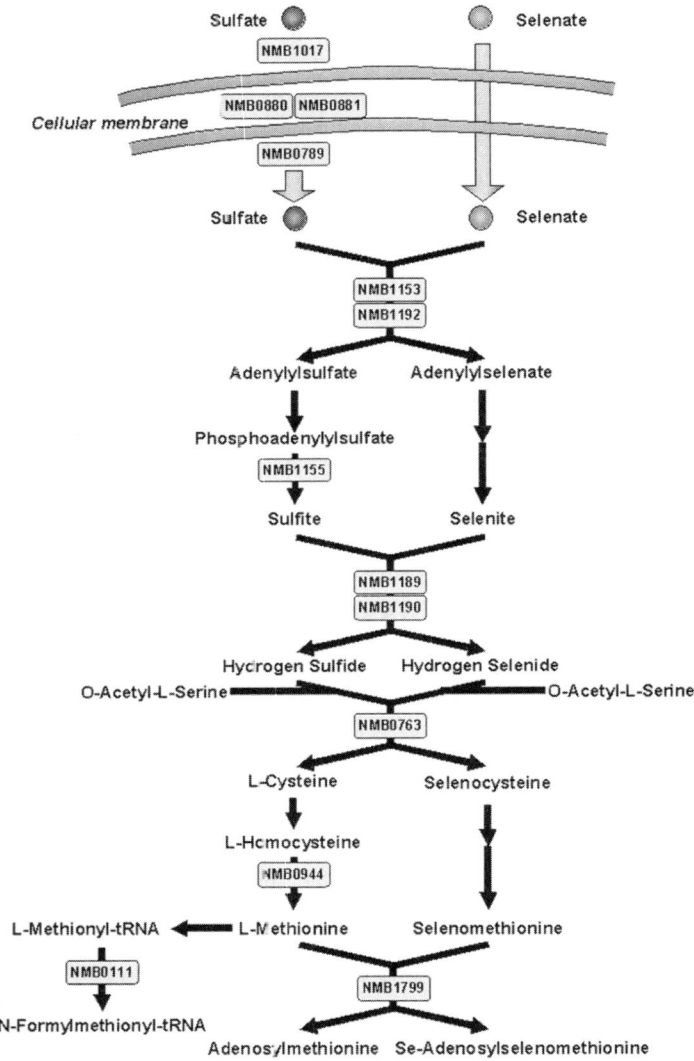

FIGURE 3. Regulation of genes involved in sulfur acquisition and metabolism. Each arrow represents a specific biochemical step in the overall sulfate and selenate up-take and metabolism of MenB. Genes involved in specific reactions and found upregulated in adhering bacteria are boxed over the corresponding arrows.

radicals[24,25] is one of the mechanisms by which eukaryotic cells try to protect themselves against pathogen aggression.

Genes involved in DNA metabolism are often critical for bacterial pathogenesis and, as for DNA restriction-modification genes, are often located within pathogenicity islands[26] or subjected to phase variation.[27-29] In *S. typhimurium*, adenine methylation influences the expression of several virulence genes.[30,31] We found that two restriction modification genes (mod (NMB1261), NMB01375), both encoding DNA methylases and genes coding for nucleases, transposases, helicases, and ligases (NMB0090, recQ (NMB0274), ligA-1 (NMB0666), NMB1251, gcr (NMB1278), and NMB1798) were upregulated during adhesion in both MenB and *N. lactamica*. In addition to these genes, in MenB interaction with epithelial cells promotes transcription of three other DNA metabolism genes (xseB (NMB0262), NMB1510 and mutS (NMB2160)) and three additional transposase genes (NMB1050, NMB1601, NMB1770).

Proteases, chaperonins and proteins involved in protein stabilization, classified as "protein fate" genes, also contribute to the virulence of several pathogens. Our analysis has shown that five genes of this class are upregulated in both *Neisseria* species (prlC (NMB0214), NMB1428, secY (NMB0162), dnaK (NMB0554), hscB (NMB1383)). Eleven "protein fate" genes are MenB-specific and, among these, the only one to be upregulated is the dsbA gene (NMB0278) encoding a periplasmic thiol:disulfide oxidoreductase. In *E. coli*, DsbA plays a role in adhesion by stabilizing type IV fimbriae,[32] and in *Shigella flexneri* it contributes to intracellular survival and propagation.[33]

Recently, Sun *et al.*[10] have developed STM to identify MenB virulence genes. Their study lead to the identification of 73 genes whose inactivation conferred an attenuated phenotype in a mouse model. Nine of the 73 genes were found to be regulated in our analysis, including three genes involved in amino acid synthesis (metF (NMB0943), metH (NMB0944) and gdhA (NMB1710)), the murein transglycosylase B gene (NMB1279), the gene coding for the Cl⁻ channel protein (NMB2006), the translation elongation factor Tu gene (tufA (NMB0139)), downregulated at 30 minutes of contact with 16HBE14, and three genes of unknown function (NMB0188 and NMB1971, both upregulated, and NMB1523 which was downregulated). Four of these nine genes were MenB-specific (metH, tufA, NMB2006, and NMB1523).

Host-Cell Contact Induces Bacterial Surface Remodeling

Among the adhesion-modulated genes, approximately 44% potentially encode peripherally located proteins suggesting that, when in contact with the host, MenB undergoes a significant remodeling of its membrane components. These biological events have important implications in vaccine design. Particularly abundant antigens or antigens specifically expressed during infection are likely to be better vaccine candidates than proteins whose concentration rapidly decreases when in contact with the host.

In order to confirm that epithelial cell interaction leads to a change in surface protein profile as inferred by microarray data, we used FACS analysis on adhering bacteria using the mouse sera against 12 recombinant proteins whose transcription was found to be particularly activated upon adhesion (see TABLE 1). All proteins were FACS positive: four of them could be detected on the bacterial surface only after

TABLE 1. MenB proteins selected for FACS and bactericidal analyses

Gene locus	Product/Function	RNA activation				Predicted location	FACS analysis[a]		Bactericidal[b] assay
		30'	1h	2h	3h		Free bacteria	Adhering bacteria	
NMBO207	glyceraldehyde 3-P DHase (gapA-1)/virulence	4.8	1.0	0.8	1.2	cytoplasm	+	++	<1/4
NMBO214	oligopeptidase A (prtC)/virulence	5.3	3.7	0.9	0.7	cytoplasm	−	+	<1/4
NMBO315		1.7	2.2	1.2	1.2	periplasmic space	+	+	1/512
NMBO655		4.2	2.8	0.8	0.8	cytoplasm	−	+	<1/4
NMBO652	mafA prt (mafA-2)/adhesion	2.7	1.5	0.8	1.1	outer membrane	+	++	1/1024
NMBO741		15.5	9.4	1.4	2.2	inner membrane	+	+	<1/4
NMBO787	AA ABC transp, periplasmic AA-binding protein	0.5	1.3	8.4	2.4	outer membrane	+	+	<1/4
NMBO995	macrophage infectivity potentiator-related protein/virulence	1.0	2.5	9.4	3.2	inner membrane	+	++	1/750
NMB1061		4.2	3.3	1.5	2.7	cytoplasm	−	+	<1/4
NMB1119		5.3	4.9	1.5	1.5	cytoplasm	−	+	1/384
NMB1875		7.4	5.5	1.2	1.1	inner membrane	+	++	<1/4
NMB1876	N-acetylglutamate synthetase biosynthesis (argA)	3.0	2.0	1.3	3.5	cytoplasm	+	++	1/1024

[a]FACS analysis was carried out on the free growing bacteria and cell-adhering bacteria using mouse sera against the selected recombinant proteins.
[b]Bactericidal activity was determined on MC58 using rabbit serum complement and mouse sera against the selected proteins. Titers were expressed as the reciprocal of serum dilution yielding at least 50% bacterial killing.

adhesion to epithelial cells, five proteins were present in nonadhering bacteria but their expression increased upon interaction with the host, and three proteins were present on the surface of both adhering and nonadhering bacteria but their expression, differently from their corresponding RNA, did not appear to vary upon epithelial cell interaction.

Taken together these data confirm that interaction with the host involves substantial modification of surface protein components, and that DNA microarrays coupled to FACS analysis with sera against recombinant proteins is an effective approach to identify surface antigens subject to adhesion-dependent modulation. Interestingly, some of these antigens could not be predicted as membrane-associated by the available computer algorithms. They include glyceraldehyde 3-P dehydrogenase, recently shown to be on the surface of some gram-positive pathogens, *N*-acetylglutamate synthetase and the products of the hypothetical genes NMB1061, NMB1119, and NMB0655.

Identification of Vaccine Candidates

Having identified 12 adhesion-induced antigens localized on the surface of adhering bacteria, we tested the ability of their corresponding antisera to mediate complement-dependent killing of MenB. Of the 12 sera analyzed, 5 showed bactericidal activity against the homologous strain MC58 (TABLE 1). Two of the bactericidal sera were against hypothetical proteins (the products of NMB0315 and NMB1119 genes) whose function remains to be elucidated. The third bactericidal serum was against the adhesin MafA, one of the two adhesin proteins homologous to gonococcal Maf adhesins.[2] The other two sera were against the MIP-related protein and the enzyme *N*-acetylglutamate synthetase (ArgA).

CONCLUSIONS

Whole-genome microarrays, together with other genomic technologies, were used to study the behavior of each bacterial gene under conditions, which were not accessible to study using previous techniques.[34] We have used these techniques to study the changes occurring in gene expression during a critical step of bacterial invasion, that is the first contact between a bacterium and the host cell. In addition, in order to identify the changes that are important for virulence, we have compared the changes in expression profile between a pathogen (MenB) and a commensal bacteria (*N. lactamica*). The interesting findings discussed in this paper may help to better understand the pathogenicity of MenB and how it differs from the commensal *N. lactamica*. In addition, by following the indication derived from the microarray data, we have investigated the fate of some antigens and confirmed that cell contact indeed promotes a remodeling of the bacterial cell surface antigenic profile. This may prove very useful in rational design of new vaccines. Indeed, 5 out of 12 surface antigens shown to be upregulated after contact to epithelial cells were capable of inducing bactericidal antibodies in the mouse model.

In conclusion, this study not only sheds light on interesting aspects of the first steps of *Neisseria* interaction with its host but also provides a first example of the possible application of DNA microarray technology in vaccine discovery.

ACKNOWLEDGMENTS

The authors thank H. Tettelin, Giulio Ratti, and R. Beltrami for their contribution to primer design, M. M. Giuliani, L. Santini, and B. Brunelli for providing mice sera and for helpful discussions, and A. Maiorino for her expert secretarial assistance.

REFERENCES

1. NASSIF, X., C. PUJOL, P. MORAND & E. EUGÈNE. 1999. Mol. Microbiol. **32:** 1121–1132.
2. MERZ, A.J. & M. So. 2000. Annu. Rev. Cell. Dev. Biol. **16:** 423–457.
3. TETTELIN, H. et al. 2000. Science **287:** 1809–1815.
4. CUMMINGS, C.A. & D.A. RELMAN. 2000. Emerg. Infect. Dis. **6:** 513–522
5. COHEN, P. et al. 2000. J. Biol. Chem. **275:** 11181–11190.
6. EKMANN, L., J.R. SMITH, M.P. HOUSLEY, et al. 2000. J. Biol. Chem. **275:** 14084–14094.
7. BELCHER, C.E. et al. Proc. Natl. Acad. Sci. USA **97:** 13847–13857.
8. RAPPUOLI, R. 2000. Proc. Natl. Acad. Sci. USA **97:** 13468–13469.
9. Pizza, M. et al. 2000. Science **287:** 1816–1820.
10. SUN, Y.-H., S. BAKSHI, R. CHALMERS & C.M. TANG. 2000. Nature Med. **6:** 1269–1273.
11. GENCO, C.A. & P.J. DESAI. 1996. Trends Microbiol. **4:** 179–184.
12. PUJOL, C., E. EUGÈNE, L. DE SAINT MARTIN & X. NASSIF. 1997. Infect. Immun. **65:** 4836–4842).
13. DEGHMANE, Al.-E. et al. 2000. EMBO J. **19:** 1068–1078.
14. PUJOL, C., E. EUGÈNE, M. MARCEAU & X. NASSIF. 1999. Proc. Nat. Acad. Sci. USA **96:** 4017–4022.
15. SUSA, M., J. HACKER & R. MARRE. 1996. Infect. Immun. **64:** 1679–1684.
16. WINTEMEYER, E., B. LUDWIG, M. STEINERT, et al. 1995. Infect. Immun. **63:** 4576–4583.
17. HORNE, S.M., T.J. KOTTOM, L.K. NOLAN & K.D. YOUNG. 1997. Infect. Immun. **65:** 806–810.
18. SHEA, J.E., J.D. SANTANGELO & R. FELDMAN. 2000. Curr. Opin. Microbiol. **3:** 451–458.
19. LOTTENBERG, R., C.C. BRODER, M.D. BOYLE, et al. 1992. J. Bacteriol. **174:** 5204–5210.
20. DE MATTEIS, M.A. et al. 1994. Proc. Natl. Acad. Sci. USA **91:** 1114–1118.
21. CASH, P., E. ARGO, L. FORD, et al. 1999. Electrophoresis **20:** 2259–2268.
22. PANCHOLI, V. & V.A. FISCHETTI. 1997. J. Exp. Med. **186:** 1633–1643.
23. WINRAM, S.B. & R. LOTTEMBERG. 1996. Microbiology **142:** 2311–2320.
24. KLEBANOFF, S.J., R.M. LOCKSLEY, E.C. JONG & H. ROSEN. 1983. Ciba Found. Symp. **99:** 92–112.
25. RAMARAO, N., S.D. GRAY-OWEN & T.F. MEYER. 2000. Mol. Microbiol. **38:** 103–113.
26. SALAMA, N., K. GUILLEMIN, T.K. MCDANIEL, et al. 2000. Proc. Natl. Acad. Sci. USA **97:** 14668–14673.
27. GE, Z. & D.E. TAYLO. 1999. Annu. Rev. Microbiol. **53:** 353–387.
28. SAUNDERS, N. et al. 2000. Mol. Microbiol. **37:** 207–215.
29. BRAATEN, B., Y. NOU, L. KALTENBACH & D. LOW. 1994. Cell **76:** 577–588
30. HEITHOFF, D.M., R.L. SINSHEIMER, D.A. LOW & M.J. MAHAN. 1999. Science **284:** 967–970.
31. GARCIA-DEL PORTILLO, F., M.G. PUCCIARELLI & J. CASADESUS. 1999. Proc. Natl. Acad. Sci. USA **96:** 11578–11583.
32. ZHANG, H.Z. & M.S. DONNENBERG. 1996. Mol. Microbiol. **21:** 787–797.
33. YU, I., B. EDWARDS-JONES, O. NEYROLLES & J.S. KROLL. 2000. Infect. Immun. **68:** 6449–6456.
34. GRANDI, G. 2001. Trends Biotechnol. **19:** 181–188.

Prognosis of Breast Cancer and Gene Expression Profiling Using DNA Arrays

FRANÇOIS BERTUCCI,[a,b,e] RÉMI HOULGATTE,[c] SAMUEL GRANJEAUD,[c] VALÉRY NASSER,[a] BÉATRICE LORIOD,[c] EMMANUEL BEAUDOING,[c] PASCAL HINGAMP,[c] JOCELYNE JACQUEMIER,[d] PATRICE VIENS,[b,e] DANIEL BIRNBAUM,[a,f] AND CATHERINE NGUYEN[c]

[a]Département d'Oncologie Moléculaire, TAGC, Institut Paoli-Calmettes (IPC), IFR57, Marseille, France

[b]Département d'Oncologie Médicale, IPC, Marseille, France

[c]TAGC, ERM-206 INSERM, IFR57, Marseille, France

[d]Département d'Anatomopathologie, IPC, Marseille, France

[e]Université de la Méditerranée, Marseille, France

[f]Laboratoire d'Oncologie Moléculaire, U.119 INSERM, IFR57, Marseille, France

ABSTRACT: Breast cancer is a complex genetic disease characterized by the accumulation of multiple molecular alterations. The resulting clinical heterogeneity makes current therapeutic strategies—based on clinicopathological factors—less than perfectly adapted to each patient. Today, DNA arrays, by allowing the simultaneous and quantitative analysis of the mRNA expression levels of thousands of genes in a single assay, provide novel tools to tackle this complexity. Potential applications are multiple in the cancer field and the first research results are promising. Using home-made DNA arrays in an approach easily compatible with academic research—nylon support and radioactive detection—we identified a predictor set of 23 genes whose expression patterns differentiated two groups of breast cancer patients with different survival after adjuvant chemotherapy. We then validated and further extended these results in a larger, independent and homogeneous series of poor prognosis primary breast cancers treated with adjuvant anthracyclin-based chemotherapy. We confirmed the prognostic classification provided by the 23-gene set predictor. We then improved the predictor set and refined the classification by sorting the tumors into three classes with significantly different long-term survival. These results show the potential of the technology with an accessible approach for academic research teams. We also showed that nylon DNA arrays with radioactive detection are associated with excellent sensitivity, an advantage in clinical situations where the amount of available material is limited.

KEYWORDS: breast cancer; DNA microarray; gene expression; prognosis

Breast cancer is a major public health concern in Western countries. Despite recent progress, long-term survival levels off at 70%. Currently, a handful of clinical,

Address for correspondence: F. Bertucci, Département d'Oncologie Médicale, Institut Paoli-Calmettes, IFR57, 232, Bd Ste-Marguerite, 13273 Marseille Cedex 9, France. Voice: 04 91 26 93 19; fax: 04 91 26 94 60.
bertucci@ciml.univ-mrs.fr

pathological and molecular parameters enable clinicians to class individual tumors in a given prognostic category and to select therapies. However, these classification systems are insufficient to capture the extensive clinical heterogeneity of disease, making current therapeutic strategies less than perfectly adapted to each patient. In a number of cases, the response to treatment and the clinical outcome vary widely between apparently similar tumors, suggesting the existence of important yet unrecognized subclasses.

Breast cancer is a complex genetic disease characterized by the accumulation and the combination of multiple molecular alterations. These anomalies disturb the expression of genes controlling critical regulatory processes, causing tumorogenesis and genetic instability, and leading to an increasingly invasive and resistant phenotype. Metastatic process and response to treatment are not likely to be associated with the disturbance of a single gene, but rather with the combined influence of many genes. Comprehensive, systematic and unbiased molecular analyses are thus required to capture the complex cascade of events that sustain the clinical behavior of tumors

Today the emerging high-throughput molecular technologies, direct consequences of the Human Genome Project and of various technological developments, can provide real molecular portraits of complex biological samples. In particular, DNA arrays allow for the simultaneous and quantitative measurement of the mRNA expression levels of thousands of genes in a single assay.[1,2] Potential applications are multiple in oncology.[3] Detailed molecular characterization of tumors should allow a better understanding of mammary oncogenesis, the improvement of the diagnostic and prognostic classification of the disease, and the development of new more specific anticancer therapeutics.

Four years ago, we initiated a program of molecular profiling of breast cancer using DNA arrays in an approach compatible with academic research. Our main objective was and remains primarily clinical; we are looking to identify new prognostic subclasses of breast cancer unrecognized with classical parameters. This paper presents a summary of our work so far. Finally we discuss an issue important for future and reliable applications of DNA arrays in clinical oncology, the sensitivity of the technology.

DNA ARRAY TECHNOLOGY

The general approach uses arrays of DNA probes for hybridization to a labeled target prepared with RNA extracted from a biological sample. The target is produced by reverse transcription of RNA and simultaneous labeling; it contains many different sequences in various amounts, corresponding to the numbers of copies of the original mRNA species in the sample. After hybridization, the signal present on each probe is automatically detected and quantified; it is proportional to the concentration of the corresponding mRNA species in the target; that is, to the expression level of the concerned gene. Intensities are then normalized for the experimental differences between independent hybridizations. Each experiment thus provides an indication of the expression level of each of the genes represented on the array in the original sample. Thousands of data points can be collected simultaneously. During data analysis, profiles of different samples are compared with each other, for instance profiles from normal and tumor tissues, or profiles from morphologically similar tumors with different clinical outcomes.

Briefly, two main implementations of DNA arrays have been developed. The first one uses arrays of cDNA clones (double-strand) robotically spotted on a solid support in the form of PCR products. Several versions exist depending on the type of support (nylon, glass) and type of target labeling (radioactivity, colorimetry, fluorescence).[4–6] The second implementation of DNA arrays uses arrays of oligonucleotides (single-strand) either directly synthesized *in situ* on a support[7] or presynthesized and subsequently robotically spotted.[8] Commercial sets of arrays are now available for both techniques.

Our aim was to use an approach compatible with existing academic laboratory methods and equipment. We initially focused on the oldest version of nylon DNA arrays known as "macroarrays," in use in the laboratory for a long time.[9–11] "Macroarrays" are high-density filters made on large nylon membranes (typically one hundred cm^2) in which PCR products representing hundreds or thousands of genes are regularly arranged with a spot spacing of one or two millimeters. Targets are generally labeled with radioactivity (^{33}P). Expression levels can be measured using less

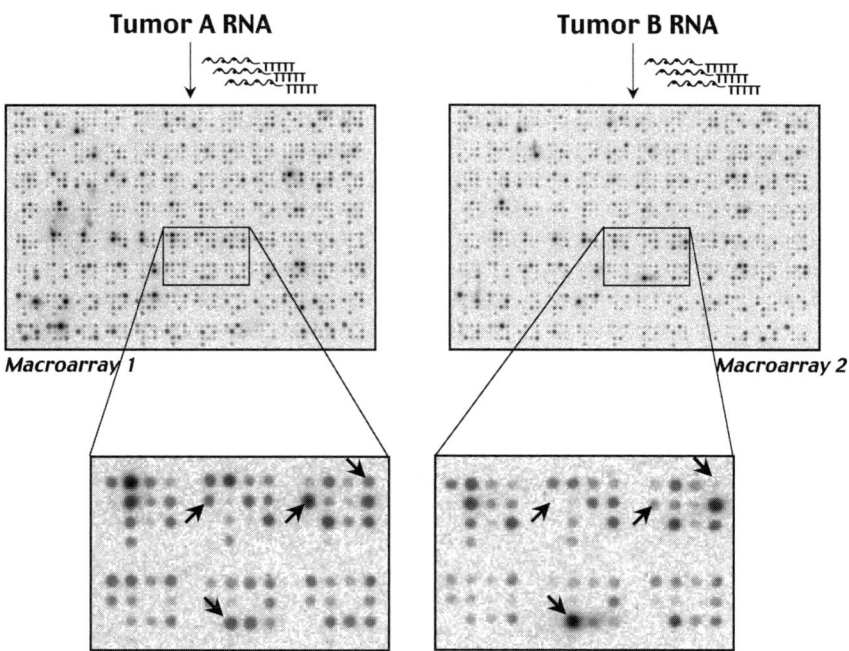

FIGURE 1. Differential gene expression between two tumors. DNA arrays are 8×12 cm^2 nylon "macroarrays" containing PCR products of ~1,000 cDNA clones. *Top:* membrane images after hybridization with complex targets made from total RNA (5 µg) from mammary carcinoma samples A and B. *Bottom:* four differentially expressed genes are indicated by *arrows*.

than a microgram of mRNA, with a linear response for over three decades. Nylon "macroarrays" can be readily produced (in particular, the purification of PCR products before spotting is not needed) and hybridized using current laboratory conditions; and the results are acquired with imaging plate systems and adapted software. Furthermore, after hybridizations, filters can be stripped and reused four to six times (personal observation). The system is thus cheap and compatible with the equipment present in most academic laboratories. It is also very flexible, allowing the laboratory to design and assemble custom sets adapted to each particular project using available IMAGE cDNA clones and relatively simple robotic equipment. FIGURE 1 shows hybridization images of nylon "macroarrays" containing about 1,000 genes and hybridized with radioactive targets prepared with RNA from two breast tumors.

GENE EXPRESSION PROFILING OF BREAST CANCER

Our project was initiated in 1997. The objective was to use the comprehensive gene expression profiles of breast tumors to identify new prognostic subgroups within clinically and morphologically similar groups of tumors.

Gene expression measurements with DNA arrays require attention to a number of parameters, from the quality of the clone set to the control of hybridization artifacts as well as the procedures of handling, normalization, and analysis of data. Therefore, our first study intended to validate our approach by profiling cancer cell lines with known molecular alterations. These lines provided a readily available and homogeneous material for technological set up, before the analysis of more precious clinical cancer samples. Total RNA from six cancer cell lines (25 µg each), including four breast cell lines, was hybridized using nylon "macroarrays" ($8 \times 12 \, cm^2$) representing about 200 genes selected for a proven or putative implication in mammary oncogenesis.[12] The achievement of good-quality quantitative data was verified: low background-to-signal ratio, negative controls, positive controls (ubiquitous genes as well as genes known to be overexpressed in certain cell lines), linear and dynamic range of values (three to four orders of magnitude), and reproducibility of hybridizations. Several differences were observed between tested cell lines: some of them were expected according to literature, while many provided novel information. For example, the GATA3 transcription factor gene was overexpressed in the estrogen receptor (ER)-positive mammary cell lines as compared to ER-negative lines. Hierarchical clustering[13] based on gene expression levels clustered the breast cancer cell lines together, suggesting the capacity of expression profiles to classify samples in a relevant way. Finally, we demonstrated the feasibility of analyzing small tumor samples, using only 5 µg of total RNA

In two subsequent studies, we used this system for profiling tumors from patients treated in our institution. All tested tissue samples were invasive breast carcinomas collected during surgery for a localized form of disease. After resection, the tumors were macrodissected: a section was taken for the pathologist's diagnosis and an adjacent piece was quickly frozen in liquid nitrogen for molecular analyses. We first analyzed 34 unselected tumor samples and a normal breast tissue sample (Clontech, Palo Alto, CA) using "macroarrays" with about 200 candidate genes.[14] We observed extensive heterogeneity of tumors at the transcriptional level. Analysis was conducted along three directions.

We first compared the expression profiles of normal tissue and 34 tumors. Among the differentially expressed genes (see TABLE 1), some were known to be involved in disease progression (*MYBL2, STMY3, MUC1, ERBB2*...), whereas others such as *GATA3* were potential new markers.

We then searched for genes whose expression levels correlated with conventional prognostic parameters: age of patients, axillary lymph node status, pathological tumor size, grade, and ER status. These features are insufficient to reflect the whole heterogeneity of disease. Each of them depends on the expression of several hundreds of genes and it is likely that subtle differences important for clinical outcome are hidden by these rough factors. Identification of these subtleties using DNA arrays might provide new prognostic or predictive markers and help to decipher the complex biological pathways which control these phenotypic features. No significant correlation was found with age, tumor size and grade. However, the expression of some genes correlated with axillary node involvement and ER status. By comparing the expression profiles of node-negative tumors to profiles of tumors with massive axillary extension (10 or more positive nodes), we found a positive correlation between the expression level of *ERBB2*—a known cancer villain—and the number of tumor-involved nodes. Amongst other differentially expressed genes (TABLE 1), some have a function in agreement with a potential role in invasion (*CDH1, CD44*...), while for others, such as *SOX4* and *GSTP1*, the connection is not clear and calls for further investigation. We then compared the expression profiles of ER-positive tumors and ER-negative tumors. Several genes were identified with expression associated with the ER status (TABLE 1). In particular, we found a strong correlation between the mRNA expression of *GATA3* and the protein expression of ER as measured with immunohistochemistry (IHC), confirming the data obtained with cell lines. A Northern blot analysis of 79 tumors with a *GATA3* probe both confirmed the validity of our DNA array data and the correlation between these two transcription factors.

Finally, using a hierarchical clustering algorithm, we identified, among tumors with poor prognosis, two molecularly distinct subgroups with different survival after adjuvant anthracyclin-based chemotherapy. This separation could not be obtained using the commonly used prognostic features. It resulted from the differential expression of 23 genes, which included genes already associated with the prognosis of disease such as *ERBB2, CDH1*, and *MYC* as well as other genes not yet recognized as important for prognosis, such as *GATA3, CRABP2*, and *EFNA1*. This study was the first to demonstrate the potential prognostic value of gene expression profiling in breast cancer.

Such prognostic discrimination which might identify the patients who benefit from standard adjuvant chemotherapy is clinically relevant for several reasons. First, the recent consensus conference led by the US National Cancer Institute has recommended the enlargement of the criteria of use of adjuvant anthracyclin-based chemotherapy for localized breast cancer.[15] Second, even if the benefit of such therapy on survival is proven, its efficiency remains relatively limited (about 60% of five-year metastasis-free survival) and no clinical or pathological factor is able to predict the clinical outcome. Third, alternative systemic therapies with promising results in

TABLE 1. Genes differentially expressed in breast cancer

Symbol	Gene/Protein Identity	T/NB
MYBL2	MYB-related protein B	(a)
GATA3	GATA-binding protein 3	17.8
STMY3	stromelysin 3	15.9
GZMH	granzyme H	9.5
CD2	T-lymphocyte surface CD2 antigen	7.5
CRABP2	cellular retinoic acid-binding protein 2	7.2
CREBBP	CREB-binding protein	5.1
GRB2	EGFR-binding protein GRB2	5.0
Symbol	Gene/Protein Identity	10N+/N−
ERBB2	ERBB2 receptor protein-tyrosine kinase	6.5
PPP2R2C	protein phosphatase 2, regulatory subunit B (PR 52), gamma isoform	4.0
GSTP1	glutathione S transferase Pi	2.7
SOX4	SOX4 protein	2.7
IL2RB	interleukin 2 receptor beta chain	2.4
ZNF144	zinc finger protein 144	1.9
MUC1	mucin 1	1.8
CD44	CD44 antigen, epithelial form	1.7
Symbol	Gene/Protein Identity	ER+/ER−
GATA3	GATA-binding protein 3	28.6
GZMA	granzyme A	5.7
MYB	MYB proto-oncogene	3.4
KIAA1075	KIAA1075 protein	3.3
STMY3	stromelysin 3	3.1
MST1	macrophage-stimulating 1	2.8
CRABP2	cellular retinoic acid-binding protein 2	2.7
XBP1	X-box-binding protein 1	2.7

NOTES: T/NB, ratio of median expression level in 34 tumors to expression level in normal breast; (a), expression level undetectable in NB; 10N+/N−, ratio of median expression level in tumors with 10 or more involved axillary lymph nodes to median expression level in node-negative tumors; ER+/ER−, ratio of median expression level in ER-positive tumors to median expression level in ER-negative tumors (adapted from ref. 14)

19. ZHANG, W., P.M. LABORDE, K.R. COOMBES, et al. 2001. Cancer genomics: promises and complexities. Clin. Cancer Res. **7:** 2159–2167.
20. RAMASWAMY, S. & T.R. GOLUB. 2002. DNA microarrays in clinical oncology. J. Clin. Oncol. **20:** 1932–1941.
21. LUO, L., R.C. SALUNGA, H. GUO, et al. 1999. Gene expression profiles of laser-captured adjacent neuronal subtypes. Nat. Med. **5:** 117–122.
22. WANG, E., L.D. MILLER, G.A. OHNMACHT, et al. 2000. High-fidelity mRNA amplification for gene profiling. Nat Biotechnol. 18: 457–459.
23. BERTUCCI, F., K. BERNARD, B. LORIOD, et al. 1999. Sensitivity issues in DNA array-based expression measurements and performance of nylon microarrays for small samples. Hum. Mol. Genet. **8:** 1715–1722.

Identifying Immunotherapeutic Targets for Prostate Carcinoma through the Analysis of Gene Expression Profiles

PETER S. NELSON

The Divisions of Human Biology and Clinical Research
Fred Hutchinson Cancer Research Center
Seattle, Washington 98109-1024, USA

ABSTRACT: Carcinoma of the prostate represents one of the most frequently diagnosed cancers in men. If detected at an early stage, prostate cancer is highly treatable. However, cancers identified at a late stage are rarely cured with contemporary medical therapies. Early detection strategies presently center on the identification of prostate-specific proteins in the serum, and emerging therapeutics have utilized genes and proteins with prostate-restricted expression for tissue-selective immunological regimens incorporating vaccines, dendritic cell therapy, gene therapy, and antibody-based cell targeting. In order to develop improved therapeutic procedures, efforts have been directed toward the identification of genes exhibiting prostate-restricted expression profiles, or altered expression levels in neoplastic cells relative to their normal counterparts. Comprehensive expression profiling approaches such as the analysis of oligonucleotide- or complementary DNA (cDNA)-microarrays have greatly enhanced these efforts. Genes and their cognate proteins identified using such methods offer additional diagnostic and therapeutic targets that may aid in the understanding and treatment of prostate carcinoma.

KEYWORDS: prostate carcinoma; gene expression profiles; immunotherapy

INTRODUCTION: PROSTATE CARCINOMA

Prostate carcinoma is the most common malignant tumor diagnosed in men and the second leading cause of cancer related mortality. In the United States alone, more than 39,000 men are projected to die of prostate cancer in 2002.[1] Early cancer diagnosis offers the best chance for cure, though the available medical regimens, surgery and radiotherapy, have significant associated morbidities. The progression of prostate cancer to sites outside the prostate represents a disease state that is rarely cured with currently available treatments including hormone manipulation and chemotherapy. While the exquisite sensitivity of prostate cancer cells to the requirement for circulating androgenic hormones provides a temporizing treatment through surgical or chemical castration, the disease will predictably progress to an androgen-independent disease, and an associated median life expectancy of one year.[2] At the time of

---

Address for correspondence: Peter S. Nelson, The Divisions of Human Biology and Clinical Research, Fred Hutchinson Cancer Research Center, 1100 Fairview Ave. North, 04-100, Seattle, Washington 98109-1024, USA. Voice: 206-667-3377; fax: 206-667-2917.
pnelson@fhcrc.org

hormone independence, there are no therapeutic modalities for prostate carcinoma with a proven survival benefit.[2–4]

IMMUNOTHERAPY STRATEGIES

As a result of the limited efficacy of conventional radiotherapy and chemotherapy regimens for treating advanced prostate cancer and the significant morbidities associated with surgical treatment of localized disease, other approaches for treating prostate carcinoma are actively under investigation. Among these, immunotherapeutics represent a spectrum of alternative modalities that have proven to be effective in other malignancies such as renal cell carcinoma and malignant melanoma.[5,6] In general, immunotherapies are designed to augment or manipulate the host immune response to eradicate neoplastic cells. One major hurdle for this approach involves the high similarity between the genome and proteome of a normal cell and it's corresponding malignant counterpart. Not surprisingly, very few cancer-specific genes or proteins have been identified. This is in sharp contrast to immunotherapies targeted toward microbial pathogens in which many proteins are unique to the infectious agent. The practical ramifications of the high genotypic and phenotypic identity exhibited between normal and neoplastic cells involves the ability of an immune-based therapy to break immunological tolerance and to avoid toxicity directed toward normal host cells. Nonetheless, the immune system does exert significant anticancer effects as demonstrated by the presence of cytotoxic lymphocytes infiltrating tumors,[7] the increased incidence of malignancies such as cervical carcinoma in immunocompromised individuals,[8] and the graft-versus-leukemia effect observed in allogeneic bone marrow transplantation.[9] However, the very existence of neoplastic diseases and the almost certain progression without intervention underscores the failure of the natural surveillance systems to effectively police every tumorigenic event. The result of allowing even one critical transforming incident to progress unimpeded can be catastrophic for the human host. Thus, the primary objective of oncological immunotherapeutic approaches is to enhance the potency and effectiveness of the immune response toward the recognition and eradication of neoplastic disease.

Cancer immunotherapies can be broadly categorized into those utilizing active or passive mechanisms. Active immunotherapy entails vaccinating patients with antigens and adjuvants that activate tumor-specific T cells, the major cellular immune effector component. T cells identify target cells through a membrane-bound protein known as the T-cell receptor (TCR). The TCR recognizes short peptide antigens in association with major histocompatibility complex (MHC) molecules displayed by antigen-presenting cells (APCs). Thus, generating tumor-specific immunity is consequently dependent on an appropriate target antigen and the effective presentation of that antigen to the patient's immune system. The critical roles for APCs in this process have recently been appreciated as APCs such as dendritic cells are responsible for the uptake, processing, and presentation of antigens to cytolytic–T (CD8) and helper-T (CD4) cells in the context of MHC class I and class II molecules.[10]

To generate an immune response, initial efforts to produce cancer vaccines utilized irradiated neoplastic cells derived from the patient (autologous) or from other individuals (allogeneic) to inoculate cancer patients.[11] The advantage of this approach is that multiple potential target antigens may be present in the tumor inoculum, and the specific identity of any particular antigen is not required. However, this approach could be expected to have greater side effects due to cross-reactivity with normal host antigens, and the immune response may not be optimized due to the potential low expression level of any particular target. Subsequently, for some malignancies, focused efforts to identify and characterize cancer-specific antigens have distinguished well-defined targets for T cell recognition.[12,13] For most cancers, ideal targets represent antigens expressed by neoplastic cells (cancer-specific antigens) but not by normal cells. These often represent products of mutated oncogenes or tumor suppressor genes (e.g., mutated ras or p53 peptides). However, most human cancer antigens identified to date are also expressed at lower levels by normal cells (cancer-associated antigens). For some malignancies such as prostate carcinoma, the normal organ (prostate) is not essential to life, and is thus expendable if immunotherapy cross-reactivity occurs. Thus, tissue-specific rather than tumor-specific antigens can be viewed as viable therapeutic targets. One may debate that immune tolerance for these "self" antigens acquired during development could reduce the effectiveness of normal tissue-specific antigens as cancer vaccine candidates. However, as described below, creative vaccine approaches using prostate-specific proteins with immunostimulatory molecules have been shown to elicit antitumor immune responses. For example, studies have shown that gene-modified tumor vaccines expressing specific cytokines, including interleukin 2, IFN-gamma[14] and GM-CSF,[15] induce T-cell-specific responses that can result in antitumor effects.

In contrast to active immunotherapy, passive immunotherapy relies on the administration of immune-mediating effector cells (e.g., lymphokine-activated killer cells, tumor-infiltrating lymphocytes), or tumor antigen-targeted monoclonal antibodies (mAb). These approaches are often combined with nonspecific immune-enhancing agents such as cytokines (e.g., interleukin-2, interferon, or GM-CSF) administered either systemically or intratumorally.[7] Recently, mAb therapy has proven efficacious in clinical cancer treatment. These successes include the anti-CD20 mAb (Rituxan) for B cell lymphoma[16] and anti-Her2/neu mAb (Herceptin) for metastatic breast cancer.[17] As with many other tumor types, the development of antibody therapeutics for prostate cancer has been limited by a paucity of antigens known to be expressed at a high frequency and at a significant level in prostate-cancer patients. However, as described below, large-scale approaches designed to identify prostate tissue-specific antigens, and cancer-specific molecular alterations, have yielded many new potential targets.

Targets and Approaches for Prostate Cancer Immunotherapy

To date, the most extensively studied antigens for prostate cancer immunotherapy have been prostate-specific antigen (PSA), prostate acid phosphatase (PAP), and prostate-specific membrane antigen (PSMA). While not prostate cancer-specific, the high expression levels of these proteins in normal and neoplastic prostate epithelial cells, relative to all other normal human tissues, has propelled studies designed to exploit this tissue compartmentalization to provide a favorable therapeutic index. The following description of ongoing immunotherapy studies for prostate cancer is not meant to be comprehensive in nature, but rather to provide an introduction to the variety of approaches and types of targets currently under evaluation.

Prostate-specific antigen (PSA) is a serine protease secreted by luminal epithelial cells lining prostatic ducts.[18,19] The normal function of PSA appears to be the cleavage and inactivation of semenogelin, a protein involved in seminal fluid coagulation.[19] Elevated levels of PSA are found in the serum of men with prostate carcinoma, and the protein is expressed in both androgen-dependent and advanced androgen-independent cancers.[20,21] The identification of T-cell specific epitopes within the protein sequence of PSA led to studies demonstrating that PSA peptides could stimulate human cytotoxic T lymphocytes (CTL) *in vitro*.[22] Studies using various immunization protocols have shown that anti-PSA antibody responses can be induced by PSA vaccination.[23] In addition, studies of PSA vaccines in men with advanced cancers resulted in the stabilization of serum PSA levels and the induction of a T-cell proliferative response to a PSA peptide.[24] Additional mechanisms of PSA-vaccine efficacy are suggested by a recent study providing evidence of epitope determinant spreading in the antibody responses to prostate cell surface antigens in patients immunized with PSA.[25] This effect is thought to be enhanced by local inflammatory reaction with subsequent elaboration and recognition of auto- and neoantigens associated with the prostate tumor.[25] Further efforts to modulate anti-PSA immunity with cytokines, costimulatory molecules and other immune enhancing agents may improve the therapeutic efficacy of PSA vaccines. Clinical trials designed to evaluate vaccine potency in different disease stages using various vectors and administration routes need to be performed to determine the ultimate utility of PSA as a therapeutic target.

Prostate acid phosphatase (PAP) is a protein expressed in normal and neoplastic prostate luminal epithelial cells and exemplifies another prostate tumor-associated target antigen currently being exploited using a variety of strategies.[26] In support of these studies are preclinical rodent models that demonstrate the induction of a destructive prostatitis by PAP-specific CTLs.[27] Naturally occurring PAP-specific T-helper cell responses have been detected in men with prostate cancer, albeit at low levels (11%).[28] This suggests that an immune environment capable of supporting antigen-specific CTL may exist *in vivo*.[28] Dendritic cells loaded with an engineered antigen-cytokine fusion protein consisting of PAP and GM-CSF are capable of inducing a potent cellular immune response *in vivo* to rodent tissues and tumors that express PAP.[29] In this model system, the importance of the GM-CSF protein and dendritic cells for antigen presentation and enhanced immune responses was determined. Based on these preclinical observations, a dendritic cell product consisting of autologous dendritic cells loaded with the human PAP-GM-CSF fusion protein was developed, and clinical testing was undertaken through a phase I/II trial in patients with advanced androgen-independent prostate cancer.[29] The study demonstrated that all patients developed specific immune responses to the recombinant fusion protein, and 38% developed immune responses to PAP. The time to disease progression correlated with the development of an immune response to PAP and with the dose of dendritic cells received. Minimal side effects of the therapy were observed. The clinical efficacy of this strategy is now under evaluation in Phase III trials.

Prostate specific membrane antigen (PSMA) encodes a folate hydrolase of 100 kDa that is localized to the cell surface of normal and neoplastic prostate epithelial cells.[30] PSMA is also expressed in the neovasculature endothelial cells of many non-prostatic primary tumors.[31] A radioimmunoconjugate form of anti-PSMA monoclonal antibody is currently being used to diagnose prostate cancer metastases and recurrent disease.[30] A phase I study using autologous dendritic cells pulsed with PSMA peptides reported significant clinical responses in 7 out of 51 advanced stage prostate carcinoma patients without significant acute or chronic side-effects.[32] Thirty-three patients with metastatic prostate cancer completed a phase II trial using the same treatment approach and 27% were identified as partial responders, 33% had no significant change in tumor markers or tumor size, and 39% exhibited disease progression.[33] A phase III clinical trial in patients with late-stage prostate cancer was recently announced.[34] Clinical trials using immunizations with "naked" PSMA DNA and PSMA sequences cloned into replication-deficient viral vectors have also been initiated,[35] and phase I/II toxicity dose-escalation results indicate that the approach is safe. Several patients achieved clinical responses as evidenced by a change in the local disease, distant metastases, and PSA levels. Phase II clinical studies to evaluate the effectiveness of the therapy are underway.[35]

Prostate stem cell antigen (PSCA) is a cell-surface protein with 30% homology to stem cell antigen 2, a member of the Thy-1/Ly-6 family of glycosylphosphatidylinositol (GPI)-anchored cell surface antigens highly restricted in expression in normal and neoplastic prostate epithelium.[36] In situ hybridization (ISH) and immunohistochemistry (IHC) studies demonstrate PSCA expression in more than 80% of localized prostate cancers and in all metastatic bone lesions examined.[37] Elevated PSCA expression has been shown to correlate with increased tumor stage, grade, and progression to androgen-independent disease.[37] Two recent studies demonstrated that a passive immunotherapy approach using anti-PSCA monoclonal antibody therapy inhibits prostate tumor growth and metastasis formation, and further prolongs survival of mice bearing human prostate cancer xenografts.[38,39] In addition, PSCA may also be an appropriate target for T cell-based immunotherapy.[40] Based upon these preclinical studies, PSCA represents another prostate protein target that may be suitable for immunotherapeutic trials.

Additional Targets and Approaches

Several other genes and proteins have been identified with prostate restricted or enhanced expression profiles. These include prostase/KLK4,[41] PATE,[42] GDEB,[43] PRAC,[44] DD3,[45] and STEAP,[46] as well as others described below. By virtue of their compartmentalized tissue and cellular distribution patterns, many prostate-specific genes are in various stages of evaluation for immune-based therapeutic strategies. Other cancer-related molecular alterations such as the amplified Her-2/neu oncoprotein have also been suggested as viable immunotherapy targets in prostate carcinoma.[47] Clinical trials indicate that T-cell immunity can be generated toward the HER-2/neu protein after active immunization with HER-2/neu peptide-based vaccines in patients with solid tumors. In addition to the vaccine schemas described for specific proteins such as PSA and PSMA, autologous whole prostate cell vaccines have been developed that are modified to secrete immunostimulatory proteins such as GM-CSF by *ex vivo* gene transfer.[48] These "personalized" whole cell vaccines represent an approach to circumvent the significant tumor heterogeneity that is evident when comparing the expression levels of individual antigens in tumors derived from different patients. A strategy complimentary to this "whole cell" approach entails the development of polyvalent vaccines employing multiple highly specific and highly antigenic targets. Such a strategy mandates the discovery of many new prostate cancer antigens.

IDENTIFICATION OF NOVEL IMMUNOTHERAPY TARGETS THROUGH MICROARRAY-BASED GENE EXPRESSION STUDIES OF PROSTATE CARCINOMA

Microarray-based studies of gene expression in a large number of tumor types have repeatedly revealed novel features of human cancers and allowed for the molecular classification and stratification of tumor characteristics that are predictive of tumor behavior.[49] In addition to profiles of gene expression, microarray studies also identify specific differences in the expression of individual genes in a comparative fashion (e.g., tumor vs. normal) that serves to identify candidate therapeutic targets. The methodology and attributes of microarray technology have been described previously and will not be detailed here.[50,51] In the context of large-scale efforts designed to identify tumor- or tissue-specific therapeutic targets, microarrays are ideally suited by virtue of their ability to simultaneously analyze the expression of thousands of genes in parallel, and the high reproducibility of array platforms that facilitates the comparative analysis of hundreds of samples.

Several studies employing microarrays to characterize prostate cancer gene expression profiles have recently been published.[52–56] Microarrays comprised of oligonucleotides and others comprised of spotted cDNAs were used to comparatively analyze gene expression differences between normal prostate tissues and well-characterized samples of prostate carcinoma. Some of these investigations have analyzed as few as 11 tumor samples[52] while others have characterized more than 50 tumor samples.[53] Strikingly, of 5 studies reviewed, all identified the transcript encoding Hepsin as a gene overexpressed in prostate carcinoma relative to benign epithelium (see TABLE 1). Hepsin is a type II integral membrane serine protease without a defined functional role.[57] Other differentially expressed genes reported in the studies include: fatty acid synthase, the TGF-beta superfamily member MIC-1, the phosphoglucomutase PGM5, and the protein kinase encoded by the PIM1 proto-oncogene (TABLE 1).

While gene expression profiling studies of prostate carcinomas may identify genes overexpressed or underexpressed in neoplastic cells relative to normal cells, the suitability of these genes and cognate gene products as therapeutic targets may be limited due to expression in other normal cells that could produce significant systemic toxicities. Our group and others have modified differential expression studies to identify genes with expression profiles restricted to the prostate gland.[41,58] As the prostate is an expendable organ, therapeutics targeted to prostate-specific cellular pathways would be expected to have a high therapeutic index. We have previously identified the gene encoding prostase/KLK4 as a serine protease with expression highly restricted to normal and neoplastic prostate cells.[41] Other groups incorporating combinations of subtractive hybridization and microarray analysis have identified several additional genes including prostein,[59] STEAP,[46] and p504S/Alpha-

TABLE 1. Identification of differentially expressed genes in prostate carcinoma by microarray analysis

Study	Number of Tumors Analyzed	Number of Genes Analyzed (Approximate)	Number of Genes Differentially Expressed	Examples of Differentially Expressed Genes	Array Platform
Magee, J.A. et al. 2001. Cancer Res. **61**: 5692–5696.	11	4,712	4 (>3-fold)	Hepsin serotonin receptor 2B	Affymetrix
Luo, J. et al. 2001. Cancer Res. **61**: 4683–4688.	16	3,215	210 ($P < 0.001$)	Hepsin E2F transcription factor 5	Spotted cDNA
Luo, J.H. et al. 2002. Mol. Carcinogen. **33**: 25–35.	15	40,000	84 ($P < 0.05$)	Hepsin AMACR	Affymetrix
Dhanasekaran, S.M. et al. 2001. Nature **412**: 822–826.	36	9,984	>200	Hepsin PIM1	Spotted cDNA
Welsh, J.B. et al. 2001. Cancer Res. **61**: 5974–5978.	24	8,900	about 400	Hepsin MIC-1	Affymetrix

Methylacyl-CoA-Racemase.[58,60] The prostate cancer-enhanced expression pattern of these genes makes them potential candidates for immunomodulatory therapy. Prostase/KLK4 is a member of the kallikrein gene family that was shown to be highly restricted in expression to human prostate epithelium and regulated by androgenic hormones.[41] Prostase/KLK4 exhibits approximately 35% amino acid identity with PSA.[41] In view of the tissue-specific expression profile, studies have been undertaken to evaluate the utility of prostase/KLK4 as a vaccine candidate. It has recently been shown that a CD4 T cell repertoire specific for prostase/KLK4 is present and is potentially expandable in prostate cancer patients.[61] These preliminary studies support the further evaluation of whole gene-, protein-, or peptide-based prostase/KLK4 cancer vaccine strategies.

IDENTIFICATION OF POTENTIAL IMMUNOTHERAPY TARGETS THROUGH MICROARRAY-BASED GENE EXPRESSION STUDIES OF THE PROSTATE ANDROGEN-RESPONSE PROGRAM

Identifying therapeutic targets that would have minimal cross-reactivity and minimal impact toward normal cells and tissues is an important consideration. Conceptually, one approach for identifying such targets would exploit an attribute, such as a metabolic pathway, used exclusively or predominantly in the tissue or cell type of interest. For example, immunotherapies developed toward malignant melanoma exploit the melanocyte-specific expression of proteins involved in melanin biosynthesis such as tyrosinase.[13] Thus, an alternative approach for identifying potential therapeutic targets expressed in the prostate entails exploiting the androgen-response pathway (ARP). Androgens and the androgen receptor (AR) mediate critical processes involved in the normal development, organizational structure, mature function, and cellular viability of the prostate gland.[62,63] During early development, the AR is expressed in mesenchymal cells of the urogenital sinus with subsequent temporal expression in prostate epithelial cells. Exposure of these cells to androgens results in a mature differentiated epithelial phenotype and the production of prostate-specific proteins. In the adult prostate gland, androgens promote cell division, proliferation, and maintenance of the epithelial cell compartment. However, androgens also appear to modulate an apoptotic program and a "proliferative shut-off" function that results in a state of cell quiescence.[64,65] In addition, androgens influence several aspects of prostate cellular metabolism including lipid biosynthesis.[66] Androgens also regulate the production of specialized secretory proteins such as prostate specific antigen (PSA) and human glandular kallikrein 2 (hK2) that exhibit a prostate-restricted expression profile.[67]

Our efforts have focused on the characterization of the temporal program of transcription that reflects the prostate cellular response to androgens, and the identification of specific androgen-regulated genes (ARGs) or gene networks that participate in these responses. To facilitate the assessment of androgen-responsive genes in the human prostate, we first assembled a cDNA clone set representative of the prostate transcriptome. cDNA libraries were constructed from a variety of normal and neoplastic prostate tissue sources that included normal basal and secretory epithelium, primary prostate carcinoma, metastatic prostate carcinoma, and a variety of prostate cancer cell lines. Clones were randomly selected, subjected to single-pass sequencing to generate Expressed Sequence Tags (ESTs)[68] and assembled into distinct clusters based on nucleotide homology. The individual ESTs and their assemblies have been deposited in a publicly available data repository named the Prostate Expression Database (PEDB) (www.pedb.org).[69] Individual cDNAs corresponding to each of approximately 6,300 putative unique transcripts were selected, relocated into 384-well microtiter plates, amplified by the PCR and arrayed onto glass slides in duplicate as we have previously described.[70] This prostate microarray was supplemented with a generic microarray comprised of 17,630 commercially available cDNAs (Research Genetics; RG array). Overall, approximately 3,000 genes overlapped on both arrays.

To assess the transcriptional response of prostate epithelial cells to androgen, hormone-responsive LNCaP prostate cancer cells were exposed to the synthetic androgen R1881 for specific time periods. The LNCaP cell line was chosen because it is the most widely used model for the study of prostate carcinoma and has also shown great utility for characterizing the direct effects of androgens on human cells.[71,72] Overall, 4,439 of the 6,388 genes on the prostate array (69%) and 5,642 of the 17,630 genes on the RG array (32%) exhibited detectable transcripts in the LNCaP cells for a total assessable LNCaP transcriptome representing approximately 8,000 genes (approximately 2,000 detectable cDNAs were in common between the two clone sets).[73] A comparison of the expression profiles at specific time points after androgen stimulation demonstrated that the vast majority of transcripts (more than 96%) did not change by more than twofold compared to untreated cells. In contrast, approximately 4% of the expressed transcripts were reproducibly altered more than twofold at one or more time points.[73] After 24 hours of stimulation, the expression of 262 genes changed by more than twofold. After either 24 or 48 hours of androgen exposure, the expression of 146 genes changed by at least threefold. Of these, 102 represent genes with described functional roles and 46 represent transcripts, putative proteins, or novel sequences with undetermined functions.[73]

In the context of identifying potential immunotherapeutic targets, our criteria for prioritizing ARGs for further characterization centered on those with a tissue distribution profile enhanced or specific to prostate tissue. To identify those genes with enhanced expression in the prostate, we selected ARGs with a temporal pattern of expression corresponding to that of PSA; a gene shown to be highly restricted in expression to prostate epithelium and directly regulated by androgens. Hierarchical cluster analysis grouped 24 genes with PSA including the well-described prostate specific ARGs KLK2 and NKX3.1.[67,74] The systematic analysis of the other PSA-associated genes is in progress. To date, we have published studies further describing three of these ARGs—TMPRSS2,[70] PART1,[75] and PSDR1[76]—and have shown that each exhibits a high level of expression in prostate tissue. TMPRSS2 is a modular type II integral membrane serine protease that is predicted to be expressed on the cell surface.[77] PART1 encodes a putative polypeptide without homology to known protein sequences in the public databases, and has been shown to be upregulated in prostate carcinoma relative to normal prostate epithelium.[78] PSDR1 encodes a short-chain dehydrogenase reductase which biochemically functions as a retinal reductase.[79]

Seventeen uncharacterized ARGs exhibited temporal expression profiles corresponding to KLK3/PSA.[73] Northern analysis using RNAs from eight different human tissues demonstrated that five genes exhibited exclusive or high expression levels in the prostate relative to all other tissues studied. KIAA0056 encodes a putative protein of 1498 residues and was originally identified through large-scale sequencing of cDNA clones from the immature myeloid cell line KG-1.[80] The cDNA represented by Unigene Hs.256301 maps to chromosome 19q13.3, a region harboring several androgen-regulated prostate proteases including PSA/KLK3, KLK2, and KLK4/ prostase. The gene represented by Hs.288821 encodes a putative WD-domain containing protein that has significant homology to proteins predicted in the *Drosophila melanogaster* and *Caenorhabditis elegans* genomes. The cDNA corresponding to Unigene sequence Hs.55028 maps to chromosome 16 and encodes a predicted polypeptide of 33 amino acids with similarity to a protein candidate for x-linked retinopathies. The cDNA for PEDB8 was derived from a library constructed from normal prostate tissue and does not exhibit significant homology with sequences in the public nucleotide databases.[73] Further work will determine the suitability of targeting these and other components of the prostate androgen-response network using immunomodulatory approaches.

CONCLUDING REMARKS

Immunotherapeutic strategies represent a growing presence in clinical trials for prostate cancer. Of paramount importance for the design of tumor vaccines is the selection of therapeutic antigens. A critical factor remains defining those antigens that will provide selected killing of tumor cells while sparing non-cancerous bystander cells. Most tumor vaccine schemas require that potential antigens be highly cancer cell specific, and thus a relatively small number of mutant or highly expressed oncoproteins such as p53 and Her2/neu are viewed as reasonable targets. However, solid tumors are often represented by heterogeneous cell populations with variable expression levels of any particular oncoprotein. Thus, while tumor cells expressing the protein under immune attack may be eliminated, the surviving cells will continue to expand and manifest their growth as clinical resistance. For some cancers, the organ or tissue of origin is not essential to human life. For these cancers, including cancer of the prostate, proteins restricted to both normal and neoplastic cells are viable targets, a fact that greatly expands the repertoire of potential antigens that can be exploited. Several of these prostate tissue-specific antigens such as PSA, PAP, and PSMA are currently being evaluated using a variety of innovative clinical trials. Newly identified prostate proteins such as PSCA, prostase/KLK4, and others are in pre-clinical testing. However, it remains a great challenge for immune-based therapies to eradicate advanced stage disease. Large tumor burdens can inhibit both global and tumor-specific T-cell responses. As with vaccine strategies designed for infectious diseases, tumor vaccines are likely to have the greatest efficacy in the setting of small tumor amounts, or prior to the development of disease. As a result, promising tumor immunotherapies should be rapidly moved into the adjuvant setting to truly evaluate their utility.

ACKNOWLEDGMENTS

This work was supported by the CaPCURE foundation, grant CA75173 from the National Cancer Institute (NIH), and a scholar award from the Cancer Research Fund of the Damon Runyon Cancer Research Foundation.

REFERENCES

1. GREENLEE, R.T. *et al.* 2001. Cancer statistics, 2001. CA Cancer J Clin. **51**(1): 15–36.
2. SCHER, H.I., G. STEINECK & W.K. KELLY. 1995. Hormone-refractory (D3) prostate cancer: refining the concept. Urology **46**(2): 142–148.
3. TANNOCK, I.F., *et al.* 1996. Chemotherapy with mitoxantrone plus prednisone or prednisone alone for symptomatic hormone-resistant prostate cancer: a Canadian randomized trial with palliative end points [see comments]. J. Clin. Oncol. **14**(6): p. 1756–1764.
4. OLSON, K.B. & K.J. PIENTA. 2000. Recent advances in chemotherapy for advanced prostate cancer. Curr. Urol. Rep. **1**(1): 48–56.
5. PARMIANI, G., et al., 2002. Cancer immunotherapy with peptide-based vaccines: what have we achieved? Where are we going? J. Natl. Cancer Inst. **94**(11): 805–818.
6. GLASPY, J.A. 2002. Therapeutic options in the management of renal cell carcinoma. Semin. Oncol. **29**(3, Suppl. 7): 41–46.
7. ROSENBERG, S.A. 2001. Progress in human tumour immunology and immunotherapy. Nature **411**(6835): 380–384.
8. ABOULAFIA, D.M. 1994. Human immunodeficiency virus-associated neoplasms: epidemiology, pathogenesis, and review of current therapy. Cancer Pract. **2**(4): 297–306.
9. WEIDEN, P.L. *et al.* 1981. Antileukemic effect of chronic graft-versus-host disease: contribution to improved survival after allogeneic marrow transplantation. N. Engl. J. Med. **304**(25): 1529–1533.
10. GUERMONPREZ, P. *et al.* 2002. Antigen presentation and T cell stimulation by dendritic cells. Annu. Rev. Immunol. 20: 621–667.
11. SEDLACEK, H.H. 1994. Vaccination for treatment of tumors: a critical comment. Crit. Rev. Oncog. **5**(6): 555–587.
12. SCANLAN, M.J. *et al.* 2002. Cancer-related serological recognition of human colon cancer: identification of potential diagnostic and immunotherapeutic targets. Cancer Res. **62**(14): 4041–4047.
13. MULLINS, D.W. *et al.* 2001. Immune responses to the HLA-A*0201-restricted epitopes of tyrosinase and glycoprotein 100 enable control of melanoma outgrowth in HLA-A*0201-transgenic mice. J. Immunol. **167**(9): 4853–4860.
14. MAIO, M. *et al.* 2002. Vaccination of stage IV patients with allogeneic IL-4- or IL-2-gene-transduced melanoma cells generates functional antibodies against vaccinating and autologous melanoma cells. Cancer Immunol. Immunother. **51**(1): 9–14.
15. LIM, M. & J.W. SIMONS. 1999. Emerging concepts in GM-CSF gene-transduced tumor vaccines for human prostate cancer. Curr. Opin. Mol. Ther. **1**(1): 64–71.
16. GRILLO-LOPEZ, A.J. *et al.* 2002. Rituximab: ongoing and future clinical development. Semin. Oncol. **29**(1, Suppl. 2): 105–112.
17. LOHRISCH, C. & M. PICCART. 2001. An overview of HER2. Semin. Oncol. **28**(6, Suppl. 18): 3–11.
18. WANG, M.C. *et al.* 1981. Prostate antigen: a new potential marker for prostatic cancer. Prostate **2**(1): 89–96.
19. LILJA, H. 1993. Structure, function, and regulation of the enzyme activity of prostate-specific antigen. World J. Urol. **11**(4): 188–191.
20. HUDSON, M.A., R.R. BAHNSON & W.J. CATALONA. 1989. Clinical use of prostate specific antigen in patients with prostate cancer. J. Urol. **142**(4): 1011–1017.
21. CATALONA, J.J. *et al.* 1991. Measurement of prostate-specific antigen as a screening test for prostate cancer. N. Engl. J. Med. **324**: 1156–1161.

22. CORREALE, P. et al. 1997. In vitro generation of human cytotoxic T lymphocytes specific for peptides derived from prostate-specific antigen. J. Natl. Cancer Inst. **89**(4): 293–300.
23. HARRIS, D.T. et al. 1999. Immunologic approaches to the treatment of prostate cancer. Semin. Oncol. **26**(4): 439–447.
24. EDER, J.P. et al. 2000. A phase I trial of a recombinant vaccinia virus expressing prostate-specific antigen in advanced prostate cancer. Clin. Cancer Res. **6**(5): 1632–1638.
25. CAVACINI, L.A. et al. 2002. Evidence of determinant spreading in the antibody responses to prostate cell surface antigens in patients immunized with prostate-specific antigen. Clin. Cancer Res. **8**(2): 368–373.
26. OSTROWSKI, W.S. & R. KUCIEL. 1994. Human prostatic acid phosphatase: selected properties and practical applications. Clin. Chim. Acta **226**(2): 121–129.
27. FONG, L. et al. 1997. Induction of tissue-specific autoimmune prostatitis with prostatic acid phosphatase immunization: implications for immunotherapy of prostate cancer. J. Immunol. **159**(7): 3113–3117.
28. MCNEEL, D.G. et al. 2001. Naturally occurring prostate cancer antigen-specific T cell responses of a Th1 phenotype can be detected in patients with prostate cancer. Prostate **47**(3): 222–229.
29. SMALL, E.J. et al. 2000. Immunotherapy of hormone-refractory prostate cancer with antigen-loaded dendritic cells. J. Clin. Oncol. **18**(23): 3894–3903.
30. CHANG, S.S. et al. 1999. Prostate-specific membrane antigen: much more than a prostate cancer marker. Mol. Urol. **3**(3): 313–320.
31. CHANG, S.S. et al. 1999. Prostate-specific membrane antigen is produced in tumor-associated neovasculature. Clin. Cancer Res. **5**(10): 2674–2681.
32. MURPHY, G.P. et al. 1999. Infusion of dendritic cells pulsed with HLA-A2-specific prostate-specific membrane antigen peptides: a phase II prostate cancer vaccine trial involving patients with hormone-refractory metastatic disease. Prostate **38**(1): 73–78.
33. TJOA, B.A. et al. 1998. Evaluation of phase I/II clinical trials in prostate cancer with dendritic cells and PSMA peptides. Prostate **36**(1): 39–44.
34. Prostate Cancer Vaccine–Northwest Biotherapeutics: CaPVax, DC1/HRPC, DCVax-Prostate. 2002. BioDrugs **16**(3): 226–227.
35. MINCHEFF, M. et al. 2000. Naked DNA and adenoviral immunizations for immunotherapy of prostate cancer: a phase I/II clinical trial. Eur. Urol. **38**(2): 208–217.
36. REITER, R.E. et al. 1998. Prostate stem cell antigen: a cell surface marker overexpressed in prostate cancer. Proc. Natl. Acad. Sci. USA **95**(4): 1735–1740.
37. GU, Z. et al. 2000. Prostate stem cell antigen (PSCA) expression increases with high gleason score, advanced stage and bone metastasis in prostate cancer. Oncogene **19**(10): 1288–1296.
38. ROSS, S. et al. 2002. Prostate stem cell antigen as therapy target: tissue expression and in vivo efficacy of an immunoconjugate. Cancer Res. **62**(9): 2546–2553.
39. SAFFRAN, D.C. et al. 2001. Anti-PSCA mAbs inhibit tumor growth and metastasis formation and prolong the survival of mice bearing human prostate cancer xenografts. Proc. Natl. Acad. Sci. USA **98**(5): 2658–2663.
40. DANNULL, J. et al. 2000. Prostate stem cell antigen is a promising candidate for immunotherapy of advanced prostate cancer. Cancer Res. **60**(19): 5522–5528.
41. NELSON, P.S. et al. 1999. Molecular cloning and characterization of prostase, an androgen-regulated serine protease with prostate-restricted expression. Proc. Natl. Acad. Sci. USA **96**(6): 3114–3119.
42. BERA, T.K. et al. 2002. PATE, a gene expressed in prostate cancer, normal prostate, and testis, identified by a functional genomic approach. Proc. Natl. Acad. Sci. USA **99**(5): 3058–3063.
43. OLSSON, P. et al. 2001. GDEP, a new gene differentially expressed in normal prostate and prostate cancer. Prostate **48**(4): 231–241.
44. LIU, X.F. et al. 2001. PRAC: A novel small nuclear protein that is specifically expressed in human prostate and colon. Prostate **47**(2): 125–1231.
45. DE KOK, J.B. et al. 2002. DD3(PCA3), a very sensitive and specific marker to detect prostate tumors. Cancer Res. **62**(9): p. 2695–2698.

46. HUBERT, R.S. et al. 1999. STEAP: a prostate-specific cell-surface antigen highly expressed in human prostate tumors. Proc. Natl. Acad. Sci. USA **96**(25): 14523–14528.
47. DISIS, M.L. et al. 2001. Clinical translation of peptide-based vaccine trials: the HER-2/neu model. Crit. Rev. Immunol. **21**(1-3): 263–273.
48. SIMONS, J.W. et al. 1999. Induction of immunity to prostate cancer antigens: results of a clinical trial of vaccination with irradiated autologous prostate tumor cells engineered to secrete granulocyte-macrophage colony-stimulating factor using ex vivo gene transfer. Cancer Res. **59**(20): 5160–5168.
49. MOHR, S. et al. 2002. Microarrays as cancer keys: an array of possibilities. J. Clin. Oncol. **20**(14): 3165–3175.
50. SCHENA, M. et al. 1995. Quantitative monitoring of gene expression patterns with a complementary DNA microarray. Science **270**: 467–470.
51. CHEE, M. et al. 1996. Accessing genetic information with high-density DNA arrays. Science **274**(5287): 610–614.
52. MAGEE, J.A. et al. 2001. Expression profiling reveals hepsin overexpression in prostate cancer. Cancer Res. **61**(15): 5692–5696.
53. DHANASEKARAN, S.M. et al. 2001. Delineation of prognostic biomarkers in prostate cancer. Nature **412**(6849): 822–826.
54. LUO, J. et al. 2001. Human prostate cancer and benign prostatic hyperplasia: molecular dissection by gene expression profiling. Cancer Res. **61**(12): 4683–4688.
55. WELSH, J.B. et al. 2001. Analysis of gene expression identifies candidate markers and pharmacological targets in prostate cancer. Cancer Res. **61**(16): 5974–5978.
56. LUO, J.H. et al. 2002. Gene expression analysis of prostate cancers. Mol. Carcinog. **33**(1): 25–35.
57. WU, Q. 2001. Gene targeting in hemostasis. Hepsin. Front Biosci. **6**: D192–D200.
58. XU, J. et al. 2000. Identification of differentially expressed genes in human prostate cancer using subtraction and microarray. Cancer Res. **60**(6): 1677–1682.
59. XU, J. et al. 2001. Identification and characterization of prostein, a novel prostate-specific protein. Cancer Res. **61**(4): 1563–1568.
60. JIANG, Z. et al. 2001. P504S: a new molecular marker for the detection of prostate carcinoma. Am. J. Surg. Pathol. **25**(11): 1397–1404.
61. HURAL, J.A. et al. 2002. Identification of naturally processed CD4 T cell epitopes from the prostate-specific antigen kallikrein 4 using peptide-based in vitro stimulation. J. Immunol. **169**(1): 557–565.
62. PRINS, G.S. 2000. Molecular biology of the androgen receptor. Mayo Clin. Proc. **75**(Suppl): S32–S35.
63. COFFEY, D.S. & K.J. PIENTA. 1987. New concepts in studying the control of normal and cancer growth of the prostate. Prog. Clin. Biol. Res. **239**: 1–73.
64. ISAACS, J.T. et al. 1992. Androgen regulation of programmed death of normal and malignant prostatic cells. J. Androl. **13**(6): 457–464.
65. GECK, P. et al. 1997. Expression of novel genes linked to the androgen-induced, proliferative shutoff in prostate cancer cells. J. Steroid Biochem. Mol. Biol. **63**(4–6): 211–218.
66. SWINNEN, J.V. & G. VERHOEVEN. 1998. Androgens and the control of lipid metabolism in human prostate cancer cells. J. Steroid Biochem. Mol. Biol. **65**(1-6): 191–198.
67. RITTENHOUSE, H.G. et al. 1998. Human kallikrein 2 (hK2) and prostate-specific antigen (PSA): two closely related, but distinct, kallikreins in the prostate. Crit. Rev. Clin. Lab. Sci. **35**(4): 275–368.
68. NELSON, P.S. et al. 1998. An expressed-sequence-tag database of the human prostate: sequence analysis of 1168 cDNA clones [In Process Citation]. Genomics **47**(1): 12–25.
69. HAWKINS, V. et al. 1999. PEDB: the Prostate Expression Database. Nucleic Acids Res. **27**(1): 204–208.
70. LIN, B. et al. 1999. Prostate-localized and androgen-regulated expression of the membrane-bound serine protease TMPRSS2. Cancer Res. **59**(17): 4180–4184.
71. HOROSZEWICZ, J.S. et al. 1983. LNCaP model of human prostatic carcinoma. Cancer Res. **43**(4): 1809–1818.
72. CLEGG, N. et al. 2002. Digital expression profiles of the prostate androgen-response program. J. Steroid Biochem. Mol. Biol. **80**(1): 13–23.

73. NELSON, P.S. *et al.* 2002. The program of androgen-responsive genes in neoplastic prostate epithelium. Proc. Natl. Acad. Sci. USA **99:** 11890–11895.
74. BIEBERICH, C.J. *et al.* 1996. Prostate-specific and androgen-dependent expression of a novel homeobox gene. J. Biol. Chem. **271**(50): 31779–31782.
75. LIN, B. *et al.* 2000. PART-1: a novel human prostate-specific, androgen-regulated gene that maps to chromosome 5q12 [In Process Citation]. Cancer Res. **60**(4): 858–863.
76. LIN, B. *et al.* 2001. Prostate short-chain dehydrogenase reductase 1 (PSDR1): a new member of the short-chain steroid dehydrogenase/reductase family highly expressed in normal and neoplastic prostate epithelium. Cancer Res. **61**(4): 1611–1618.
77. PAOLONI-GIACOBINO, A. *et al.* 1997. Cloning of the TMPRSS2 gene, which encodes a novel serine protease with transmembrane, LDLRA, and SRCR domains and maps to 21q22.3. Genomics **44**(3): 309–320.
78. SIDIROPOULOS, M. *et al.* 2001. Expression and regulation of prostate androgen regulated transcript-1 (PART-1) and identification of differential expression in prostatic cancer. Br. J. Cancer **85**(3): 393–397.
79. KEDISHVILI, N.Y. *et al.* 2002. Evidence that the human gene for prostate short-chain dehydrogenase/reductase (PSDR1) encodes a novel retinal reductase (RalR1). J. Biol. Chem. **29:** 29.
80. NOMURA, N. *et al.* 1994. Prediction of the coding sequences of unidentified human genes. II. The coding sequences of 40 new genes (KIAA0041-KIAA0080) deduced by analysis of cDNA clones from human cell line KG-1. DNA Res. **1**(5): 223–229.

Index of Contributors

Aujame, L., 1–23
Auphan-Anezin, N., 68–76

Bandman, O., 77–90
Bartolini, E., 202–216
Beaudoing, E., 217–231
Bell, Y.C., 180–191
Bender, J., 114–131
Beretta, L., 91–100
Berger, J., 202–216
Bertucci, F., 217–231
Bienvenu, J.-G., 148–159
Birnbaum, D., 217–231
Buckley, J., 169–179
Burdin, N., 1–23

Casella, C.R., 132–147
Catalfamo, M., 46–56
Cavallo, J., 148–159
Cocks, B.G., 77–90
Coleman, R.T., 77–90
Connolly, T., 148–159
Cook, M.C., 33–45
Cooke, M.P., 33–45

Daheshia, M., 148–159
De Sanctis, G.T., 148–159
Dodet, B., ix
Draghi, M., 202–216
Drawid, A., 148–159
Druker, B.J., 180–191

Frigimelica, E., 202–216
Früh, K., 180–191

Goodnow, C.C., 33–45
Grandi, G., 202–216
Granjeaud, S., 217–231

Grifantini, R., 202–216
Griffith, D.J., 180–191

Hanash, S., 91–100
Heinrich, M.C., 180–191
Henkart, P.A., 46–56
Hildeman, D.A., 114–131
Hingamp, P., 217–231
Houlgatte, R., 217–231

Jacquemier, J., 217–231
Jarvis, M.A., 180–191
Jordan, B., 24–32
Jupp, R., 148–159

Kappler, J.W., 114–131
Katze, M.G., 160–168
Kedl, R.M., 114–131
Korth, M.J., 160–168

Le Naour, F., 91–100
Li, Y., 46–56
Liu, K., 46–56
Loring, J.F., 77–90
Loriod, B., 217–231
Luo, H., 169–179
Luukkonen, B.G.M., 180–191

MacLennan, I.C.M., 33–45
Mahony, J.B., 192–201
Marrack, P., 114–131
McManus, B.M., 169–179
Minnich, A., 148–159
Mitchell, T.C., 114–131, 132–147
Moses, A.V., 180–191
Muta, H., 101–113
Muzzi, A., 202–216

Nasser, V., 217–231
Nelson, J.A., 180–191
Nelson, P.S., 232–245
Nguyen, C., 68–76, 217–231

Podack, E.R., 101–113
Puthier, D., 68–76

Raggo, C., 180–191
Randazzo, F., 202–216
Rees, W.A., 114–131
Rezai, N., 169–179
Richards, J., 91–100
Rogge, L., 57–67
Ruhl, R., 180–191

Schmitt-Verhulst, A.-M., 68–76
Schreiner, G., 169–179
Seilhamer, J.J., 77–90
Sotosec, V., 101–113
Strbo, N., 101–113
Swanson, B., 114–131

Taylor, L., 169–179
Teague, T.K., 114–131
Thompson, B.S., 132–147
Tian, N., 148–159
Trent, J.O., 132–147
Triche, T., 169–179

Verdeil, G., 68–76
Vicari, M., ix, 1–23
Viens, P., 217–231
Vinuesa, C.G., 33–45

Wait, C.L., 180–191
Weng, N.-p., 46–56
Wu, Q., 148–159

Yanagawa, B., 169–179
Yang, D., 169–179
Yuan, J., 169–179

Zhang, M., 169–179

OHIO UNIVERSITY LIBRARY

Please return this book as soon as you have finished with it. In order to avoid a fine it must be returned by the latest date stamped below. All books are subject to recall after two weeks or immediately if needed for reserve.

CF